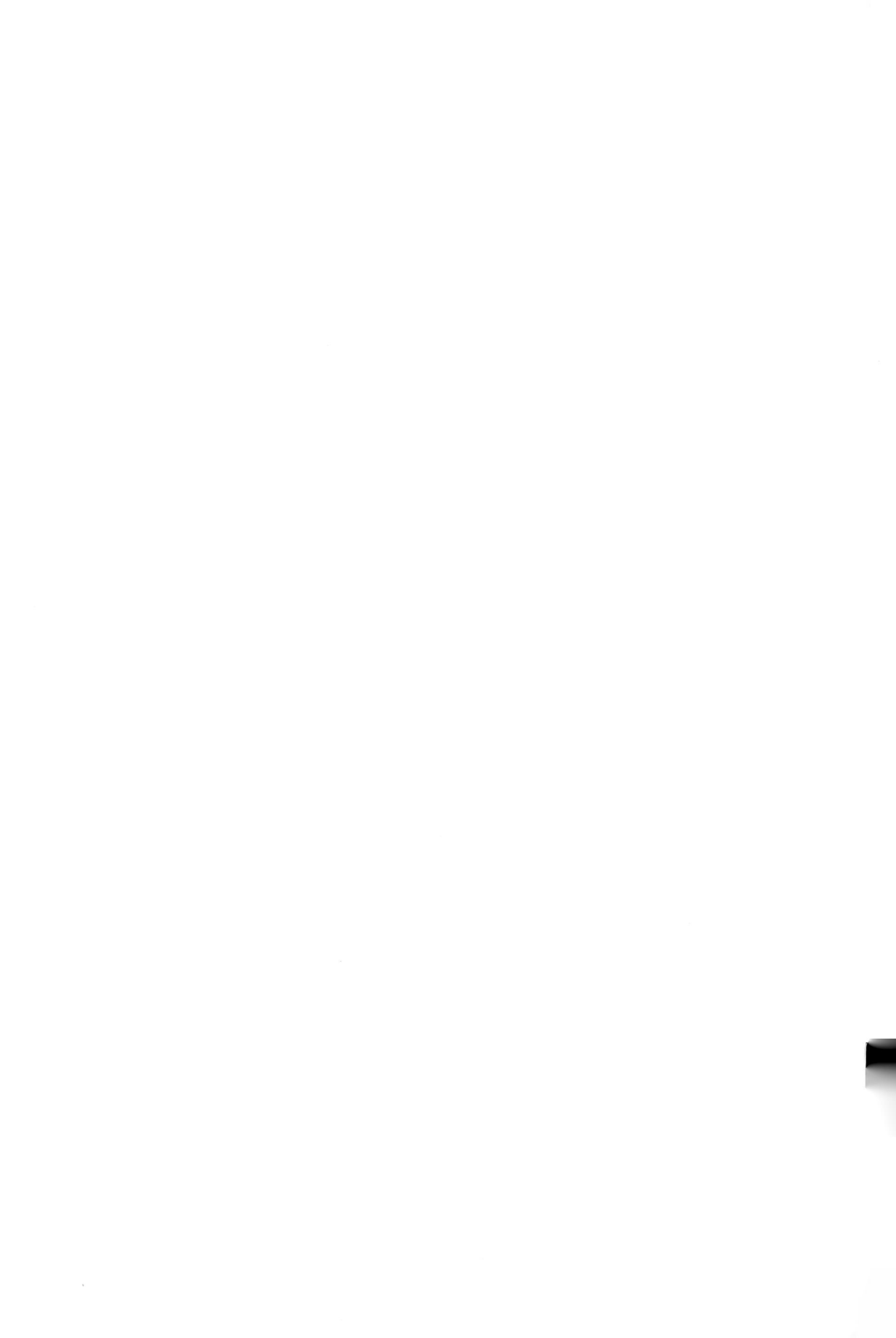

# Impact of Diet Composition on Insulin Resistance

# Impact of Diet Composition on Insulin Resistance

Editors

**Silvia V. Conde**
**Fatima O. Martins**

MDPI • Basel • Beijing • Wuhan • Barcelona • Belgrade • Manchester • Tokyo • Cluj • Tianjin

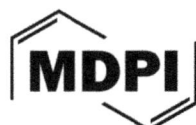

*Editors*
Silvia V. Conde
Universidade NOVA de
Lisboa
Portugal

Fatima O. Martins
Universidade NOVA de
Lisboa
Portugal

*Editorial Office*
MDPI
St. Alban-Anlage 66
4052 Basel, Switzerland

This is a reprint of articles from the Special Issue published online in the open access journal *Nutrients* (ISSN 2072-6643) (available at: https://www.mdpi.com/journal/nutrients/special_issues/Impact_Diet_Composition_Insulin_Resistance).

For citation purposes, cite each article independently as indicated on the article page online and as indicated below:

LastName, A.A.; LastName, B.B.; LastName, C.C. Article Title. *Journal Name* **Year**, *Volume Number*, Page Range.

**ISBN 978-3-0365-5405-1 (Hbk)**
**ISBN 978-3-0365-5406-8 (PDF)**

© 2022 by the authors. Articles in this book are Open Access and distributed under the Creative Commons Attribution (CC BY) license, which allows users to download, copy and build upon published articles, as long as the author and publisher are properly credited, which ensures maximum dissemination and a wider impact of our publications.

The book as a whole is distributed by MDPI under the terms and conditions of the Creative Commons license CC BY-NC-ND.

# Contents

**About the Editors** . . . . . . . . . . . . . . . . . . . . . . . . . . . . . . . . . . . . . . . . . . . . . . . . . . . . . . . . vii

**Fátima O. Martins and Silvia V. Conde**
Impact of Diet Composition on Insulin Resistance
Reprinted from: *Nutrients* 2022, 14, 3716, doi:10.3390/nu14183716 . . . . . . . . . . . . . . . . . 1

**Helena Tiekou Lorinczova, Sanjoy Deb, Gulshanara Begum, Derek Renshaw and Mohammed Gulrez Zariwala**
Comparative Assessment of the Acute Effects of Whey, Rice and Potato Protein Isolate Intake on Markers of Glycaemic Regulation and Appetite in Healthy Males Using a Randomised Study Design
Reprinted from: *Nutrients* 2021, 13, 2157, doi:10.3390/nu13072157 . . . . . . . . . . . . . . . . . 9

**Tamaeh Monteiro-Alfredo, Beatriz Caramelo, Daniela Arbeláez, Andreia Amaro, Cátia Barra, Daniela Silva, Sara Oliveira, Raquel Seiça and Paulo Matafome**
Distinct Impact of Natural Sugars from Fruit Juices and Added Sugars on Caloric Intake, Body Weight, Glycaemia, Oxidative Stress and Glycation in Diabetic Rats
Reprinted from: *Nutrients* 2021, 13, 2956, doi:10.3390/nu13092956 . . . . . . . . . . . . . . . . . 23

**Mohamad Hizami Mohamad Nor, Nurainina Ayob, Norfilza M. Mokhtar, Raja Affendi Raja Ali, Geok Chin Tan, Zhiqin Wong, Nor Hamizah Shafiee, Yin Ping Wong, Muaatamarulain Mustangin and Khairul Najmi Muhammad Nawawi**
The Effect of Probiotics (MCP® BCMC® Strains) on Hepatic Steatosis, Small Intestinal Mucosal Immune Function, and Intestinal Barrier in Patients with Non-Alcoholic Fatty Liver Disease
Reprinted from: *Nutrients* 2021, 13, 3192, doi:10.3390/nu13093192 . . . . . . . . . . . . . . . . . 43

**Francesca Tettamanzi, Vincenzo Bagnardi, Panayiotis Louca, Ana Nogal, Gianna Serafina Monti, Sara P. Mambrini, Elisa Lucchetti, Sabrina Maestrini, Silvia Mazza, Ana Rodriguez-Mateos, Massimo Scacchi, Ana M. Valdes, Cecilia Invitti and Cristina Menni**
A High Protein Diet Is More Effective in Improving Insulin Resistance and Glycemic Variability Compared to a Mediterranean Diet—A Cross-Over Controlled Inpatient Dietary Study
Reprinted from: *Nutrients* 2021, 13, 4380, doi:10.3390/nu13124380 . . . . . . . . . . . . . . . . . 61

**Amisha Pandya, Mira Mehta and Kavitha Sankavaram**
The Relationship between Macronutrient Distribution and Type 2 Diabetes in Asian Indians
Reprinted from: *Nutrients* 2021, 13, 4406, doi:10.3390/nu13124406 . . . . . . . . . . . . . . . . . 73

**Ryota Kobayashi, Miki Sakazaki, Yukie Nagai, Kenji Asaki, Takeo Hashiguchi and Hideyuki Negoro**
Effects of Different Types of Carbohydrates on Arterial Stiffness: A Comparison of Isomaltulose and Sucrose
Reprinted from: *Nutrients* 2021, 13, 4493, doi:10.3390/nu13124493 . . . . . . . . . . . . . . . . . 89

**Larry A. Tucker**
Macronutrient Intake and Insulin Resistance in 5665 Randomly Selected, Non-Diabetic U.S. Adults
Reprinted from: *Nutrients* 2022, 14, 918, doi:10.3390/nu14050918 . . . . . . . . . . . . . . . . . 99

**Zeinab Rafiee, Alba M. García-Serrano and João M. N. Duarte**
Taurine Supplementation as a Neuroprotective Strategy upon Brain Dysfunction in Metabolic Syndrome and Diabetes
Reprinted from: *Nutrients* 2022, 14, 1292, doi:10.3390/nu14061292 . . . . . . . . . . . . . . . . . 119

**Sílvia V. Conde, Fátima O. Martins, Sara S. Dias, Paula Pinto, Cristina Bárbara and Emília C. Monteiro**
Dysmetabolism and Sleep Fragmentation in Obstructive Sleep Apnea Patients Run Independently of High Caffeine Consumption
Reprinted from: *Nutrients* **2022**, *14*, 1382, doi:10.3390/nu14071382 . . . . . . . . . . . . . . . . . . **139**

**Michalina Banaszak, Ilona Górna and Juliusz Przysławski**
Non-Pharmacological Treatments for Insulin Resistance: Effective Intervention of Plant-Based Diets—A Critical Review
Reprinted from: *Nutrients* **2022**, *14*, 1400, doi:10.3390/nu14071400 . . . . . . . . . . . . . . . . . . **149**

**Adriana M. Capucho, Ana Chegão, Fátima O. Martins, Hugo Vicente Miranda and Sílvia V. Conde**
Dysmetabolism and Neurodegeneration: Trick or Treat?
Reprinted from: *Nutrients* **2022**, *14*, 1425, doi:10.3390/nu14071425 . . . . . . . . . . . . . . . . . . **163**

**Abdullatif Azab**
D-Pinitol—Active Natural Product from Carob with Notable Insulin Regulation
Reprinted from: *Nutrients* **2022**, *14*, 1453, doi:10.3390/nu14071453 . . . . . . . . . . . . . . . . . . **193**

**Marlene Lages, Renata Barros, Pedro Moreira and Maria P. Guarino**
Metabolic Effects of an Oral Glucose Tolerance Test Compared to the Mixed Meal Tolerance Tests: A Narrative Review
Reprinted from: *Nutrients* **2022**, *14*, 2032, doi:10.3390/nu14102032 . . . . . . . . . . . . . . . . . . **211**

# About the Editors

**Silvia V. Conde**

Silvia V. Conde is Assistant Professor and Principal Investigator at Nova Medical School, New University of Lisbon. Silvia has developed a new line of research on carotid body (CB) and dysmetabolism based on the pioneering idea that CB controls glucose homeostasis. She is dedicated to the characterization of pathophysiological biosignals, disease signatures and fingerprints that will allow the identification of targets for therapy, particularly bioelectronic targets, as her group has described that the high frequency electrical stimulation of the carotid sinus nerve restores glucose homeostasis in type 2 diabetes models. In 2009, Silvia was awarded with the L'Oreal Medals Honor for Women in Science Portugal and, since then, her group has won several prizes from the Portuguese Society of Diabetes and the Pulido Valente Foundation.

**Fatima O. Martins**

Fatima O. Martins is Junior Researcher and Affiliated Professor at Nova Medical School, New University of Lisbon. Fatima is interested in studying the mechanisms involved in metabolic diseases, and both the peripheral and central signals and the molecular pathways behind them. She has won many prizes for best communication and project from the Portuguese Society of Diabetes, best student at the University of Coimbra, etc . In 2015, Fatima created a biotech startup, LifeTag Diagnostics, which is currently developing a new methodology for the diagnostic of intestinal permeability alterations.

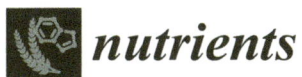

*Editorial*

# Impact of Diet Composition on Insulin Resistance

Fátima O. Martins * and Silvia V. Conde *

iNOVA4Health, NOVA Medical School, Faculdade de Ciências Médicas, Universidade Nova de Lisboa, Campo Mártires da Pátria, 1169-056 Lisboa, Portugal
* Correspondence: fatima.martins@nms.unl.pt (F.O.M.); silvia.conde@nms.unl.pt (S.V.C.)

Insulin resistance is a complex condition in which the body does not respond adequately to insulin, a hormone secreted by the pancreas with an essential role in the regulation of blood sugar levels. This condition is one of the major factors in the pathology of cardiometabolic diseases, which are commonly associated with peripheral insulin resistance. Peripheral insulin resistance consists of an impaired biologic response to insulin stimulation of peripheral target tissues, namely the liver, muscle and fat tissue [1]. More recently, central insulin resistance has been highlighted as fundamental also in cardiometabolic diseases since insulin plays an important role at brain circuitries that control food behavior and autonomic activity [1,2]. Moreover, brain insulin resistance is associated with cognition impairment and important neurodegenerative diseases such as Alzheimer's Disease and Parkinson Disease [3].

Several genetic and lifestyle factors can contribute to insulin resistance, with disruptions in diet composition being one of the major factors contributing to this condition. In contrast, different feed regimens and some nutrients have beneficial impacts on insulin resistance and disease development.

This Special Issue was developed to compile studies that highlight the beneficial or deleterious impact of different nutritional plans on insulin sensitivity and metabolism and that unravel mechanistic links between diet composition and nutritional status and the development of insulin resistance, both peripherally and centrally.

One of the most consumed food components worldwide is caffeine. This xanthine is the most widely consumed psychoactive substance in the world and is present in several dietary sources regularly consumed, such as tea, coffee, cocoa beverages, chocolate bars, and soft drinks [4]. In recent decades, physicians have advised hypertensive and diabetic patients to limit caffeine intake, based on several studies stating that caffeine acutely increases blood pressure [5] and lowers insulin sensitivity [6–8]. More recently, chronic coffee/caffeine intake was associated with an improved insulin sensitivity and glucose metabolism [9,10] and a lower risk of type 2 diabetes [11], clearly suggesting that acute and chronic caffeine intake have opposite effects on metabolism. However, obstructive sleep apnea (OSA) patients that frequently exhibit cardiometabolic dysfunction and insulin resistance [12,13] consume on average three times more caffeine than control subjects [14]. In this issue, Conde and colleagues [15] studied the impact of caffeine intake on OSA severity and OSA association with dysmetabolism and sympathetic nervous system dysfunction. They found that OSA patients consume more caffeine, but this was not associated with OSA severity or with dysmetabolism and sleep fragmentation, which rejects the common clinical recommendation for caffeine avoidance in OSA patients. The only parameter that these authors highlighted to be somehow disrupted by high caffeine levels in OSA patients, and therefore should be taken in account for clinical recommendations, is the overactivation of the sympathetic nervous system, which is frequently associated with some cardiovascular conditions [16,17] but also with insulin resistance.

Several different diet patterns are being adopted by an increasing proportion of the world population. Diet patterns can be defined as the quantities, proportions, variety, or combination of different foods, drinks, and nutrients in diets, and the frequency with

**Citation:** Martins, F.O.; Conde, S.V. Impact of Diet Composition on Insulin Resistance. *Nutrients* **2022**, *14*, 3716. https://doi.org/10.3390/nu14183716

Received: 29 August 2022
Accepted: 5 September 2022
Published: 9 September 2022

**Publisher's Note:** MDPI stays neutral with regard to jurisdictional claims in published maps and institutional affiliations.

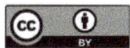

**Copyright:** © 2022 by the authors. Licensee MDPI, Basel, Switzerland. This article is an open access article distributed under the terms and conditions of the Creative Commons Attribution (CC BY) license (https://creativecommons.org/licenses/by/4.0/).

which they are habitually consumed [18]. While some of these have been described to have deleterious impacts on health, e.g., hypercaloric diets [19], others have been described as beneficial, e.g., the Mediterranean diet [20]. However, the effects of such diet patterns on physiology and pathology are surrounded by controversy due to the different results between populations and pathological conditions. For example, discussions about the impact of different regimens for the prevention of chronic diseases related with insulin resistance such as type 2 diabetes, obesity, and non-alcoholic fatty liver disease (NAFLD) among others, form the basis of a number of studies that can be found in the literature.

In this Special Issue, this discussion occupies an important space. Banaszak and colleagues reviewed the positive effects of vegetarian and vegan diets on insulin resistance [21]. These authors concluded that vegetarian and vegan populations have better blood parameters, and that more plant-based foods and fewer animal foods in a diet result in lower insulin resistance and a lower risk of prediabetes and type 2 diabetes. Additionally, they discussed the possible use of these plant-based diets in clinical applications for the treatment and prevention of chronic diseases since parameters such as body weight, body fat, BMI and lipid profile improve under this type of diet. They also showed that meat-free diets are suitable for everyone, regardless of age or health, but improperly balanced plant-based diets may carry a risk of nutritional deficiencies; in particular, deficiencies in protein, B vitamins, iron, zinc, and omega 3 fatty acids have been noted. They recommend further clinical research and provide guidance on future research directions.

Another study in this Special Issue discussing the impact of a plant-based diet on insulin resistance was conducted by Lorinczova and colleagues [22]. In this original study, the authors tested the impact of plant-derived proteins from rice, potato and of whey on insulin secretion, glucose maintenance and appetite perception in a group of healthy males in a single-blind, randomized study. They found differing glycemic and insulinemic properties between potato, rice and whey proteins following ingestion, with whey promoting a higher increase in insulin and GLP-1 secretion with a consequent higher decrease in glucose levels than plant-derived proteins. Moreover, dampened insulin and GLP-1 responses with better glycemic regulation after the ingestion of plant proteins compared to whey, with no significant differences in average appetite perception, was observed. Taken together, the results of the study suggest that the characteristics of each protein, irrespective of plant or animal origin, result in differing metabolic responses and that plant-based protein regimens may have benefits for populations where tighter control of glycemic and insulinemic regulation may be beneficial while maintaining total protein intake.

It is agreed upon that high sugar intake is associated with insulin resistance and with an increased incidence of metabolic diseases, such as obesity and metabolic syndrome. Sugars can be categorized as intrinsic/natural and extrinsic/added sugars depending on if they are naturally present in the structure or matrix of whole fresh fruits and vegetables, milk, and dairy products without further processing, or if they are added to food. Added sugars include sucrose, fructose, glucose, starch hydrolysates and other isolated sugar preparations added during food preparation and manufacturing [23]. These intrinsic and added sugars have been described to have different impacts on these pathological conditions, with the added sugars being highly associated with metabolic diseases. However, there is still controversy about whether the intrinsic sugars from fruit juices have a similar harmful effect as sugars added to beverages. The work of Monteiro-Alfredo and colleagues [24] contributes to the knowledge in this field by comparing the impact of four different fruit juices administered across four weeks with sugary solutions having a similar sugar profile and concentration on weight, hyperglycemia, glycation and oxidative stress in control and diabetic animal models. They demonstrated that sugars naturally present in fruit juices have a less severe impact in terms of metabolic control than the added sugars in foods that promote a poorer glycemic profile and increased levels of glycation and oxidative stress, particularly in tissues such as the heart and the kidney [24]. Taken together, these results reinforce the evidence supporting a noxious role for added sugars and a harmless effect of moderate intakes of fruit sugars, even in diabetic models. Nevertheless, the authors stress that more research should be performed to investigate the long-term effect of fruit juices in metabolism as well as in animal models.

A comparison between two carbohydrates, isomaltulose—a disaccharide carbohydrate composed of glucose and fructose—and sucrose, in arterial stiffness in response to acute hyperglycemia was also performed in this Special Issue by Kobayashi et al. [25]. With the knowledge that an increased arterial stiffness in response to acute hyperglycemia is associated with high cardiovascular risk [26], this study investigated the efficacy of low-glycemic-index isomaltulose on arterial stiffness during hyperglycemia in ten middle-aged and older adults. They found that arterial stiffness and systolic blood pressure did not change following isomaltulose intake in middle-age and older adults, in contrast with sucrose ingestion, suggesting that isomaltulose could be used as an alternative to sucrose.

The Mediterranean diet has been referenced for decades as a diversified diet with a beneficial impact on cardiometabolic diseases. Interest in this diet began in the 1950s/1960s, when it was realized that Mediterranean countries had lower rates of heart disease than other countries worldwide [20]. However, the impact of the Mediterranean diet is broader as there is robust evidence suggesting that it improves HbA1c and insulin sensitivity [27,28], which are benefits that have been associated with the presence of large number of functional foods and nutraceuticals. Such a diet, predominantly plant-based, is characterized by a high consumption of extra-virgin olive oil, nuts, red wine, vegetables, and other polyphenol-rich elements, with a moderate consumption of fish, poultry, and eggs and a low consumption of red meat [20]. High-protein diets have also been shown to be efficacious in promoting weight loss along with improvements in insulin sensitivity [19]. The comparison between a diversified diet pattern, such as the Mediterranean diet, and a high protein diet can be observed in the original article from Tettamanzi et al. [29] where they found that a high protein diet was more effective in reducing insulin resistance and improving glycemic control in morbidly obese women with pre-diabetes. Additionally, they assessed microbial diversity in the gut of these women, and identified a panel of microbes that explain the differences in the effect of the two diet patterns. However, further investigation is required to elucidate the links between dietary interventions, the microbiome and insulin action regulation.

Still related to products from Mediterranean countries, Azab and colleagues reviewed the impact of carob, one of the major food trees for people of Mediterranean origin, on the regulation of metabolism [30]. They described the nutritional composition of carob, highlighting that D-Pinitol as one of the most important components. D-pinitol has been used for decades as a medicinal product with antidiabetic, anti-Alzheimer, anticancer, antioxidant, anti-inflammatory, and immune- and hepato-protective properties. The authors state that more studies are needed to define the exact mechanisms of D-pinitol in insulin regulation as well as to establish the clinical applications of this compound and others found in carob.

Along with the beneficial impact of some diet components and patterns on metabolism [e.g., potato and rice—[22]] and the deleterious effects of others [e.g., added sugars—[24]] described in this Special Issue, the original work of Mohamad Hizami et al. introduces new results on the impact of probiotics on hepatic steatosis, fibrosis and biochemical blood tests related with NAFLD [31]. Probiotics are foods or supplements containing live microorganisms aiming to maintain or improve microbiota. Given that insulin resistance relates to the increased incidence of NAFLD and that the gut microbiota, by being part of the gut-liver axis, can be a target for NAFLD related problems, the authors performed a randomized, double-blind, placebo-controlled trial with 39 NAFLD patients supplemented with either a probiotics sachet (MCP® BCMC® strains) or a placebo for a total of 6 months. They did not find clinical improvements in NAFLD patients after the use of probiotics, but this treatment was shown to stabilize the mucosal immune function. These results led them to state that probiotics usage can protect NAFLD patients against the increase in intestinal permeability and suggest the need of additional studies with larger sample sizes, a longer duration, and different probiotic strains to evaluate the real benefit of probiotics in the management of NAFLD.

The impact of diet patterns on the regulation of the metabolism and in the pathological conditions related with insulin resistance is also known to be dependent not only on different cultural behaviors between different populations but also on their genetic background. Pandya and colleagues studied the Asian Indian (AI) population from Mangal Mandir, a Hindu temple in the Baltimore/Washington Metropolitan Area [32]. AI populations are at an increased risk of developing type 2 diabetes mellitus compared to other ethnic groups, even though they have a lower body mass index, for a number of reasons. These include that the age of onset for T2DM in AI populations is estimated to occur 10 years earlier than in Europeans; AI populations require lower BMI cut-offs for the effective identification of T2DM risk; and AI individuals may be predisposed to IR and T2DM because AI children are born smaller, have more fat, and less lean muscle [33]. The authors performed a descriptive statistical analysis where they found that weight loss may not be the recommendation for diabetes management in this population, yet an increase in protein and insoluble fiber consumption could play a critical role.

Tucker studied the relationship between several macronutrients and insulin resistance in 5665 non-diabetic U.S. adults and the author determined the extent to which these associations were influenced by multiple potential confounding variables [34]. The study was a cross-sectional design of 8 years of data from 2011 to 2018 from the U.S. National Health and Nutrition Examination Survey (NHANES) database. The author found that macronutrient intake was predictive of insulin resistance in this population with higher intakes of carbohydrates, leading to a worse scenario in terms of insulin resistance. Additionally, the author described that a higher intake of protein or unsaturated fat leads to lower levels of insulin resistance.

Additionally, in this Special Issue the thematic of methodologies to assess metabolic dysfunction is debated. The oral glucose tolerance test (OGTT) is recognized as the gold standard test for diagnosing diabetes [35]. However, even though it provides important information about glucose tolerance, it does not replicate the physiological effect of a complete meal and the impact of it this insulin secretion and insulin action [36]. Therefore, Lages and colleagues [37] reviewed clinical data that shows the importance of a mixed meal tolerance test (MMTT) as a method that is more reliable and better resembles physiological prandial changes when diagnosing metabolic alterations. They concluded that a complete nutritional challenge performed in the MMTT seems to be more physiological but the divergency in results highlights the need to compare this method and the OGTT in the diagnosis of diseases such as type 2 diabetes in larger clinical trials.

Finally, and with the knowledge that insulin does not only act in the periphery but is also present in the brain where it has an important role in the regulation of food behavior and cognition, this Special Issue also highlights the impact of central insulin resistance in the link between metabolic and neurodegenerative diseases.

Rafiee and colleagues debated the role of taurine in neurodegeneration-metabolic diseases [38]. Taurine is a sulfur-containing amino acid naturally found in meat, fish, dairy products, and human milk, and is also available as a dietary supplement. While it is generally accepted that taurine supplementation has beneficial effects in the peripheral dysmetabolism in animals and humans [39–41], several studies have also proposed that the deregulation of brain taurine homeostasis may play a role in dysmetabolism-neurodegeneration. Although taurine concentration is decreased in the brains of models of neurodegenerative disorders [42], diet-induced obesity leads to taurine accumulation in the hippocampus [43]. Therefore, the authors speculate that the cerebral accumulation of taurine might constitute a compensatory mechanism that attempts to prevent neurodegeneration, due to its cytoprotective effect. By reviewing the literature, they debated the role of cerebral taurine in obese and diabetic individuals and concluded that taurine contributes to brain health improvements in those subjects by various mechanisms including the modulation of inhibitory neurotransmission, the stimulation of antioxidant systems, and the stabilization of mitochondria and thus of energy production and Ca2+ homeostasis. They also suggest that further studies are needed to unravel the exact mechanisms of taurine action in metabolic disorders with an impact on brain function.

Finally, the study by Capucho and colleagues reviews the literature supporting the link between metabolic syndrome and neurodegeneration [44]. They discuss the impact of aging and dietary habits as important hallmarks for the development of neurodegeneration, focusing on two of the most prevalent neurodegenerative diseases, Alzheimer Disease and Parkinson's Disease. They provide evidence for a central role of insulin in cognitive function regulation and food behavior control and review the mechanisms behind hypercaloric diet intake and brain insulin deregulation on neurodegenerative processes. They conclude by proposing new targets of therapeutic interventions to control these epidemics of metabolic and neurodegenerative diseases.

The studies compiled in this Special Issue are representative of the numerous studies focusing on the association between diet composition, dietary patterns and insulin resistance that have been conducted to date with controversial results. Therefore, more investigations are certainly needed to untangle the complex associations between diet composition and insulin resistance, both peripherally and centrally, to better understand the mechanisms behind the connection between different diet patterns and the development of metabolic and neurodegenerative disorders and to establish new methodologies to correctly diagnose these pathologies.

This Special Issue will open new doors to manage insulin-resistance associated diseases by appropriately and individually modulating nutritional strategies.

**Funding:** FO Martins is supported by Portuguese Science and Technology Foundation (CEECIND/04266/2017).

**Conflicts of Interest:** The authors declare no conflict of interest.

# References

1. Huang, X.; Liu, G.; Guo, J.; Su, Z. The PI3K/AKT pathway in obesity and type 2 diabetes. *Int. J. Biol. Sci.* **2018**, *14*, 1483–1496. [CrossRef]
2. Taouis, M.; Torres-Aleman, I. Editorial: Insulin and the brain. *Front. Endocrinol.* **2019**, *10*, 299. [CrossRef]
3. Hölscher, C. Brain insulin resistance: Role in neurodegenerative disease and potential for targeting. *Expert Opin. Investig. Drugs* **2020**, *29*, 333–348. [CrossRef]
4. Fredholm, B.B.; Bättig, K.; Holmén, J.; Nehlig, A.; Zvartau, E.E. Actions of caffeine in the brain with special reference to factors that contribute to its widespread use. *Pharmacol. Rev.* **1999**, *51*, 83–133. Available online: http://pharmrev.aspetjournals.org/content/51/1/83.abstract (accessed on 28 August 2022).
5. Riksen, N.P.; Rongen, G.A.; Smits, P. Acute and long-term cardiovascular effects of coffee: Implications for coronary heart disease. *Pharmacol. Ther.* **2009**, *121*, 185–191. [CrossRef]
6. Moisey, L.L.; Kacker, S.; Bickerton, A.C.; E Robinson, L.; E Graham, T. Caffeinated coffee consumption impairs blood glucose homeostasis in response to high and low glycemic index meals in healthy men. *Am. J. Clin. Nutr.* **2008**, *87*, 1254–1261. [CrossRef]
7. Keijzers, G.B.; De Galan, B.E.; Tack, C.J.; Smits, P. Caffeine can decrease insulin sensitivity in humans. *Diabetes Care* **2002**, *25*, 364–369. [CrossRef]
8. Sacramento, J.F.; Ribeiro, M.J.; Yubero, S.; Melo, B.F.; Obeso, A.; Guarino, M.P.; Gonzalez, C.; Conde, S.V. Disclosing caffeine action on insulin sensitivity: Effects on rat skeletal muscle. *Eur. J. Pharm. Sci.* **2015**, *70*, 107–116. [CrossRef]
9. Conde, S.V.; Nunes Da Silva, T.; Gonzalez, C.; Mota Carmo, M.; Monteiro, E.C.; Guarino, M.P. Chronic caffeine intake decreases circulating catecholamines and prevents diet-induced insulin resistance and hypertension in rats. *Br. J. Nutr.* **2012**, *107*, 86–95. [CrossRef]
10. Reis, C.E.; Dórea, J.G.; da Costa, T.H. Effects of coffee consumption on glucose metabolism: A systematic review of clinical trials. *J. Tradit. Complement. Med.* **2018**, *9*, 184–191. [CrossRef]
11. Hubert, K.; Stephan, M.; Kerstin, K. Coffee and Lower Risk of Type 2 Diabetes: Arguments for a Causal Relationship. *Nutrients* **2021**, *13*, 1144.
12. Bonsignore, M.R.; Borel, A.L.; Machan, E.; Grunstein, R. Sleep apnoea and metabolic dysfunction. *Eur. Respir. Rev.* **2013**, *22*, 353–364. [CrossRef] [PubMed]
13. Almendros, I.; Basoglu, Ö.K.; Conde, S.V.; Liguori, C.; Saaresranta, T. Metabolic dysfunction in OSA: Is there something new under the sun? *J. Sleep Res.* **2022**, *31*, 1–16. [CrossRef] [PubMed]
14. Bardwell, W.A.; Ziegler, M.G.; Ancoli-Israel, S.; Berry, C.C.; Nelesen, R.A.; Durning, A.; Dimsdale, J.E. Does caffeine confound relationships among adrenergic tone, blood pressure and sleep apnoea? *J. Sleep Res.* **2000**, *9*, 269–272. [CrossRef]

15. Conde, S.V.; Martins, F.O.; Dias, S.S.; Pinto, P.; Bárbara, C.; Monteiro, E.C. Dysmetabolism and Sleep Fragmentation in Obstructive Sleep Apnea Patients Run Independently of High Caffeine Consumption. *Nutrients* **2022**, *14*, 1382. [CrossRef]
16. Iqbal, M.; Shah, S.; Fernandez, S.; Karam, J.; Jean-Louis, G.; McFarlane, S.I. Obesity, obstructive sleep apnea, and cardiovascular risk. *Curr. Cardiovasc. Risk Rep.* **2008**, *2*, 101–106. [CrossRef]
17. Narkiewicz, K.; Van De Borne, P.J.H.; Montano, N.; Dyken, M.E.; Phillips, B.G.; Somers, V.K. Contribution of tonic chemoreflex activation to sympathetic activity and blood pressure in patients with obstructive sleep apnea. *Circulation* **1998**, *97*, 943–945. [CrossRef]
18. United States Department of Agriculture. *A Series of Systematic Reviews on the Relationship Between Dietary Patterns and Health Outcomes*; U.S. Department of Health and Human Services: Virginia, USA, 2014; p. 501.
19. McAuley, K.A.; Hopkins, C.M.; Smith, K.J.; McLay, R.T.; Williams, S.M.; Taylor, R.W.; Mann, J.I. Comparison of high-fat and high-protein diets with a high-carbohydrate diet in insulin-resistant obese women. *Diabetologia* **2005**, *48*, 8–16. [CrossRef]
20. Widmer, R.J.; Flammer, A.J.; Lerman, L.O.; Lerman, A. The Mediterranean diet, its components, and cardiovascular disease. *Am. J. Med.* **2015**, *128*, 229–238. [CrossRef]
21. Banaszak, M.; Górna, I.; Przysławski, J. Non-Pharmacological Treatments for Insulin Resistance: Effective Intervention of Plant-Based Diets—A Critical Review. *Nutrients* **2022**, *14*, 1400. [CrossRef]
22. Tiekou Lorinczova, H.; Deb, S.; Begum, G.; Renshaw, D.; Zariwala, M.G. Comparative assessment of the acute effects of whey, rice and potato protein isolate intake on markers of glycaemic regulation and appetite in healthy males using a randomised study design. *Nutrients* **2021**, *13*, 2157. [CrossRef]
23. Agostoni, C.V.; Bresson, J.L.; Tait, S.F.; Flynn, A.; Golly, I.; Korhonen, H.; Lagiou, P.; Løvik, M.; Marchelli, R.; Martin, A.; et al. Scientific Opinion on Dietary Reference Values for carbohydrates and dietary fibre. *EFSA J.* **2016**, *8*, 1462.
24. Monteiro-Alfredo, T.; Caramelo, B.; Arbeláez, D.; Amaro, A.; Barra, C.; Silva, D.; Oliveira, S.; Seiça, R.; Matafome, P. Distinct Impact of Natural Sugars from Fruit Juices and Added Sugars on Caloric Intake, Body Weight, Glycaemia, Oxidative Stress and Glycation in Diabetic Rats. *Nutrients* **2021**, *13*, 2956. [CrossRef]
25. Kobayashi, R.; Sakazaki, M.; Nagai, Y.; Asaki, K.; Hashiguchi, T.; Negoro, H. Effects of Different Types of Carbohydrates on Arterial Stiffness: A Comparison of Isomaltulose and Sucrose. *Nutrients* **2021**, *13*, 4493. [CrossRef]
26. Tominaga, M.; Eguchi, H.; Manaka, H.; Igarashi, K.; Kato, T.; Sekikawa, A. Impaired glucose tolerance is a risk factor for cardiovascular disease, but not impaired fasting glucose. The Funagata Diabetes Study. *Diabetes Care* **1999**, *22*, 920–924. [CrossRef]
27. Shai, I.; Schwarzfuchs, D.; Henkin, Y.; Shahar, D.R.; Witkow, S.; Greenberg, I.; Golan, R.; Fraser, D.; Bolotin, A.; Vardi, H.; et al. Weight Loss with a Low-Carbohydrate, Mediterranean, or Low-Fat Diet. *N. Engl. J. Med.* **2008**, *359*, 229–241. [CrossRef]
28. Greco, M.; Chiefari, E.; Montalcini, T.; Accattato, F.; Costanzo, F.S.; Pujia, A.; Foti, D.; Brunetti, A.; Gulletta, E. Early Effects of a Hypocaloric, Mediterranean Diet on Laboratory Parameters in Obese Individuals. *Mediat. Inflamm.* **2014**, *2014*, 750860. [CrossRef]
29. Tettamanzi, F.; Bagnardi, V.; Louca, P.; Nogal, A.; Monti, G.S.; Mambrini, S.P.; Lucchetti, E.; Maestrini, S.; Mazza, S.; Rodriguez-Mateos, A.; et al. A High Protein Diet Is More Effective in Improving Insulin Resistance and Glycemic Variability Compared to a Mediterranean Diet—A Cross-Over Controlled Inpatient Dietary Study. *Nutrients* **2021**, *13*, 4380. [CrossRef]
30. Azab, A. D-Pinitol—Active Natural Product from Carob with Notable Insulin Regulation. *Nutrients* **2022**, *14*, 1453. [CrossRef]
31. Nor, M.H.M.; Ayob, N.; Mokhtar, N.M.; Ali, R.A.R.; Tan, G.C.; Wong, Z.; Shafiee, N.H.; Wong, Y.P.; Mustangin, M.; Nawawi, K.N.M. The Effect of Probiotics (MCP® BCMC® Strains) on Hepatic Steatosis, Small Intestinal Mucosal Immune Function, and Intestinal Barrier in Patients with Non-Alcoholic Fatty Liver Disease. *Nutrients* **2021**, *13*, 3192.
32. Pandya, A.; Mehta, M.; Sankavaram, K. The Relationship between Macronutrient Distribution and Type 2 Diabetes in Asian Indians. *Nutrients* **2021**, *13*, 4406. [CrossRef] [PubMed]
33. Bhopal, R.S. A four-stage model explaining the higher risk of Type 2 diabetes mellitus in South Asians compared with European populations. *Diabet. Med.* **2012**, *30*, 35–42. [CrossRef] [PubMed]
34. Tucker, L.A. Macronutrient Intake and Insulin Resistance in 5665 Randomly Selected, Non-Diabetic U.S. Adults. *Nutrients* **2022**, *14*, 918. [CrossRef] [PubMed]
35. World Health Organization. *Definition and Diagnosis of Diabetes Mellitus and Intermediate Hyperglycaemia: Report of a WHO/IDF Consultation*; World Health Organization: Geneva, Switzerland, 2006; Available online: https://apps.who.int/iris/handle/10665/43588 (accessed on 20 August 2022).
36. Meier, J.J.; Baller, B.; Menge, B.A.; Gallwitz, B.; Schmidt, W.E.; Nauck, M.A. Excess glycaemic excursions after an oral glucose tolerance test compared with a mixed meal challenge and self-measured home glucose profiles: Is the OGTT a valid predictor of postprandial hyperglycaemia and vice versa? *Diabetes Obes. Metab.* **2009**, *11*, 213–222. [CrossRef] [PubMed]
37. Lages, M.; Barros, R.; Moreira, P.; Guarino, M.P. Metabolic Effects of an Oral Glucose Tolerance Test Compared to the Mixed Meal Tolerance Tests: A Narrative Review. *Nutrients* **2022**, *14*, 2032. [CrossRef]
38. Rafiee, Z.; García-Serrano, A.M.; Duarte, J.M.N. Taurine Supplementation as a Neuroprotective Strategy upon Brain Dysfunction in Metabolic Syndrome and Diabetes. *Nutrients* **2022**, *14*, 1292. [CrossRef]
39. De Carvalho, F.G.; Brandao, C.F.C.; Muñoz, V.R.; Batitucci, G.; Tavares, M.E.d.A.; Teixeira, G.R.; Pauli, J.R.; De Moura, L.P.; Ropelle, E.R.; Cintra, D.E.; et al. Taurine supplementation in conjunction with exercise modulated cytokines and improved subcutaneous white adipose tissue plasticity in obese women. *Amino Acids* **2021**, *53*, 1391–1403. [CrossRef]

40. Kim, K.S.; Oh, D.H.; Kim, J.Y.; Lee, B.G.; You, J.S.; Chang, K.J.; Chung, H.; Yoo, M.C.; Yang, H.-I.; Kang, J.-H.; et al. Taurine ameliorates hyperglycemia and dyslipidemia by reducing insulin resistance and leptin level in Otsuka Long-Evans Tokushima fatty (OLETF) rats with long-term diabetes. *Exp. Mol. Med.* **2012**, *44*, 665–673. [CrossRef]
41. Tao, X.; Zhang, Z.; Yang, Z.; Rao, B. The effects of taurine supplementation on diabetes mellitus in humans: A systematic review and meta-analysis. *Food Chem. Mol. Sci.* **2022**, *4*, 100106. Available online: https://www.sciencedirect.com/science/article/pii/S266656622200034X (accessed on 29 August 2022). [CrossRef]
42. Aquilani, R.; Costa, A.; Maestri, R.; Cotta Ramusino, M.; Pierobon, A.; Dossena, M.; Solerte, S.B.; Condino, A.M.; Torlaschi, V.; Bini, P.; et al. Mini Nutritional Assessment May Identify a Dual Pattern of Perturbed Plasma Amino Acids in Patients with Alzheimer's Disease: A Window to Metabolic and Physical Rehabilitation? *Nutrients* **2020**, *12*, 1845. [CrossRef]
43. Lizarbe, B.; Soares, A.F.; Larsson, S.; Duarte, J.M.N. Neurochemical modifications in the hippocampus, cortex and hypothalamus of mice exposed to long-term high-fat diet. *Front. Neurosci.* **2019**, *13*, 985. [CrossRef] [PubMed]
44. Capucho, A.M.; Chegão, A.; Martins, F.O.; Miranda, H.V.; Conde, S.V. Dysmetabolism and Neurodegeneration: Trick or Treat? *Nutrients* **2022**, *14*, 1425. [CrossRef] [PubMed]

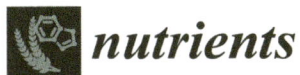

Article

# Comparative Assessment of the Acute Effects of Whey, Rice and Potato Protein Isolate Intake on Markers of Glycaemic Regulation and Appetite in Healthy Males Using a Randomised Study Design

Helena Tiekou Lorinczova [1], Sanjoy Deb [1], Gulshanara Begum [1], Derek Renshaw [2,†] and Mohammed Gulrez Zariwala [1,*,†]

1. Centre for Nutraceuticals, School of Life Sciences, University of Westminster, 115 New Cavendish Street, London W1W 6UW, UK; w1505041@my.westminster.ac.uk (H.T.L.); S.Deb@westminster.ac.uk (S.D.); begumru@westminster.ac.uk (G.B.)
2. Centre for Sport, Exercise and Life Sciences, Institute of Health & Wellbeing, Coventry University, Priory Street, Coventry CV1 5FB, UK; derek.renshaw@coventry.ac.uk
* Correspondence: zariwam@wmin.ac.uk; Tel.: +44-20-7911-5000 (ext. 65086)
† These authors contributed equally to this work.

**Abstract:** Global protein consumption has been increasing for decades due to changes in demographics and consumer shifts towards higher protein intake to gain health benefits in performance nutrition and appetite regulation. Plant-derived proteins may provide a more environmentally sustainable alternative to animal-derived proteins. This study, therefore, aimed to investigate, for the first time, the acute effects on glycaemic indices, gut hormones, and subjective appetite ratings of two high-quality, plant-derived protein isolates (potato and rice), in comparison to a whey protein isolate in a single-blind, triple-crossover design study with nine male participants (30.8 ± 9.3 yrs). Following a 12 h overnight fast, participants consumed an equal volume of the three isocaloric protein shakes on different days, with at least a one-week washout period. Glycaemic indices and gut hormones were measured at baseline, then at 30, 60, 120, 180 min at each visit. Subjective palatability and appetite ratings were measured using visual analogue scales (VAS) over the 3 h, at each visit. This data showed significant differences in insulin secretion with an increase in whey (+141.8 ± 35.1 pmol/L; $p$ = 0.011) and rice (−64.4 ± 20.9 pmol/L; $p$ = 0.046) at 30 min compared to potato protein. A significantly larger total incremental area under the curve (iAUC) was observed with whey versus potato and rice with $p$ < 0.001 and $p$ = 0.010, respectively. There was no significant difference observed in average appetite perception between the different proteins. In conclusion, this study suggests that both plant-derived proteins had a lower insulinaemic response and improved glucose maintenance compared to whey protein.

**Keywords:** protein; animal-derived proteins; plant-derived proteins; whey protein; potato protein; rice protein; insulin; GLP-1; appetite; glucose homeostasis; type 2 diabetes mellitus (T2DM)

## 1. Introduction

Global protein consumption has been increasing steadily for decades [1] and is expected to continue to rise due to a combination of factors, which include changing socio-economic demographics [2] and changing consumer trends towards higher protein intake [3]. Health benefits frequently reported include improved free fat mass [4]; strength [5,6] and physical function [7] in adults. Furthermore, the satiating effects of protein have been well established [8–10]. In addition to reports describing a reduction in energy intake, protein consumption has the potential to impact weight loss [11]. The mechanisms responsible for protein-mediated appetite suppression include an alteration in gastric emptying [12] and modulation of regulation of gut-derived satiety hormones, including peptide YY (PYY), glucagon-like peptide-1 (GLP-1) and cholecystokinin (CCK) [13–15]. Furthermore, protein meals, and more prominently those containing whey protein, have been shown to have greater insulinaemic responses and improved regulation of postprandial glucose homeostasis [16]. Taken together, these observations suggest that dietary protein intake may have a positive association with metabolic and physical health.

Dairy foods are a rich source of proteins (e.g., whey and casein), which provide the necessary amino acids that the human body cannot synthesise [17]. Animal-derived proteins such as whey, are often cited as being of high quality due to their favourable rates of absorption, comprehensive amino acid profile and high levels of branched-chain amino acids (BCAA; leucine, isoleucine and valine); particularly leucine (~3 g/25 g whey protein), which stimulates muscle protein synthesis [18]. Whey and casein have also been shown to regulate appetite by increasing satiety and delaying the return of the feeling of hunger [19]. In addition, whey and casein have been reported to reduce subsequent energy intake [20,21], with an inclination towards whey having a superior effect [22]. These factors have led to an exponential growth in the adoption of whey protein in consumer products such as beverages and functional foods for appetite regulation and performance nutrition applications [23].

In parallel to the commercial growth of whey protein fortified functional foods and supplements, there has also been greater interest and adoption of plant-based eating patterns, such as vegetarian and veganism [24]. Various non-animal derived protein sources such as soy protein, rice protein and wheat protein have been explored scientifically and commercially in recent years, demonstrating varying levels of benefits and drawbacks [25,26]. Potato protein is a relatively novel source of plant-derived protein that provides a promising alternative to milk proteins [27]. Potato protein isolate is derived as a byproduct of starch manufacture and is therefore relatively cost-efficient compared to other protein sources. Furthermore, its nonallergenic, gluten and lactose-free characteristics make it an attractive dietary ingredient [28]. Interestingly, evidence from previous studies demonstrate that proteins from varied sources may differ significantly in their quality and consequently their satiating capacity [12,16,28]. It remains to be fully elucidated whether proteins from alternative sources can provide the identical metabolic benefits as those associated with milk proteins.

Towards this end, several assessments of protein quality have been put forward and various scales devised. Scales such as the protein digestibility–corrected amino acid score (PDCAAS), adopted by the World Health Organisation (WHO) [29] and the digestible Indispensable Amino Acid Score (DIAAS) [30] have been reviewed extensively elsewhere [30]. However, protein quality also needs to be balanced with effects on human health, at least in certain groups. Recent evidence from obese, insulin resistant groups indicate that the BCAA metabolite signature, indicative of increased catabolism of BCAA, were present and may be associated with the pathogenesis of obesity-associated insulin resistance [31]. In addition, the work of Rigamonti et al. [32] has implicated specific amino acids as having appetite suppressant and GLP-1 stimulating effects mediated via nutrient-sensing receptors in the gastrointestinal (GI) wall. Given the differing structural compositions and variable metabolic effects, it would be prudent to compare the appetite-regulating effects of proteins from differing sources.

To date, acute comparisons of appetite and glycaemic responses between animal and plant-derived protein have only focused on soy and pea protein isolates compared to whey [33–35]. These studies have suggested that soy and pea protein isolates elicit comparable effects on insulin, glucose and appetite regulation; however, to the authors' knowledge, the evidence comparing plant-derived protein isolates, such as potato and rice protein, to whey protein appears to be sparse. The current study was designed to investigate the acute effects on glycaemic indices, gut hormones and subjective palatability and appetite ratings of two high-quality, plant-derived protein isolates; potato protein isolate (Solanic®100, ProteinmiXer.com®, Bonn, Germany) and rice protein isolate (Organic Oryzatein® Silk 90, Axiom Foods/Growing Naturals, Inc., Los Angeles, CA, USA), against a high quality whey protein isolate-*BiPRO*® (Davisco Foods International, Inc., Eden Prairie, MN, USA) using a randomised, blinded cross-over design study. To the best knowledge of the authors, this is the first study of its kind that compares the above parameters between these protein isolates.

## 2. Materials and Methods

### 2.1. Participants

A total of 9 (from the randomized 12, Figure S1) male participants between the ages of 21 and 47 years completed the study. Participants' suitability for the study was assessed using a Health Screening Questionnaire, completed on the first laboratory visit. Questions on pre-existing health conditions such as diabetes, high blood pressure and coronary heart disease (including whether on medication) were asked. In addition, dietary and supplementation aspects were captured. Individuals consuming more than 21 units of alcohol/week, having allergies to ingredients in the test shakes, suffering from illnesses that affect taste or appetite, gastrointestinal disorders, eating disorders, depression and/or smokers were not suitable for participation. Baseline anthropometric measurements were also collected on the same day by trained research staff. Height was measured using a Seca Leicester Height Measure (Seca GmbH & Co. KG, Hamburg, Germany). Weight, body mass index (BMI) and body fat % were measured using the Seca 515 medical Body Composition Analyser (Seca GmbH & Co. KG, Hamburg, Germany) and Bod Pod® (Life Measurement, Concord, CA, USA). Participants signed written informed consent forms prior to participation. Ethical approval (ID: VRE1516-1375) was granted by the Faculty of Science and Technology Ethics Committee, University of Westminster, in accordance with the ethical standards of the Helsinki Declaration of 1975.

### 2.2. Study Design

A single-blind (blinding of participants), randomised, triple cross-over study design was employed. Participants received three different protein shakes in a random order which was generated using the online service by Randomization.com [36]. Equal volume of the three isocaloric protein shakes prepared using whey, rice and potato protein powders were administered on different days, with at least a one-week washout period (Figure 1).

### 2.3. Study Protocol

Prior to the experimental trial days, the participants were instructed to attend the laboratory having abstained from caffeine intake and following a 12 h overnight fast. On arrival, a cannula was inserted in the antecubital fossa via an Introcan Safety® IV catheter (20G) (B. Braun, Sheffield, UK), after which a baseline blood sample was collected (Time 0; T0). Participants were presented with one of the randomly assigned protein shakes (detailed below) from identical dark bottles and were instructed to drink the full amount within 5 min. Further blood samples were then drawn at timepoints T30, T60, T120 and T180 during each visit. Approximately 10 mL of blood was collected from each participant per timepoint using Becton Dickinson (BD) Vacutainer® EDTA tubes (BD, Oxford, UK). Blood in the EDTA (ethylenediaminetetraacetic acid) tubes was kept on ice and centrifuged (Hettich 340r, Hettich GmbH & Co. KG, Tuttlingen, Germany) within 2 h of collection, for 10 min at 3857 g. Plasma supernatants were aliquoted into 1.5 mL microcentrifuge tubes immediately post-centrifugation and stored at $-80$ °C. Furthermore, visual analogue scales (VAS) [37] were completed by all participants to measure subjective aspects such as palatability (measured during consumption of test shake) and satiety (measured at T0, T30, T60, T90, T120, T150 and T180).

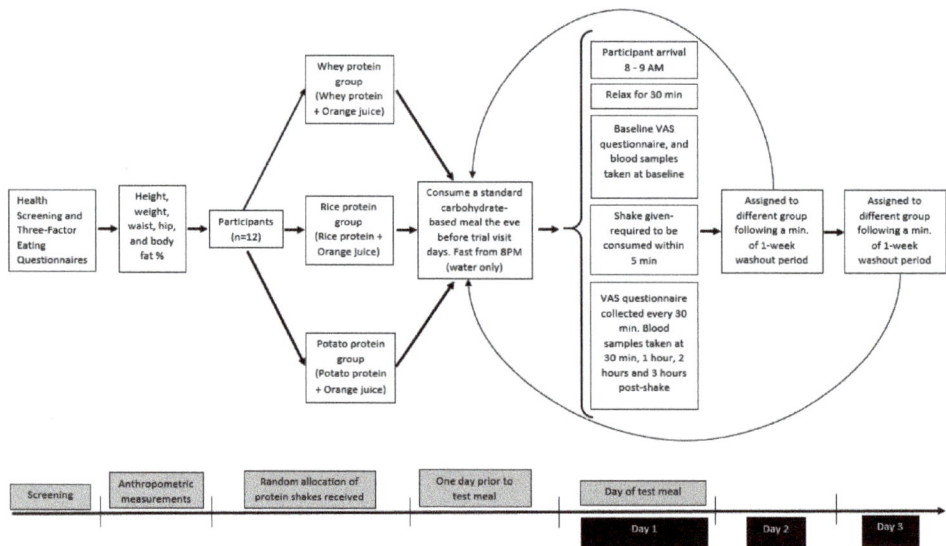

**Figure 1.** Overview of study design.

*2.4. Protein Shake Intervention*

Participants were provided with the same volume of three different (whey, rice and potato) isocaloric protein shakes with an equal weight of protein content (Table 1). Protein content in each condition equated to approximately 45 g protein, as this had previously been shown to elicit satiating effects in a plant-derived protein (soy; [38]) and was above the threshold to elicit satiating effects from whey protein [39].

**Table 1.** Composition of protein shakes.

| Protein Product | Product (g) in Shake | Protein (g) in Shake | Nutritional Composition of Orange Juice | Water (mL) | Total Energy Per Drink (Kcal) |
|---|---|---|---|---|---|
| Instantized *BiPRO*® (Whey Protein Isolate) | 50 | 45.5 | Volume: 207 mL<br>Calories: 43.5 kcal<br>Carbohydrates: 8.0 g<br>Protein: 0.6 g | 43 | 233.5 |
| Oryzatein™ 90 (Rice Protein Isolate) | 50 | 45.5 | Volume: 183 mL<br>Calories: 43.5 kcal<br>Carbohydrates: 7.1 g<br>Protein: 0.5 g | 67 | 233.4 |
| Solanic®100 (Potato Protein Isolate) | 48 | 45.3 | Volume: 250 mL<br>Calories: 52.4 kcal<br>Carbohydrates: 9.8 g<br>Protein: 0.75 g | 0 | 233.5 |

The shakes were prepared freshly on the visit day by mixing the required amount of the specific protein powder in 250 mL of liquid consisting of low sugar orange juice (Tropicana Trop50, Tropicana UK LTD, Leicester, UK) to improve palatability and water in predefined ratios. The orange juice allowed for the overall calorie and protein content to be matched across the three trials, to mitigate for their confounding effects on markers of appetite regulation. The composition of carbohydrates was within 2.7 g across the three conditions, which may result in a typical 0.5–0.8 mmol/L difference in blood glucose [40]. The three protein powders used were whey protein isolate (WPI; Instantized *BiPRO*®, Davisco Foods International, Inc., Eden Prairie, MN, USA), rice protein isolate (RPI; Organic

Oryzatein® Silk 90, Axiom Foods/Growing Naturals, Inc., Los Angeles, CA, USA), and potato protein isolate (PPI; Solanic®100, ProteinmiXer.com®, Bonn, Germany). The WPI used was a dairy protein of high dispersibility [41] and high purity, with a 91% protein content (nutritional information provided by Davisco Foods International, Inc., Eden Prairie, MN, USA). The RPI used was sourced from whole rice grain, which is a suspendable food grade product with a protein content of 91% [42]. The PPI used was a product of protein absorption technology that enables the coagulation of protein from potato juice. The PPI is of high protein quality based on its DIAAS [27], with a protein content of 94% (nutritional information provided by Avebe, Veendam, The Netherlands) [27,43]. The full amino acid profiles of the protein powders are outlined in Table 2.

**Table 2.** Typical amino acid profile expressed per 100 g protein.

| Amino Acids (AA) | Whey Protein Isolate (%) | Rice Protein Concentrate (%) | Potato Protein Isolate (%) |
|---|---|---|---|
| Histidine * | 2.0 | 2.2 | 1.8 |
| Isoleucine *,+ | 5.6 | 4.2 | 5.9 |
| Leucine *,+ | 12.7 | 8.3 | 9.8 |
| Lysine * | 10.2 | 2.9 | 7.6 |
| Methionine * | 2.3 | 3.0 | 1.1 |
| Phenylalanine * | 3.5 | 5.6 | 7.0 |
| Threonine * | 4.7 | 3.7 | 4.7 |
| Tryptophan * | 2.9 | 1.5 | 1.5 |
| Valine *,+ | 5.4 | 5.6 | 8.6 |
| Arginine | 2.4 | 8.3 | 4.8 |
| Cysteine | 2.8 | 2.4 | 2.4 |
| Glutamic Acid/Glutamine | 16.1 | 17.9 | 7.9 |
| Glycine | 1.7 | 4.5 | 5.7 |
| Proline | 4.7 | 4.8 | 5.4 |
| Tyrosine | 3.6 | 5.6 | 5.4 |
| Alanine | 4.9 | 5.7 | 2.5 |
| Aspartic Acid/Asparagine | 11.4 | 8.9 | 13.1 |
| Serine | 3.3 | 5.1 | 4.8 |
| **Total EAA** | 49.3 | 37 | 48 |
| **Total BCAA** | 23.7 | 18.1 | 24.3 |

* Essential Amino Acid (EAA), + branch-chain amino acids (BCAA).

### 2.5. Plasma Analysis

Plasma was analysed to determine the primary outcomes of this study, which was to assess the acute effects of whey, rice and potato protein isolates on glucose, insulin, Homoeostasis Model Assessment–Estimated Insulin Resistance (HOMA–IR), total GLP-1 (amount of GLP-1, 7–36 and 9–36 forms), PYY and ghrelin. For each biomarker, assay kits were from the same Lot number and all samples were measured on the same day.

Plasma glucose concentrations were detected using a YSI 2300 STAT Plus Glucose Lactate Analyzer (YSI, Inc., Yellow Springs, OH, USA) and this is considered to be a gold standard method [44]. The YSI analyser utilises a steady-state measurement methodology based on the glucose oxidase technique (YSI STAT 2300 Plus laboratory manual). Plasma insulin concentration was analysed using an insulin ELISA (enzyme-linked immunosorbent assay) kit (DRG Insulin Elisa kit, DRG Instruments GmbH, Marburg, Germany). The measurement involved a solid phase enzyme-linked immunosorbent assay based on the sandwich principle. The analytical sensitivity was 0.076 ng/mL and the assay range was 0.076–4.33 ng/mL, and an intra-assay coefficient of variation (CV) of 2.5%, and inter-assay CV of 4.8% were determined. The measured plasma glucose and insulin levels were used to calculate HOMA–IR, a method for assessing β-cell function, using the following formula: fasting serum insulin (μU/mL) × fasting plasma glucose (mmol/L)/22.5 [45]. Total plasma GLP-1 was analysed using GLP-1 Total ELISA (Millipore Corporation, Billerica, MA, USA), a sandwich ELISA assay. The limit of sensitivity was 1.5 pM, and the assay range was

4.1 pM to 1000 pM GLP-1 Total/50 µl sample respectively, and an intra-assay CV of 2.1% and inter-assay CV of 9.8% were determined. Plasma peptide YY (PYY) was analysed using the Human PYY ELISA Kit (FineTest, Wuhan Fine Biological Technology Co., Ltd., Wuhan, Hubei, China). The kit's sensitivity and detection range were 18.75 pg/mL and 31.25–2000 pg/mL, respectively, with an intra-assay CV of 6.6% and inter-assay CV of 9.4%. Total plasma ghrelin was detected using a competitive Millipore Human Ghrelin (Total) ELISA kit (Sigma-Aldrich, Darmstadt, Germany). The kit's sensitivity was 9 pmol/L (20 µl sample size), with an intra-assay CV of 2.2% and inter-assay CV of 6.3%. All assay procedures were performed according to the manufacturer's instructions and plates were read using a microplate reader (SPECTROstar® Nano, BMG Labtech GmbH, Ortenberg, Germany).

### 2.6. Satiety and Palatability

The palatability of the protein shakes was assessed using VAS [37], consisting of five characteristics related to visual appeal, smell, taste, aftertaste and palatability (where 0 = good and 100 = bad). The satiety effects of the protein shakes were evaluated using a VAS measurement tool (a psychometric response scale using a 100 mm line with anchor statements at either end of the line). The satiety VAS contained eight characteristics of interest and included levels of hunger (0 = not hungry at all, 100 = never been hungrier), satisfaction (0 = completely empty, 100 = cannot eat another bite), fullness (0 = not at all full, 100 = totally full) and prospective food intake (0 = nothing at all, 100 = a lot). This data was used to calculate an average appetite response across the measurement period, using an adapted equation from Zafar et al. [46]:

Average appetite = [prospective food intake + hunger + (100 − fullness) + (100 − satisfaction)]/4

### 2.7. Statistical Analysis

The Shapiro–Wilk test provided no evidence to reject the hypothesis that all data were normally distributed. A two-way (condition (whey vs. potato vs. rice) * time) repeated measures analysis of variance (ANOVA) was used to assess differences in glucose, insulin, HOMA-IR, GLP-1, PYY, ghrelin, palatability, and average appetite. Furthermore, incremental area under the curve (iAUC) analysis was performed on glucose, insulin, GLP-1, PYY and ghrelin for each condition. Total iAUC was compared between whey, rice and potato for each variable using a one-way ANOVA. Where a significant main effect was found following the ANOVA, Bonferroni post hoc paired comparisons were performed. All analyses were carried out using IBM SPSS (v25.0 for Windows; SPSS, Chicago, IL, USA). The level of significance was set at $p < 0.05$. To establish statistical power, a post hoc power calculation was performed, with a reported power (1−β) greater than 0.8 for insulin, glucose, and GLP-1. In contrast, PYY and ghrelin had a power of 0.33 and 0.65, respectively. All descriptive data are presented as mean ± standard deviation unless otherwise stated.

## 3. Results

Nine healthy male participants volunteered for the study with the following characteristics (mean ± SD), age: 30.8 ± 9.3 years; height: 180.2 ± 7.5 cm; and bodyweight: 86.6 ± 6.7 kg.

### 3.1. Glycemic and Insulinaemic Response

There was an overall significant Condition * Time interaction for blood glucose ($p < 0.001$; Figure 2a). While these differences were not apparent at baseline, the whey condition had significantly lower blood glucose concentrations at 30 min compared to potato and rice conditions ($p = 0.05$ and $p = 0.038$, respectively), and this remained significantly different to the potato condition at 60 min ($p = 0.004$). No other differences were observed between conditions at other timepoints. Furthermore, time-related changes were also observed within all three conditions. In the whey condition, there was a significant reduction in glucose at 60 min to 4.5 ± 0.3 mmol/L compared to all other timepoints (all

$p < 0.05$). A fall in glucose concentration was observed in the potato and rice conditions but this only reached significance at 120 min in the rice condition (vs. 30 min; $p = 0.007$); while the potato condition saw significant differences at 120 and 180 min (vs. baseline and 30 min; all $p < 0.05$). Overall differences in blood glucose were also observed with total iAUC comparisons (Table 3), with the whey condition showing significantly lower iAUC compared to potato ($p = 0.048$) but not rice ($p = 0.082$).

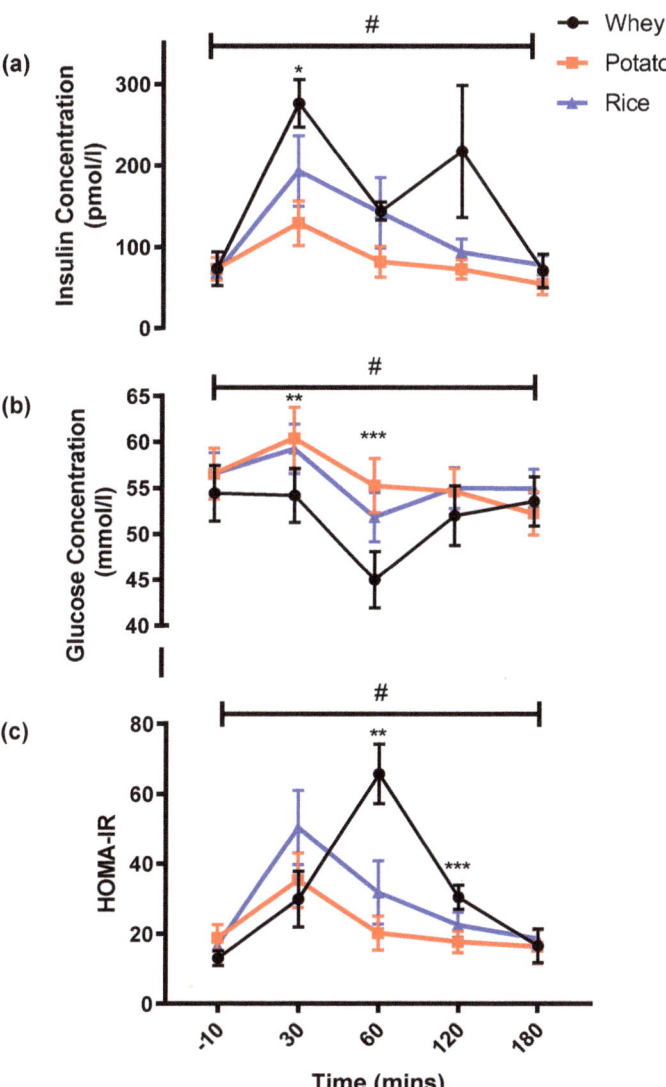

**Figure 2.** (**a**). Blood Insulin concentrations, (**b**) Blood Glucose concentrations and (**c**) HOMA-IR observed across the three experimental conditions. * Potato is significantly different to both conditions ($p < 0.05$). ** Whey is significantly different to both conditions ($p < 0.05$). *** Whey is significantly different from potato only ($p < 0.05$). # Shows that significance was present with time ($p < 0.05$).

**Table 3.** Mean (±SD) total iAUC for blood glucose, plasma insulin, GLP-1, PYY and ghrelin.

|  | Whey | Potato | Rice | Overall Significance |
|---|---|---|---|---|
| Glucose | 2.16 ± 3.8 * | 14.01 ± 11.50 | 13.24 ± 12.3 | 0.013 |
| Insulin | 20,290.71 ± 14,222.9 # | 3293.2 ± 2179.5 | 9002.8 ± 9564.8 | <0.001 |
| GLP-1 | 4248.5 ± 1323.1 # | 325.1 ± 596.7 | 1646.4 ± 1289.1 | <0.001 |
| PYY | 511.7 ± 930.1 | 794.7 ± 923.8 | 905.4 ± 1076.9 | 0.697 |
| Ghrelin | 1433.9 ± 22268.8 | 4668.3 ± 5540.3 | 17,186.1 ± 24,893.6 | 0.130 |

* Whey is statistically significant compared to Potato ($p < 0.05$); # Whey is statistically significant compared to Potato and Rice ($p < 0.05$).

Blood insulin also displayed an overall significant Condition * Time interaction ($p = 0.031$; Figure 2b), with post hoc analysis revealing significant changes only occurred at 30 min as the potato condition remained significantly lower than the rice ($-64.4 ± 20.9$ pmol/L; $p = 0.046$) and whey ($-141.8 ± 35.1$ pmol/L; $p = 0.011$) conditions. Concerning time, differences were only observed in the whey condition as blood insulin peaked at 30 min, which was significantly greater than baseline, 60 and 180 min, but not 120 min. This was also reflected in the total iAUC being higher in the whey condition than potato ($p = 0.013$) and rice ($p = 0.001$).

The HOMA-IR also reflected the changes observed with glucose and insulin as a significant Condition * Time interaction was observed ($p < 0.001$; Figure 2c). The whey condition demonstrated a significantly greater response at 60 min compared to potato ($p = 0.004$) and rice ($p = 0.009$), but this difference was only sustained at 120 min with the potato condition ($p = 0.024$). From baseline, only rice saw a significant increase at 30 min ($p = 0.026$), but this fell towards baseline levels from 60 min onwards. In comparison, the whey condition saw a peak at 60 min ($p < 0.05$), which also remained significantly elevated compared to baseline at 120 min ($p = 0.011$). No differences were seen in the potato condition during the 180 min sampling period.

### 3.2. Appetite Related Hormones

Overall differences in GLP-1 were observed with a Condition * Time interaction ($p < 0.001$; Figure 3a). The potato condition showed no change in GLP-1 throughout the measurement period and remained significantly lower compared to whey at 30 min ($p = 0.007$) and to both whey and rice at 60 min ($p = 0.001$ and $p = 0.033$, respectively), 120 min ($p < 0.001$ and $p = 0.001$, respectively), and 180 min ($p = 0.007$ and $p = 0.001$, respectively). While differences between whey and rice were present at 60 min ($p = 0.001$). The whey condition demonstrated an overall three-fold increase in concentration from baseline to 120 min ($p = 0.001$). Significant increases were present from baseline to 30 min ($p = 0.001$) and 60 min ($p < 0.001$), after which GLP1 concentrations began to plateau, as differences between 60 min and 120 min were not present ($p = 1.0$). The rice condition also exhibited a peak at 120 min, which was a significantly greater concentration than both the 30 min ($p = 0.024$) and 60 min ($p = 0.04$) timepoints. The iAUC calculations highlighted a significantly larger total iAUC in the whey condition compared to both the potato ($p < 0.001$) and rice conditions ($p = 0.010$; Table 3).

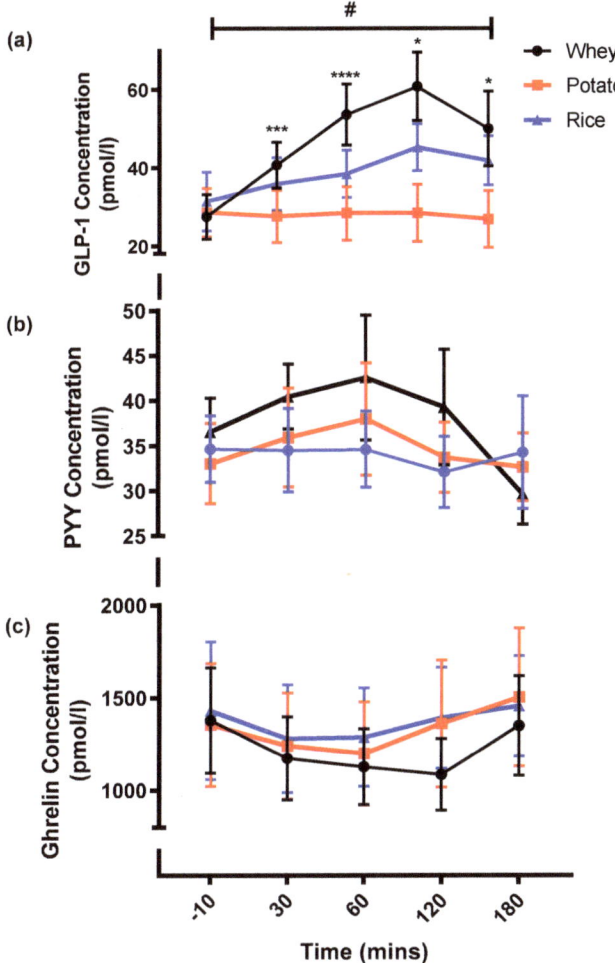

**Figure 3.** (a) Blood GLP-1 concentrations, (b) Blood PYY concentrations and (c) Blood ghrelin concentrations observed across the three experimental conditions. * Potato is significantly different to both conditions ($p < 0.05$). *** Whey is significantly different from potato only ($p < 0.05$). **** All conditions significantly different to each other ($p < 0.05$). # Shows that significance was present with time ($p < 0.05$).

Differences in PYY were not detected by time or condition (Figure 3b), with any changes throughout the measurement period remaining nonsignificant. Equally, no differences in iAUC of PYY were calculated ($p = 0.697$). Ghrelin concentrations between conditions and time were also nonsignificant (Figure 3c; $p = 0.290$). However, there was a trend for greater total iAUC in the rice condition (Table 3), but this was also nonsignificant ($p = 0.09$).

### 3.3. Palatability and Satiety

The whey beverage was reported to possess greater visual appeal ($p = 0.022$) and palatability ($p = 0.009$) compared to the rice protein beverage. There were no other differences in smell, taste, aftertaste, visual appeal, or palatability observed between the three conditions (Table 4). Average appetite perception was not different between the protein conditions, but average appetite increased, showing a trend to significance with time (Figure 4; $p = 0.013$).

**Table 4.** Mean (±SD) scores from the VAS questions on palatability.

|  | Whey | Potato | Rice | Overall Significance |
|---|---|---|---|---|
| Smell | 27.9 ± 21.8 | 38.4 ± 30.4 | 36.7 ± 18.4 | 0.102 |
| Taste | 36.9 ± 26.6 | 52.3 ± 36.2 | 53.5 ± 22.0 | 0.173 |
| Aftertaste | 44.7 ± 32.7 | 56.6 ± 31.0 | 56.1 ± 31.0 | 0.06 |
| Visual appeal | 24.3 ± 23.0 * | 37.3 ± 29.6 | 42.6 ± 27.4 | 0.022 |
| Palatability | 33.7 ± 21.9 * | 54.1 ± 35.5 | 67.0 ± 27.7 | 0.009 |

* Whey is statistically significant compared to Rice only ($p < 0.05$).

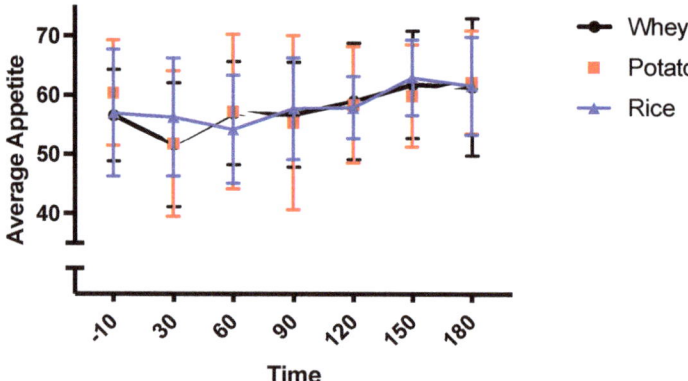

**Figure 4.** Shows average appetite perception across the three conditions.

## 4. Discussion

This study demonstrated differing glycaemic and insulinaemic properties between potato, rice and whey proteins following ingestion. The insulin and glucose responses with whey protein were more substantial than both plant-derived proteins, with an acute rise in blood insulin accompanied by a reduction in blood glucose. Conversely, the glucose and insulin responses in rice and potato conditions were smaller, with a significantly lower response to blood insulin shown at 30 min following potato ingestion compared to whey. GLP-1 changes correspond to changes in insulin levels, with potato showing no change throughout the measurement period, but both rice and whey proteins increased with time to differing extents. However, appetite perception did not change as a result of the metabolic responses. Together, this suggests that characteristics of each protein, irrespective of plant or animal origin, may result in differing metabolic responses.

Potato protein isolate compares favourably with whey protein in terms of protein quality and has been scored 0.87 and 0.85 on the PDCAAS and DIAAS compared to whey protein, which scored as 1.0 and 0.90, respectively [3]. Rice protein fares less well in comparison to whey at 0.53 and 0.52, respectively [3]; although, comparisons of whey protein and brown rice protein supplementation on indices of body composition and exercise performance in resistance-trained males found no significant differences in post-exercise recovery and changes in body composition [47]. Significant absorption of total amino acids, essential amino acids, branch chain amino acids, and leucine have previously been demonstrated following a test meal of potato protein isolate in an acute feeding study [48]; although the appearance of amino acids in the blood following the meal was blunted and occurred later than whey protein. Proteins affect insulin secretion differently and may be influenced by the amino acid composition [49,50], but also by the rate of appearance of specific amino acids in the blood, including BCAA, phenylalanine, arginine and tyrosine [51–53], and/or the release of incretin hormones after ingestion of different proteins [52]. BCAAs, in particular, are thought to be potently insulinotropic [54,55]. In the current study, the total amount of BCAAs in the whey protein isolate and the potato protein isolate are well matched; however, given the results of previous studies [48], it is likely that the rate of digestion/absorption of whey protein derived BCAAs is more rapid than the plant-derived proteins and peaks earlier [48]. Nuttall et al. [56] previously demonstrated that incretin hormone release rather than total plasma amino acid levels is responsible for stimulating insulin release, which is in agreement with the current data.

The stimulation and release of GLP-1 hormone by amino acids and dipeptides is triggered in the gut lumen on the apical surface of the entero-endocrine L cells rather than by plasma levels of absorbed amino acids [57]. L cells are located throughout the human GI tract [58], with the majority concentrated in the distal gut [59]. This luminal location of the GLP-1 sensing machinery may indicate that the rate of digestion and the appearance of specific amino acids may be key to triggering GLP-1 release rather than the rate of absorption per se. This more rapid rate of digestion of whey protein may be influential in stimulating incretin hormone release (in this case, GLP-1) in the current study. This data indicates that whey and rice protein isolates significantly increase levels of GLP-1 and insulin, whereas potato protein has no effect.

Glutamine is a potent stimulator of GLP-1 release in endocrine L cell in vitro models, such as the GLUTag cell line [57]; however, this effect has not been demonstrated in vivo in humans. Interestingly, in the current study, glutamine levels were lowest in the potato protein isolate (7.9%; see Table 2) compared to whey (16.1%) or rice protein (17.9%). Therefore, the glutamine amino acid content of proteins may go some way to explaining the lack of GLP-1 hormone release in response to potato protein ingestion in the current study.

The current data, therefore, sheds more light onto the area of amino acid digestion/absorption and suggests that as well as the amino acid composition, the rate of digestion/absorption of BCAAs, essential amino acids (EAAs), total amino acids (TAAs) or individual amino acids may influence the release of incretin hormones (in this case GLP-1), which leads to insulinotropic effects. This may suggest that a threshold exists for incretin hormone release in the presence of amino acid digestion/absorption and that the potato protein described in the current study was below this threshold for GLP-1 sensing/stimulation. In contrast, whey and rice protein isolates breached this threshold and therefore triggered GLP-1 release, which stimulated insulin release to restore glucose homeostasis. Potato protein isolate also stimulates muscle protein synthesis during rest and following resistance exercise [60], indicating anabolic properties similar to whey protein.

Palatability and sensory characteristics are known drivers of food choice [61]. Although protein isolates are known to have a relatively better palatability profile compared to protein hydrolysates, very few studies have compared palatability between different proteins isolates in humans. This study shows that although whey protein demonstrated significantly greater visual appeal and palatability than rice protein, there were no other significant changes in smell, taste, aftertaste, visual appeal, and palatability between the three protein isolates. The variability in palatability between whey protein and rice protein also suggests that the use of low sugar orange juice as a flavouring agent did not fully mask the proteins' original sensory and palatability characteristics.

## 5. Conclusions

This study is the first to observe the differing glycaemic, insulinaemic and appetite responses of potato and rice protein isolates compared to whey protein. While the metabolic effects of whey protein have been well established, the results demonstrate a dampened insulin response after the ingestion of the plant proteins, with potato protein maintaining better glycaemic regulation compared to whey. Equally, GLP-1 responses were also muted in the plant protein condition compared to whey, which included no changes in GLP-1 following potato protein ingestion. The differences in GLP-1 stimulation may be explained by the amino acid profiles of the protein isolates and, in particular, the lower concentrations of glutamine in the potato protein isolate. Taken together, this study sheds light on the implications of the protein source on glycaemic, insulinaemic and appetite regulation. These metabolic responses may elicit potential benefits for populations where tighter control of glycaemic and insulinaemic regulation may be beneficial while maintaining total protein intake.

**Supplementary Materials:** The following are available online at https://www.mdpi.com/article/10.3390/nu13072157/s1, Figure S1: CONSORT flow diagram showing number of participants through each stage of the randomised cross-over trial.

**Author Contributions:** Conceptualisation and methodology: M.G.Z., D.R., G.B. and H.T.L.; Randomisation, participants' enrolment, and treatment sequence allocation: H.T.L.; Supervision: M.G.Z., D.R. and G.B.; Investigation and data curation: H.T.L. and S.D.; Data analysis: S.D.; Writing—original draft preparation: H.T.L., D.R., S.D. and M.G.Z.; Writing—review and editing: M.G.Z., D.R., G.B., S.D. and H.T.L. All authors have read and agreed to the published version of the manuscript.

**Funding:** This research received no external funding.

**Institutional Review Board Statement:** The study was conducted according to the guidelines of the Declaration of Helsinki, and approved by the Faculty of Science and Technology Ethics Committee, University of Westminster (ID: VRE1516-1375 18 November 2016).

**Informed Consent Statement:** Informed consent was obtained from all subjects involved in the study.

**Data Availability Statement:** The data presented in this study are available on request from the corresponding author. The data are not publicly available due to ethical, legal and privacy issues.

**Acknowledgments:** We gratefully acknowledge the time and dedication of all participants who participated in this study. We thank Davisco Foods International, Inc., Eden Prairie, MN, USA, for providing us samples of Instantized BiPRO®® and Axiom Foods/Growing Naturals, Inc., Los Angeles, CA, USA, for providing us samples of Organic Oryzatein®® Silk 90. We would like to acknowledge all colleagues from The University of Westminster who contributed support and expertise to this study. We thank Bradley Elliot for his assistance and training with the cannulation protocol and Helen Lloyd for her technical assistance.

**Conflicts of Interest:** The authors declare no conflict of interest.

## References

1. Food and Agriculture Organization. *World Agriculture: Towards 2015/2030: An FAO Perspective*; FAO: Rome, Italy, 2003.
2. Henchion, M.; Hayes, M.; Mullen, A.M.; Fenelon, M.; Tiwari, B. Future protein supply and demand: Strategies and factors influencing a sustainable equilibrium. *Foods* **2017**, *6*, 53. [CrossRef]
3. Hertzler, S.R.; Lieblein-Boff, J.C.; Weiler, M.; Allgeier, C. Plant Proteins: Assessing Their Nutritional Quality and Effects on Health and Physical Function. *Nutrients* **2020**, *12*, 3704. [CrossRef] [PubMed]
4. Houston, D.K.; Nicklas, B.J.; Ding, J.; Harris, T.B.; Tylavsky, F.A.; Newman, A.B.; Jung, S.L.; Sahyoun, N.R.; Visser, M.; Kritchevsky, S.B. Dietary protein intake is associated with lean mass change in older, community-dwelling adults: The Health, Aging, and Body Composition (Health ABC) study. *Am. J. Clin. Nutr.* **2008**, *87*, 150–155. [CrossRef] [PubMed]
5. McLean, R.R.; Mangano, K.M.; Hannan, M.T.; Kiel, D.P.; Sahni, S. Dietary Protein Intake Is Protective Against Loss of Grip Strength Among Older Adults in the Framingham Offspring Cohort. *J. Gerontol. Ser. A Biol. Sci. Med. Sci.* **2016**, *71*, 356–361. [CrossRef]
6. Mishra, S.; Goldman, J.D.; Sahyoun, N.R.; Moshfegh, A.J. Association between dietary protein intake and grip strength among adults aged 51 years and over: What We Eat in America, National Health and Nutrition Examination Survey 2011–2014. *PLoS ONE* **2018**, *13*, e0191368. [CrossRef] [PubMed]
7. Mustafa, J.; Ellison, R.C.; Singer, M.R.; Bradlee, M.L.; Kalesan, B.; Holick, M.F.; Moore, L.L. Dietary Protein and Preservation of Physical Functioning among Middle-Aged and Older Adults in the Framingham Offspring Study. *Am. J. Epidemiol.* **2018**, *187*, 1411–1419. [CrossRef] [PubMed]
8. de Castro, J.M. Macronutrient relationships with meal patterns and mood in the spontaneous feeding behavior of humans. *Physiol. Behav.* **1987**, *39*, 561–569. [CrossRef]
9. Hill, A.J.; Blundell, J.E. Comparison of the Action of Macronutrients on the Expression of Appetite in Lean and Obese Human Subjects. *Ann. N. Y. Acad. Sci.* **1989**, *575*, 529–531. [CrossRef]
10. Latner, J.D.; Schwartz, M. The effects of a high-carbohydrate, high-protein or balanced lunch upon later food intake and hunger ratings. *Appetite* **1999**, *33*, 119–128. [CrossRef]

11. Paddon-Jones, D.; Westman, E.; Mattes, R.D.; Wolfe, R.R.; Astrup, A.; Westerterp-Plantenga, M. Protein, weight management, and satiety. *Am. J. Clin. Nutr.* **2008**, *87*, 1558S–1561S. [CrossRef]
12. Hall, W.L.; Millward, D.J.; Long, S.J.; Morgan, L.M. Casein and whey exert different effects on plasma amino acid profiles, gastrointestinal hormone secretion and appetite. *Br. J. Nutr.* **2003**, *89*, 239–248. [CrossRef]
13. De Graaf, C.; Blom, W.A.M.; Smeets, P.A.M.; Stafleu, A.; Hendriks, H.F.J. Biomarkers of satiation and satiety. *Am. J. Clin. Nutr.* **2004**, *79*, 946–961. [CrossRef] [PubMed]
14. Karhunen, L.J.; Juvonen, K.R.; Huotari, A.; Purhonen, A.K.; Herzig, K.H. Effect of protein, fat, carbohydrate and fibre on gastrointestinal peptide release in humans. *Regul. Pept.* **2008**, *149*, 70–78. [CrossRef] [PubMed]
15. Fromentin, G.; Darcel, N.; Chaumontet, C.; Marsset-Baglieri, A.; Nadkarni, N.; Tomé, D. Peripheral and central mechanisms involved in the control of food intake by dietary amino acids and proteins. *Nutr. Res. Rev.* **2012**, *25*, 29–39. [CrossRef]
16. Pal, S.; Ellis, V. The acute effects of four protein meals on insulin, glucose, appetite and energy intake in lean men. *Br. J. Nutr.* **2010**, *104*, 1241–1248. [CrossRef]
17. Górska-Warsewicz, H.; Laskowski, W.; Kulykovets, O.; Kudlińska-Chylak, A.; Czeczotko, M.; Rejman, K. Food products as sources of protein and amino acids—The case of Poland. *Nutrients* **2018**, *10*, 1977. [CrossRef] [PubMed]
18. Moore, D.R.; Churchward-Venne, T.A.; Witard, O.; Breen, L.; Burd, N.A.; Tipton, K.D.; Phillips, S.M. Protein Ingestion to Stimulate Myofibrillar Protein Synthesis Requires Greater Relative Protein Intakes in Healthy Older Versus Younger Men. *J. Gerontol. Ser. A Biol. Sci. Med. Sci.* **2015**, *70*, 57–62. [CrossRef]
19. Pal, S.; Radavelli-Bagatini, S.; Hagger, M.; Ellis, V. Comparative effects of whey and casein proteins on satiety in overweight and obese individuals: A randomized controlled trial. *Eur. J. Clin. Nutr.* **2014**, *68*, 980–986. [CrossRef] [PubMed]
20. Alfenas, R.C.G.; Bressan, J.; de Paiva, A.C. Efeitos da qualidade proteica no apetite e metabolismo energético de indivíduos eutróficos. *Arq. Bras. Endocrinol. Metabol.* **2010**, *54*, 45–51. [CrossRef]
21. Astbury, N.M.; Stevenson, E.J.; Morris, P.; Taylor, M.A.; MacDonald, I.A. Dose-response effect of a whey protein preload on within-day energy intake in lean subjects. *Br. J. Nutr.* **2010**, *104*, 1858–1867. [CrossRef]
22. Veldhorst, M.A.B.; Westerterp-Plantenga, M.S.; Westerterp, K.R. Gluconeogenesis and energy expenditure after a high-protein, carbohydrate-free diet. *Am. J. Clin. Nutr.* **2009**, *90*, 519–526. [CrossRef]
23. Patel, S. Emerging trends in nutraceutical applications of whey protein and its derivatives. *J. Food Sci. Technol.* **2015**, *52*, 6847–6858. [CrossRef] [PubMed]
24. Medawar, E.; Huhn, S.; Villringer, A.; Veronica Witte, A. The effects of plant-based diets on the body and the brain: A systematic review. *Transl. Psychiatry* **2019**, *9*, 1–17. [CrossRef] [PubMed]
25. Ahnen, R.T.; Jonnalagadda, S.S.; Slavin, J.L. Role of plant protein in nutrition, wellness, and health. *Nutr. Rev.* **2019**, *77*, 735–747. [CrossRef] [PubMed]
26. Gorissen, S.H.M.; Crombag, J.J.R.; Senden, J.M.G.; Waterval, W.A.H.; Bierau, J.; Verdijk, L.B.; van Loon, L.J.C. Protein content and amino acid composition of commercially available plant-based protein isolates. *Amino Acids* **2018**, *50*, 1685–1695. [CrossRef] [PubMed]
27. Levy, R.; Okun, Z.; Davidovich-Pinhas, M.; Shpigelman, A. Utilization of high-pressure homogenization of potato protein isolate for the production of dairy-free yogurt-like fermented product. *Food Hydrocoll.* **2021**, *113*, 106442. [CrossRef]
28. Acheson, K.J.; Blondel-Lubrano, A.; Oguey-Araymon, S.; Beaumont, M.; Emady-Azar, S.; Ammon-Zufferey, C.; Monnard, I.; Pinaud, S.; Nielsen-Moennoz, C.; Bovetto, L. Protein choices targeting thermogenesis and metabolism. *Am. J. Clin. Nutr.* **2011**, *93*, 525–534. [CrossRef] [PubMed]
29. Schaafsma, G. The protein digestibility-corrected amino acid score. *J. Nutr.* **2000**, *130*, 1865–1867. [CrossRef]
30. Mathai, J.K.; Liu, Y.; Stein, H.H. Values for digestible indispensable amino acid scores (DIAAS) for some dairy and plant proteins may better describe protein quality than values calculated using the concept for protein digestibility-corrected amino acid scores (PDCAAS). *Br. J. Nutr.* **2017**, *117*, 490–499. [CrossRef]
31. Newgard, C.B.; An, J.; Bain, J.R.; Muehlbauer, M.J.; Stevens, R.D.; Lien, L.F.; Haqq, A.M.; Shah, S.H.; Arlotto, M.; Slentz, C.A.; et al. A Branched-Chain Amino Acid-Related Metabolic Signature that Differentiates Obese and Lean Humans and Contributes to Insulin Resistance. *Cell Metab.* **2009**, *9*, 311–326. [CrossRef]
32. Rigamonti, A.E.; Leoncini, R.; De Col, A.; Tamini, S.; Cicolini, S.; Abbruzzese, L.; Cella, S.G.; Sartorio, A. The Appetite—Suppressant and GLP-1-Stimulating Effects of Whey Proteins in Obese Subjects are Associated with Increased Circulating Levels of Specific Amino Acids. *Nutrients* **2020**, *12*, 775. [CrossRef] [PubMed]
33. Melson, C.E.; Nepocatych, S.; Madzima, T.A. The effects of whey and soy liquid breakfast on appetite response, energy metabolism, and subsequent energy intake. *Nutrition* **2019**, *61*, 179–186. [CrossRef]
34. Crowder, C.M.; Neumann, B.L.; Baum, J.I. Breakfast Protein Source Does Not Influence Postprandial Appetite Response and Food Intake in Normal Weight and Overweight Young Women. *J. Nutr. Metab.* **2016**, *2016*. [CrossRef] [PubMed]
35. Hawley, A.L.; Gbur, E.; Tacinelli, A.M.; Walker, S.; Murphy, A.; Burgess, R.; Baum, J.I. The Short-Term Effect of Whey Compared with Pea Protein on Appetite, Food Intake, and Energy Expenditure in Young and Older Men. *Curr. Dev. Nutr.* **2020**, *4*. [CrossRef] [PubMed]
36. Randomization.com. Available online: http://www.randomization.com (accessed on 11 May 2021).
37. Flint, A.; Raben, A.; Blundell, J.E.; Astrup, A. Reproducibility, power and validity of visual analogue scales in assessment of appetite sensations in single test meal studies. *Int. J. Obes.* **2000**, *24*, 38–48. [CrossRef]

38. Nepocatych, S.; Melson, C.E.; Madzima, T.A.; Balilionis, G. Comparison of the effects of a liquid breakfast meal with varying doses of plant-based soy protein on appetite profile, energy metabolism and intake. *Appetite* **2019**, *141*. [CrossRef]
39. MacKenzie-Shalders, K.L.; Byrne, N.M.; Slater, G.J.; King, N.A. The effect of a whey protein supplement dose on satiety and food intake in resistance training athletes. *Appetite* **2015**, *92*, 178–184. [CrossRef]
40. My Diabetes My Way. Available online: https://www.mydiabetesmyway.scot.nhs.uk/#gsc.tab=0 (accessed on 28 April 2021).
41. Ohr, L.M. Proteins Pick Up the Pace. *Food Technol.* **2014**, *68*, 60–67.
42. Kalman, D.S. Amino acid composition of an organic brown rice protein concentrate and isolate compared to soy and whey concentrates and isolates. *Foods* **2014**, *3*, 394–402. [CrossRef]
43. Consultation, F.E. Dietary protein quality evaluation in human nutrition. Report of an FAQ Expert Consultation-PubMed. *FAO Food Nutr. Pap.* **2013**, *92*, 1–66.
44. Lindquist, K.A.; Chow, K.; West, A.; Pyle, L.; Isbell, T.S.; Cree-Green, M.; Nadeau, K.J. The StatStrip Glucose Monitor Is Suitable for Use During Hyperinsulinemic Euglycemic Clamps in a Pediatric Population. *Diabetes Technol. Ther.* **2014**, *16*, 298–302. [CrossRef] [PubMed]
45. Matthews, D.R.; Hosker, J.P.; Rudenski, A.S.; Naylor, B.A.; Treacher, D.F.; Turner, R.C. Homeostasis model assessment: Insulin resistance and β-cell function from fasting plasma glucose and insulin concentrations in man. *Diabetologia* **1985**, *28*, 412–419. [CrossRef] [PubMed]
46. Zafar, T.A.; Waslien, C.; AlRaefaei, A.; Alrashidi, N.; AlMahmoud, E. Whey protein sweetened beverages reduce glycemic and appetite responses and food intake in young females. *Nutr. Res.* **2013**, *33*, 303–310. [CrossRef]
47. Joy, J.M.; Lowery, R.P.; Wilson, J.M.; Purpura, M.; De Souza, E.O.; Wilson, S.M.; Kalman, D.S.; Dudeck, J.E.; Jäger, R. The effects of 8 weeks of whey or rice protein supplementation on body composition and exercise performance. *Nutr. J.* **2013**, *12*, 86. [CrossRef] [PubMed]
48. He, T.; Spelbrink, R.E.J.; Witteman, B.J.; Giuseppin, M.L.F. Digestion kinetics of potato protein isolates in vitro and in vivo. *Int. J. Food Sci. Nutr.* **2013**, *64*, 787–793. [CrossRef]
49. Tremblay, F.; Lavigne, C.; Jacques, H.; Marette, A. Role of dietary proteins and amino acids in the pathogenesis of insulin resistance. *Annu. Rev. Nutr.* **2007**, *27*, 293–310. [CrossRef] [PubMed]
50. Gannon, M.C.; Nuttall, F.Q. Amino acid ingestion and glucose metabolism-A review. *IUBMB Life* **2010**, *62*, 660–668. [CrossRef]
51. Calbet, J.A.L.; MacLean, D.A. Plasma glucagon and insulin responses depend on the rate of appearance of amino acids after ingestion of different protein solutions in humans. *J. Nutr.* **2002**, *132*, 2174–2182. [CrossRef]
52. Nilsson, M.; Stenberg, M.; Frid, A.H.; Holst, J.J.; Björck, I.M.E. Glycemia and insulinemia in healthy subjects after lactose-equivalent meals of milk and other food proteins: The role of plasma amino acids and incretins. *Am. J. Clin. Nutr.* **2004**, *80*, 1246–1253. [CrossRef]
53. Van Loon, L.J.C.; Saris, W.H.M.; Verhagen, H.; Wagenmakers, A.J.M. Plasma insulin responses after ingestion of different amino acid or protein mixtures with carbohydrate. *Am. J. Clin. Nutr.* **2000**, *72*, 96–105. [CrossRef]
54. Nair, K.S.; Short, K.R. Hormonal and signaling role of branched-chain amino acids. *J. Nutr.* **2005**, *135*, 1547S–1552S. [CrossRef] [PubMed]
55. Nilsson, M.; Holst, J.J.; Björck, I.M.E. Metabolic effects of amino acid mixtures and whey protein in healthy subjects: Studies using glucose-equivalent drinks. *Am. J. Clin. Nutr.* **2007**, *85*, 996–1004. [CrossRef]
56. Nuttall, F.Q.; Gannon, M.C.; Wald, J.L.; Ahmed, M. Plasma glucose and insulin profiles in normal subjects ingesting diets of varying carbohydrate, fat, and protein content. *J. Am. Coll. Nutr.* **1982**, *4*, 437–450. [CrossRef]
57. Reimann, F.; Ward, P.S.; Gribble, F.M. Signaling mechanisms underlying the release of glucagon-like peptide 1. *Diabetes* **2006**, *55*, S78–S85. [CrossRef]
58. Theodorakis, M.J.; Carlson, O.; Michopoulos, S.; Doyle, M.E.; Juhaszova, M.; Petraki, K.; Egan, J.M. Human duodenal enteroendocrine cells: Source of both incretin peptides, GLP-1 and GIP. *Am. J. Physiol. Endocrinol. Metab.* **2006**, *290*. [CrossRef] [PubMed]
59. Larsson, L.I.; Holst, J.; Håkanson, R.; Sundler, F. Distribution and properties of glucagon immunoreactivity in the digestive tract of various mammals: An immunohistochemical and immunochemical study. *Histochemistry* **1975**, *44*, 281–290. [CrossRef] [PubMed]
60. Oikawa, S.Y.; Bahniwal, R.; Holloway, T.M.; Lim, C.; McLeod, J.C.; McGlory, C.; Baker, S.K.; Phillips, S.M. Potato Protein Isolate Stimulates Muscle Protein Synthesis at Rest and with Resistance Exercise in Young Women. *Nutrients* **2020**, *12*, 1235. [CrossRef]
61. Blundell, J.; De Graaf, C.; Hulshof, T.; Jebb, S.; Livingstone, B.; Lluch, A.; Mela, D.; Salah, S.; Schuring, E.; Van Der Knaap, H.; et al. Appetite control: Methodological aspects of the evaluation of foods. *Obes. Rev.* **2010**, *11*, 251–270. [CrossRef]

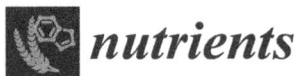

*Article*

# Distinct Impact of Natural Sugars from Fruit Juices and Added Sugars on Caloric Intake, Body Weight, Glycaemia, Oxidative Stress and Glycation in Diabetic Rats

Tamaeh Monteiro-Alfredo [1,2,3,4], Beatriz Caramelo [1,2,3], Daniela Arbeláez [1], Andreia Amaro [1,2,3], Cátia Barra [1,2,3,5], Daniela Silva [1,2,3], Sara Oliveira [1,2,3], Raquel Seiça [1] and Paulo Matafome [1,2,3,6,*]

[1] Coimbra Institute of Clinical and Biomedical Research (iCBR) and Institute of Physiology, Faculty of Medicine, University of Coimbra, 3000-548 Coimbra, Portugal; tamaehamonteiro@gmail.com (T.M.-A.); bia.caramelo@gmail.com (B.C.); daniarcha98@gmail.com (D.A.); andreia.amaro15@hotmail.com (A.A.); cat_barra@hotmail.com (C.B.); daniela.silva26@hotmail.com (D.S.); saraoliveira116@gmail.com (S.O.); rseica@fmed.uc.pt (R.S.)
[2] Center for Innovative Biomedicine and Biotechnology (CIBB), University of Coimbra, 3004-504 Coimbra, Portugal
[3] Clinical Academic Center of Coimbra, 3000-548 Coimbra, Portugal
[4] Research Group of Biotechnology and Bioprospecting Applied to Metabolism (GEBBAM), Federal University of Grande Dourados, Dourados 79825-070, MS, Brazil
[5] Universitary Hospital Center of Coimbra, 3000-548 Coimbra, Portugal
[6] Department of Complementary Sciences, Instituto Politécnico de Coimbra, Coimbra Health School (ESTeSC), 3046-854 Coimbra, Portugal
* Correspondence: paulo.matafome@uc.pt

**Citation:** Monteiro-Alfredo, T.; Caramelo, B.; Arbeláez, D.; Amaro, A.; Barra, C.; Silva, D.; Oliveira, S.; Seiça, R.; Matafome, P. Distinct Impact of Natural Sugars from Fruit Juices and Added Sugars on Caloric Intake, Body Weight, Glycaemia, Oxidative Stress and Glycation in Diabetic Rats. *Nutrients* 2021, 13, 2956. https://doi.org/10.3390/nu13092956

Academic Editor: Lindsay Brown

Received: 30 July 2021
Accepted: 21 August 2021
Published: 25 August 2021

**Publisher's Note:** MDPI stays neutral with regard to jurisdictional claims in published maps and institutional affiliations.

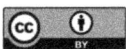

**Copyright:** © 2021 by the authors. Licensee MDPI, Basel, Switzerland. This article is an open access article distributed under the terms and conditions of the Creative Commons Attribution (CC BY) license (https://creativecommons.org/licenses/by/4.0/).

**Abstract:** Although fruit juices are a natural source of sugars, there is a controversy whether their sugar content has similar harmful effects as beverages' added-sugars. We aimed to study the role of fruit juice sugars in inducing overweight, hyperglycaemia, glycation and oxidative stress in normal and diabetic animal models. In diabetic Goto-Kakizaki (GK) rats, we compared the effects of four different fruit juices (4-weeks) with sugary solutions having a similar sugar profile and concentration. In vitro, the sugary solutions were more susceptible to AGE formation than fruit juices, also causing higher postprandial glycaemia and lower erythrocytes' antioxidant capacity in vivo (single intake). In GK rats, ad libitum fruit juice consumption (4-weeks) did not change body weight, glycaemia, oxidative stress nor glycation. Consumption of a matched volume of sugary solutions aggravated fasting glycaemia but had a moderate impact on caloric intake and oxidative stress/glycation markers in tissues of diabetic rats. Ad libitum availability of the same sugary solutions impaired energy balance regulation, leading to higher caloric intake than ad libitum fruit juices and controls, as well as weight gain, fasting hyperglycaemia, insulin intolerance and impaired oxidative stress/glycation markers in several tissues. We demonstrated the distinct role of sugars naturally present in fruit juices and added sugars in energy balance regulation, impairing oxidative stress, glycation and glucose metabolism in an animal model of type 2 diabetes.

**Keywords:** natural and added sugars; fruit juices; hyperglycaemia; oxidative stress; glycation

## 1. Introduction

Increased consumption of westernized diets, highly processed foods and sugar-sweetened beverages is associated with an increased risk for obesity and associated pathologies throughout life. Such lifestyle changes are related to the health, economic and social burden of metabolic syndrome-associated diseases, such as type 2 diabetes, non-alcoholic fatty liver disease, cardiovascular diseases, among others. Dietary changes include higher consumption of processed foods rich in long-chain saturated fatty acids and sugars (soft drinks, snacks/desserts sweets, fast food, etc.), instead of fish, fruits and vegetables, which is apparently associated to weight gain [1,2]. Added sugars contribute to an higher energy density of the diet, leading to a positive energy balance and higher waist circumference, weight gain and development of metabolic disorders [3–12]. The World Health Organization (WHO) introduced a definition of free sugars (which includes sugars naturally present in fruit beverages) and established guidelines for free sugar intake in adults and children below 5–10% of the total daily energy [13]. According to the National Portuguese Food and Physical Activity Survey report, the national average consumption of simple sugars (mono and disaccharides) is 90 g (g)/day, contributing to an average of 19.8% for the total energy value [14].

Natural or intrinsic sugars are those naturally present in foods such as fruit and vegetables (fructose), honey and the sugars present in dairy products (galactose and (lactose). Besides sugars, these foods have several other compounds in their composition, which some of them regulate sugars absorption, cell uptake and metabolism [3]. The added sugars include mono and disaccharides that are added to foods during processing, preparation or at the table, with the objective of sweetening and increasing the food palatability and shelf life, improve texture, inhibit growth of microorganisms, give functional structures or give more accessibility [4,5,9,11]. Added sugars mainly include yellow sugar, corn sweetener, corn syrup, dextrose, fructose, glucose, high fructose corn syrup, lactose, maltose, malt sugar, molasses, raw, turbined sugar, trehalose, and sucrose [12,15]. They are mostly found in sugary drinks, pastry products, cookies, energy drinks, nectars, white bread and breakfast cereals [5–7].

Hyperglycaemia is related to the increased formation of advanced glycation end-products (AGEs), which are closely associated with the development and progression of diabetes and its complications [16–20]. In addition, AGEs may also be formed in sugar-rich foods or after exposure to high temperatures and low humidity during cooking [21]. AGEs are also involved in the development of insulin resistance–associated pathologies such as cardio- and cerebrovascular diseases, non-alcoholic steatohepatitis, and central nervous system disorders [22,23]. Vascular aging due to AGEs exposure, or vascular AGEing, is related to oxidative stress due to increased generation of reactive species of oxygen and nitrogen [22,24–31], endothelial dysfunction [28–30], and changes in the extracellular matrix [29] and in inflammatory factors [31].

The main objective of this study was to determine the distinct role of naturally present sugars in fruit juices and added sugars in impairing oxidative stress, glycation, glucose metabolism and energy balance in an animal model of type 2 diabetes. Our first specific objective was to determine the post-prandial glycaemia and total antioxidant capacity of erythrocytes immediately following the intake of different fruit juices and sugary solutions with a similar profile of glucose, fructose and sucrose. Our second objective was to compare the impact of chronic ad libitum fruit juice intake with the same profile, concentration, and quantity of added sugars on glucose metabolism and oxidative stress and glycation markers in erythrocytes, liver, adipose tissue, kidney, and heart of Goto-Kakizaki (GK) rats, a model of type 2 diabetes. The third objective was to disclose the role of both sugar sources in the regulation of energy balance, comparing ad libitum fruit juice intake with ad libitum intake of the same sugary solutions with matched sugar concentrations and profiles.

## 2. Materials and Methods
### 2.1. Chemicals and Antibodies

Salts and organic solvents used in this study were all purchased from Sigma-Aldrich/Merck Portugal (Oeiras, Portugal) and Fischer Scientific (Pittsburgh, PA, USA). Antibodies were used to target catalase, GLO-1 (Ab76110, Ab96032, Abcam, Cambridge, UK), CML (KH024, TransGenic Inc, Tokyo, Japan), MG-H1 (HM5017, Hycult Biotech, Uden, Netherlands) and argpyrimidine (AGE06B, Nordic-MUbio, Susteren, the Netherlands). Calnexin (AB0037, Sicgen, Cantanhede, Portugal) was used as loading control.

## 2.2. Fruit Juice and Sugars Samples

Fruit juice samples were kindly provided by SUMOL + COMPAL S.A. (Carnaxide, Portugal) Fruit juices were prepared from 100% fruit and no sugars were added during the process. In order to avoid sample-specific effects, four distinct samples were prepared: (1) red fruits (25% red grape, 16% raspberry, 16% apple, 11% strawberry, 11% plum, 9% pear, 6.5% banana, 5.5% blueberry); (2) orange (100% orange); (3) peach (50% peach, 20% apple, 15% mango, 5% apricot, 5% banana); and (4) pear (80% pear, 13% grape, 4% orange, 3% banana). Samples were produced at industrial scale. For each sample, the sugars profile was determined (Figure 1B) and a matched sugary solution was prepared daily for each sample, with the equivalent concentration of glucose, fructose and sucrose, and with similar pH to the respective juice sample.

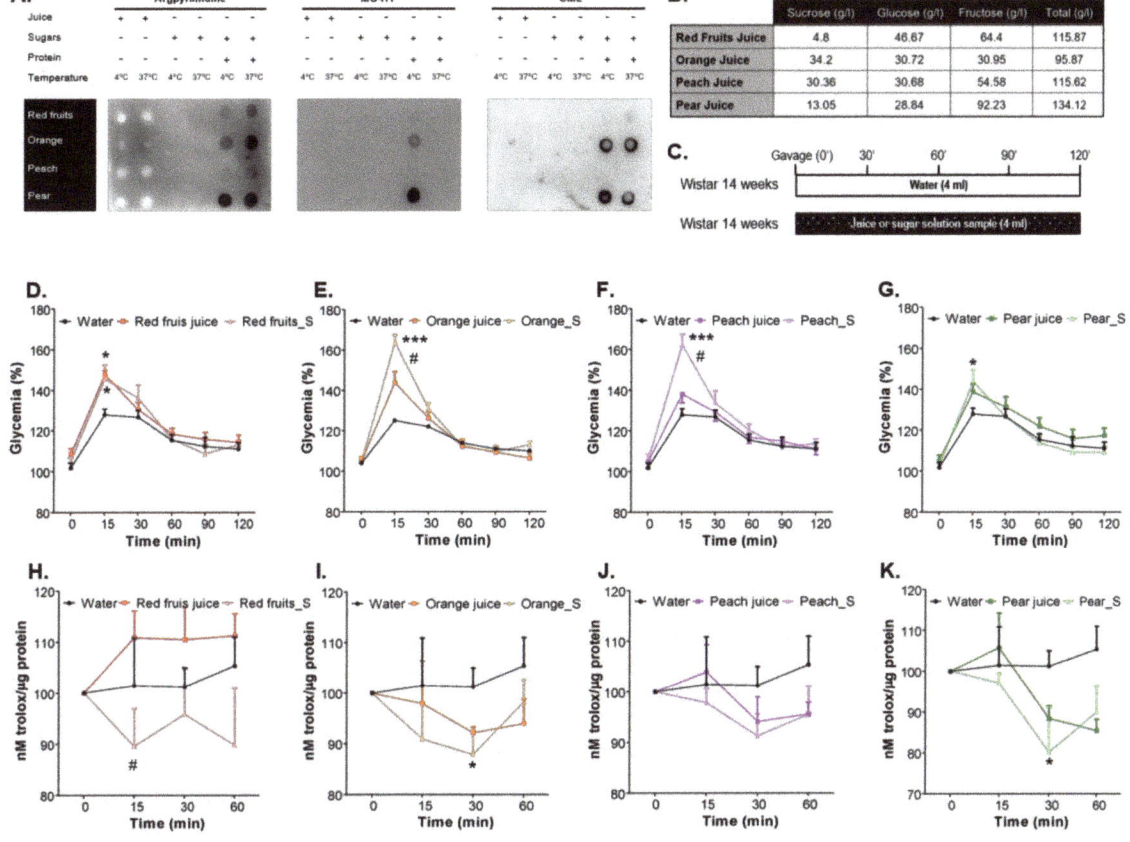

**Figure 1.** The AGEs CML, MG-H1 and Argpyrimidine were detected by dot blot (**A**) in fruit juices and sugary solutions with the same sugars profile (**B**) in the presence or absence of BSA, at 4 °C or 37 °C. In other to determine the postprandial glycaemia, an OGTT was performed (**C**) and glycaemia and total antioxidant capacity of erythrocytes was determined after intake of 4 mL of red fruits (**D,H**), orange (**E,I**), peach (**F,J**) and pear (**G,K**) fruit juices or a sugary solution with the equivalent sugars profile. * different from Water; # different from the fruit juice. 1 symbol, $p < 0.05$; 3 symbols, $p < 0.001$.

## 2.3. In Vitro Determination of AGEs Formation from Fruit Juices and Sugars' Solutions

Samples of fruit juices were incubated at 4 °C or 37 °C during 30 days in the dark. Matched sugary solutions were incubated under the same conditions, in the presence or not of BSA. The concentration of BSA used was matched with the concentration of total protein in each of the juice samples. After the period of incubation, samples were stored at −80 °C for dot blot analysis using specific antibodies.

*2.4. Determination of Post-Prandial Glycaemia and Total Antioxidant Capacity*

The study was performed according to good practices of animal handling, with the approval of the Institutional Animal Care and Use Committee (ORBEA 13/2018) and the procedures were performed by licensed users of Federation of Laboratory Animal Science Associations—FELASA, conformed to the guidelines from the Directive 2010/63/EU of the European Parliament for the Protection of Animals Used for Science Purpose. 12-week-old Wistar rats from our breeding colony (Faculty of Medicine, University of Coimbra) were fed a specific volume (4 mL) of each fruit juice sample or the same volume of matched sugary solution (Figure 1B,C). Glycaemia was determined using a glucometer and reactive test stripes (Contour Next, Bayer Portugal, Lisboa, Portugal) before and 15, 30, 60, 90 and 120 min after gavage ($n$ = 12/condition). In a different set of animals, the same protocol was followed, and blood samples were collected from the tail vein to Vacuette K3EDTA tubes (Greiner Bio-one, Kremsmünster, Austria) for evaluation of total antioxidant capacity. Blood samples were immediately centrifuged (2200× $g$, 4 °C, 15') and the cellular fraction was diluted in the same volume of ultrapure $H_2O$ and submitted to repeated cycles of freeze/thawing. Supernatant was stored at −80 °C and later used for the Total Antioxidant Capacity Assay Kit (ab65329, Abcam) according to the manufacturer's instructions.

*2.5. Animal Maintenance and Treatment*

12-week-old male Wistar rats were randomly divided in five groups ($n$ = 6–8); control, red fruits juice (Wistar Red Fruits), orange juice (Wistar Orange), peach juice (Wistar Peach) and pear juice (Wistar Pear). Rats were maintained with free (ad libitum) access to the respective fruit juice (except the control, which received water) during 4 weeks (Figure 2A). Age-matched Goto-Kakizaki (GK) rats, a non-obese model of type 2 diabetes, were randomly divided in 13 groups ($n$ = 6–8). Four groups were treated ad libitum with the same juices (GK Red Fruits, GK Orange, GK Peach, GK Pear). Four other groups were treated with a sugary solution equivalent in concentration, sugar profile and quantity the daily volume consumed by the respective groups treated with each fruit juice (GK RF_S, GK Orange_S, GK Peach_S, GK Pear_S). Another four groups were treated with sugary solutions with the same concentration and profile but with ad libitum access (GK Red Fruits_S_AL, GK Orange_S_AL, GK Peach_S_AL, GK Pear_S_AL). The last group (GK) was kept as control with free access to water and food. Animals were kept under standard conditions—2 animals per cage, with temperature at 22–24 °C, and 50–60% humidity, under standard light cycle (12 h light/12 h darkness). All animals were kept with ad libitum access to water and food (standard diet A03, Panlab, Barcelona, Spain) [32].

*2.6. In Vivo Data and Sample Collection*

Body weight, fasting glycaemia, water/juice/sugary solution and food intake were evaluated weekly. Before and after the treatment, animals were submitted to an intraperitoneal insulin tolerance test (ipITT) after 6 h of fasting. For the IIT, insulin was administered (i.p.) 0.1 U.kg$^{-1}$ (Humulin, 1000 UI/mL Lilly, Lisboa, Portugal), followed by glycaemia measurement from the tail vein with a glucometer (Contour Next, Bayer) and test strips in time 0, 15, 30, 60 and 120 min. Response to insulin tolerance was expressed by area under the curve—AUC [33].

One day after the ipITT, 6-h fasted rats were anesthetized (i.p.) with 2:1 ($v/v$) 50 mg kg$^{-1}$ ketamine (100 mg/mL)/2.5% chlorpromazine (5 mg mL$^{-1}$) and samples of blood was collected by cardiac puncture followed by cervical dislocation. Epididimal adipose tissue (EAT), liver, kidney and heart were collected for further analysis. After centrifugation of blood samples, cell fraction was diluted in the same volume of $H_2O$, submitted to freeze/thawing cycles and the supernatant was used for the determination of the total antioxidant capacity (ab65329, Abcam).

## 2.7. Western Blot and Dot Blot

Tissues were disrupted in lysis buffer (0.25 M Tris-HCl, 125 mM NaCl, 1% Triton-X-100, 0.5% SDS, 1 mM EDTA, 1 mM EGTA, 20 mM NaF, 2 mM $Na_3VO_4$, 10 mM β-glycerophosphate, 2.5 mM sodium pyrophosphate, 10 mM PMSF, 40 µL of protease inhibitor), centrifuged (14,000 rpm, 20 min, 4 °C) and denatured with Laemmli buffer (62.5 mM Tris-HCl, 10% glycerol, 2% SDS, 5% β-mercaptoethanol, 0.01% bromophenol blue). Protein was quantified through the BCA Protein Assay Kit [34]. Samples were loaded in SDS-PAGE and electroblotted onto PVDF membrane (Advansta, San Jose, CA USA). For dot blot, 1 µL of denatured samples were directly leaded to nitrocellulose membranes. All membranes were blocked with TBS-T 0.01% and BSA 5%, then incubated with the primary and respective secondary antibodies anti-mouse (GE Healthcare, Chicago, IL, USA), anti-rabbit and anti-goat (Bio-Rad Portugal, Lisboa, Portugal). Calnexin was used as loading control. Immunoblots were detected with ECL substrate and the Versadoc system (Bio-Rad).

## 2.8. Dihydroethidium (DHE) Staining

The evaluation of kidney oxidative stress was performed through the detection of dihydroethidium (DHE) in cryosections (5 mm). DAPI was used to stain nucleus and images were obtained with a fluorescence microscope (Zeiss Axio Observer Z1) equipped with an incorporated camera (Zeiss, Jena, Germany), detected with 587 nm of excitation and 610 nm of emission for DHE, and 353 nm of excitation and 465 nm of emission for DAPI. The same settings were kept constant for all analysis.

## 2.9. Statistical Analysis

Data were expressed as the mean ± standard error of the mean (SEM) and compared by analysis of variance (ANOVA) followed by Tukey post-hoc test. $p < 0.05$ was considered significant. Statistical tests were performed with GraphPad Prism 5.0 (GraphPad, San Diego, CA, USA) and IBM SPSS Statistics Software (IBM, Armonk NY, USA).

## 3. Results

### 3.1. Sugars Naturally Present in Fruit Juices Are Less Prone to AGEs Formation Than Added Sugars in Sugary Solutions and Cause a Lower Increase of Postprandial Glycaemia

The AGEs MG-H1, argpyrimidine and CML were indetectable by dot blots in all fruit juices samples incubated for 30 days at 4 °C or 37 °C (Figure 1A). On the other hand, the incubation of each sugary solution with the respective amount of BSA (the same protein content of each juice sample) resulted in immune staining of all AGEs. The intensity of the signal for each AGE depended on the type of sugar profile and temperature of incubation (Figure 1A). MG-H1 was more detected in samples incubated at 4 °C and Argpyrimidine was more detected in samples incubated at 37 °C. Such observations are consistent with the fact the MG-H1 is a more reversible product of methylglyoxal reaction with proteins, while Argpyrimidine is a more final and irreversible product of such reaction. No AGE formation was detectable when sugars were incubated without protein (Figure 1A).

The intake of a specific volume of each juice sample produced a rapid increase of glycaemia in relation to the sham rats (same volume of water). The less evident result was observed for pear, which has a lower concentration of glucose (Figure 1D–G). Nevertheless, such increase was higher for every corresponding sugary solution. Such higher increase of post-prandial glycaemia with the sugary solutions was associated with a lower total antioxidant capacity of erythrocytes at the same time-points after ingestion (Figure 1H–K).

### 3.2. Added Sugars Do Not Cause Satiety and Lead to Higher Body Weight, Caloric Intake and Impaired Glycemic Profile When Available Ad Libitum

In both normal and diabetic rats, the ad libitum consumption of fruit juices did not results in a significant body weight gain in relation to their respective controls. As well, the consumption of a matched sugary solution by diabetic rats did not change weight gain.

Weight gain was only increased in the groups of diabetic rats treated with sugary solutions ad libitum, achieving statistical significance for pear juice solution (Figure 2B–I).

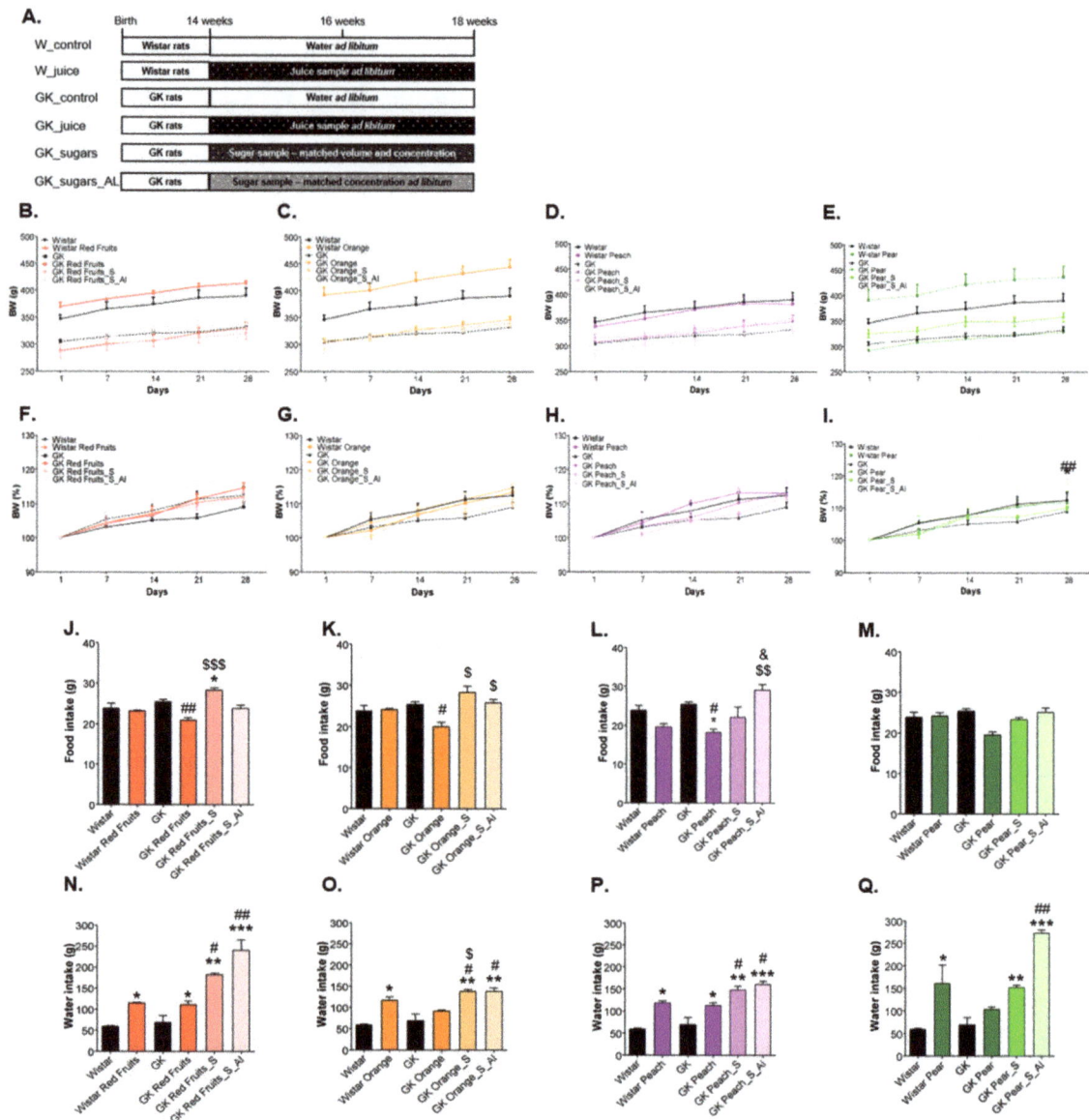

**Figure 2.** *Cont.*

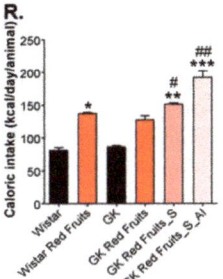 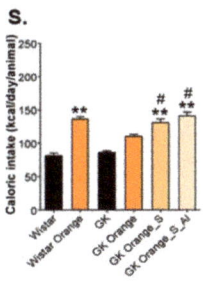 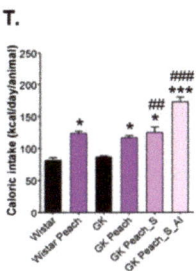 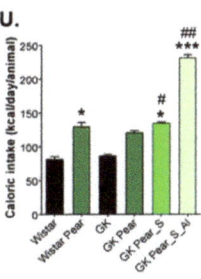

**Figure 2.** Normal and diabetic rats were treated for 4 weeks with fruit juices ad libitum. Diabetic rats were also treated during the same period with a matched sugary solution in the same volume (GK_S) or ad libitum (GK_S_AL) (**A**). Body weight was monitored during the experimental period (**B–E**) and weight gain calculated at each time-point (**F–I**). Food intake (**J–M**) and consumption of water/juice/sugary solution (**N–Q**) were monitored throughout all the experimental period. The total caloric intake/day was calculated (**R–U**). * different from Wistar; # different from GK; $ different from GK_Juice. & Different from GK_Juice_S. 1 symbol, $p < 0.05$; 2 symbols, $p < 0.01$; 3 symbols, $p < 0.001$.

This may be attributable to a poorer control of energy balance. Diabetic rats treated with fruit juices (ad libitum) drank significantly more liquid volume than controls (water) (Figure 2N–Q), but significantly reduced their food intake (Figure 2J–M), resulting in a moderate non-significant (significant only for the peach juice sample, $p < 0.05$ vs GK) increase of caloric intake (Figure 2R–U). Rats treated with the matched sugary solutions, besides drinking all the volume supplied, did not reduce their food intake (Figure 2J–M), leading to significantly higher caloric intake for almost all the samples (Figure 2R–U). When the same sugary solutions were supplied ad libitum, the water intake was further increased (Figure 2N–Q), although the food consumption was not reduced (Figure 2J–M). This resulted in a significantly higher caloric intake than GK rats maintained with water (Figure 2R–U), which was associated with increased body weight gain throughout the treatment (S_AL).

GK rats are a spontaneous model of type 2 diabetes, showing fasting hyperglycaemia and decreased insulin tolerance (higher AUC during the ITT) (Figure 3). The consumption of fruit juices did not cause significant changes in fasting (6 h) glycaemia throughout the experimental period in relation to the initial value (Figure 3A–D), nor at the end in relation to GK rats maintained with water (Figure 3E–H). In the case of orange juice, fasting glycaemia was in fact reduced in relation to GK rats at the end of the treatment (Figure 3F). Fruit juices also did not change insulin tolerance at the end of the experimental period (Figure 3I–L). The consumption of a matched (profile and volume) sugary solution slightly increased fasting glycaemia and insulin resistance at the end of the treatment, with a more significant effect being observed for red fruits sugars, possibly because they are richer in glucose (Figure 3E–H). The ad libitum consumption of the same sugary solutions produced an increase of fasting glycaemia throughout the experimental period in relation to the initial value and to the GK maintained with water (Figure 3A–D), as well as at the end of the treatment in relation to GK rats maintained with water and treated with fruit juices (Figure 3E–H). Such consumption also resulted in a significant deterioration of insulin tolerance, with higher AUC during the ITT (Figure 3I–L).

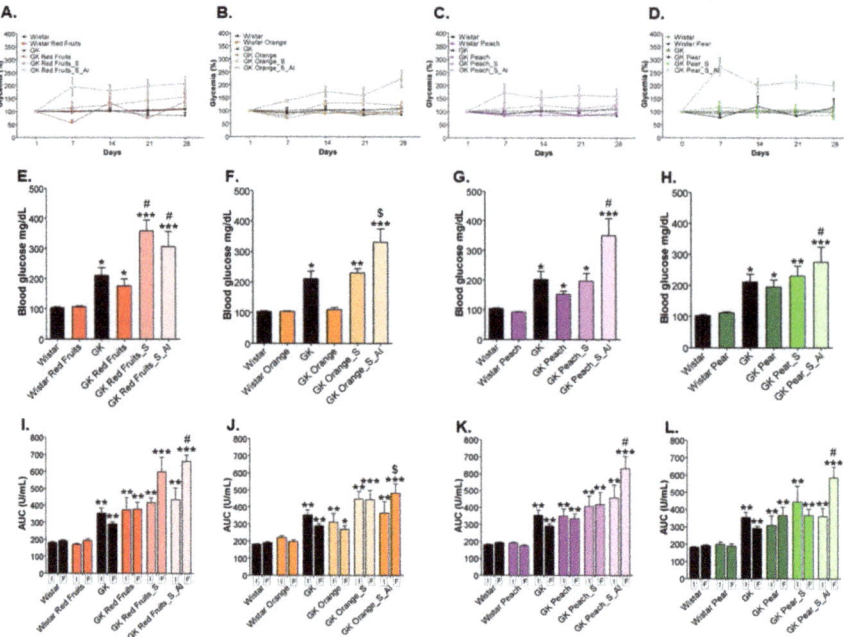

**Figure 3.** Fasting (6 h) glycaemia was evaluated weekly and calculated the percentage of the initial value (**A–D**). Fasting glycaemia at the end of the treatment is shown in (**E–H**). Before and after the experimental period an i.p. insulin tolerance test was performed and the area under the curve was calculated (**I–L**). * different from Wistar; # different from GK; $ different from GK_Juice. 1 symbol, $p < 0.05$; 2 symbols, $p < 0.01$; 3 symbols, $p < 0.001$.

### 3.3. Consumption of Added Sugars Further Impair Glycation and Oxidative Stress Markers in Liver, Adipose Tissue, Heart and Kidney

No significant differences were observed for total antioxidant capacity of erythrocytes in any group (Figure 4A–D). In erythrocytes, the levels of CML were increased in the red fruits juice group, but only in diabetic rats ($p < 0.05$ vs GK). Nevertheless, CML levels were further increased by the consumption of the sugary solution, either in the same amount of fruit juices or ad libitum ($p < 0.01$ vs GK) (Figure 4E). Such increased levels were also observed after ad libitum consumption of the sugary solution similar to pear juice (Figure 4H). Increased erythrocytes argpyrimidine was observed in diabetic rats after consumption of orange, peach and pear juice and was maintained or further increased in rats maintained with the sugary solutions either in the same amount of fruit juices or ad libitum (Figure 4I–L).

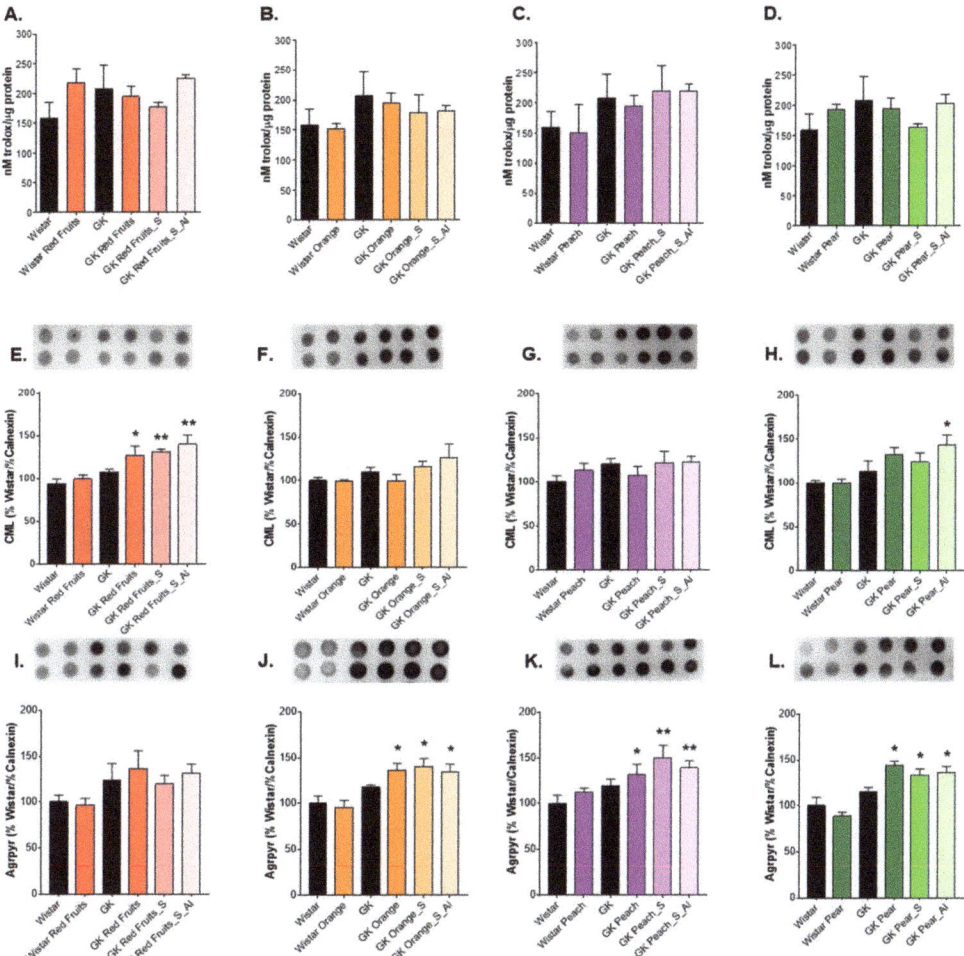

**Figure 4.** In isolated erythrocytes, total antioxidant capacity was determined (**A–D**) and CML (**E–H**) and argpyrimidine (**I–L**) were detected by dot blot. * different from Wistar. 1 symbol, $p < 0.05$; 2 symbols, $p < 0.01$.

The ad libitum consumption of sugary solutions caused an increase of liver weight in diabetic rats (Figure 5A–D). Diabetic rats showed a downregulation of catalase, which, taking all the fruit juices together, was not significantly changed by the consumption of fruit juices or sugary solutions (Figure 5E–H). Besides, there were no observed changes in GLO-1 levels, nor argpyrimidine and CML in the dot blot staining (Figure 5I).

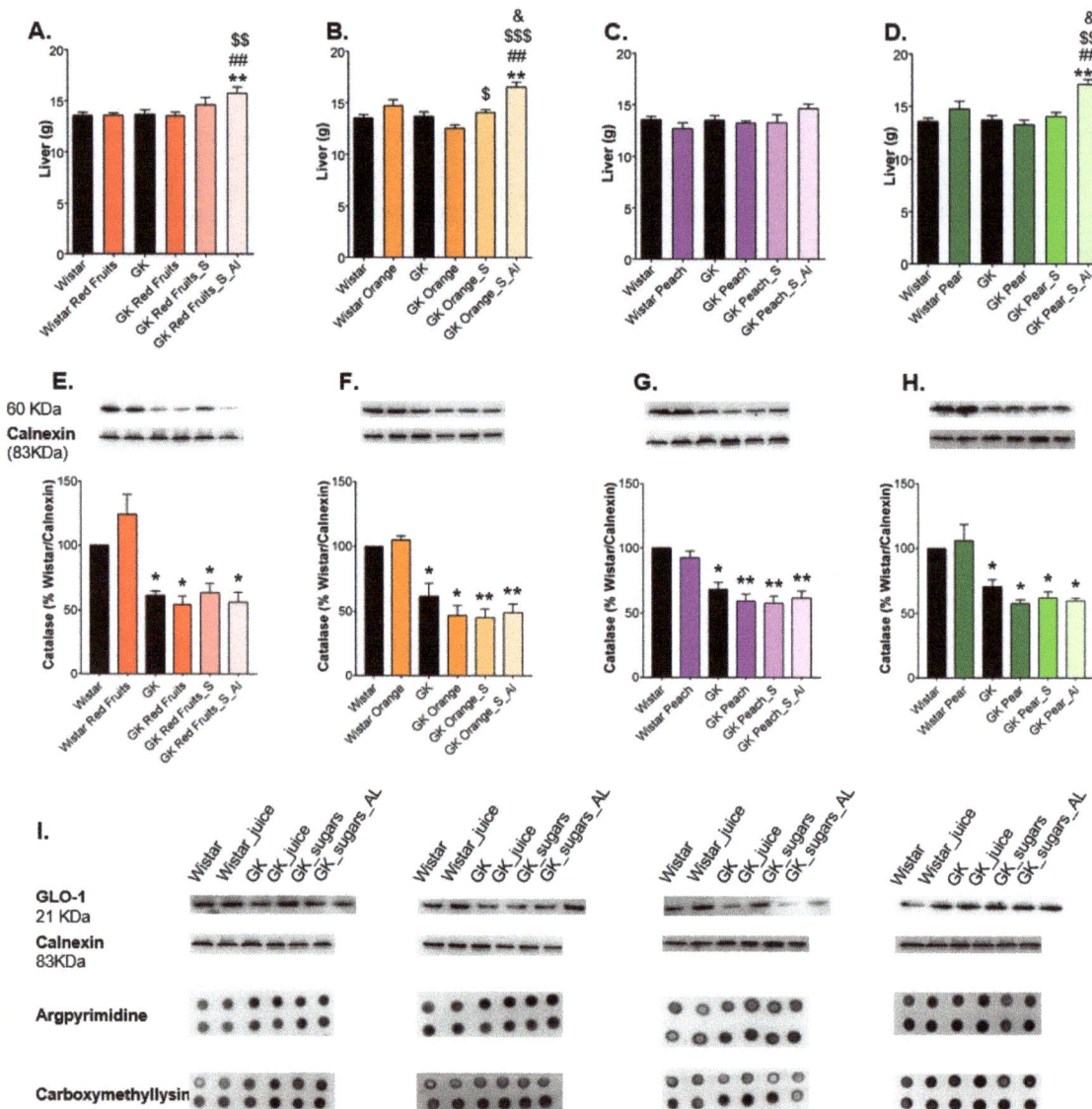

**Figure 5.** Liver weight was recorded (**A–D**) and the levels of catalase were determined by Western Blot (**E–H**). Representative western blot membranes of GLO-1 and dot blot membranes of CML and argpyrimidine in the liver are shown in (**I**). * different from Wistar; # different from GK; $ different from GK_Juice; & different from GK_S. 1 symbol, $p < 0.05$; 2 symbols, $p < 0.01$; 3 symbols, $p < 0.001$.

Similar results were observed in visceral adipose tissue, showing no significant differences between groups in argpyrimidine and CML (Figure 6M). GK rats had lower visceral adipose tissue weight (Figure 6A–D), catalase expression (Figure 6E–H) and tendentially lower GLO-1 expression (Figure 6I–L). Fruit juice consumption did not change adipose tissue weight or GLO-1 expression and induced a decrease of catalase expression in diabetic rats.

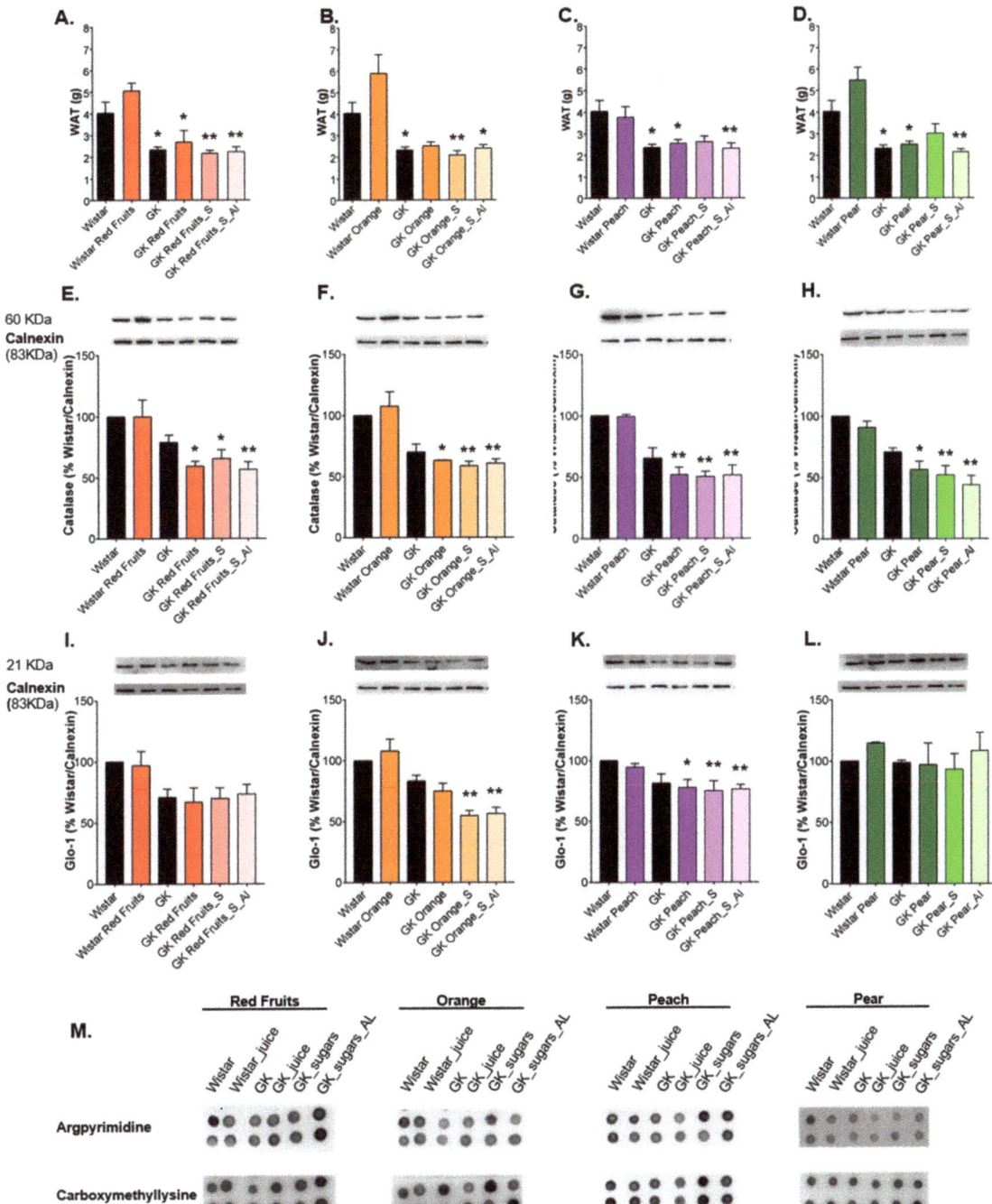

**Figure 6.** Epididymal adipose tissue weight was recorded (**A–D**) and the levels of catalase (**E–H**) and GLO-1 (**I–L**) in the tissue were determined by Western Blot. Representative dot blot membranes of CML and argpyrimidine in the adipose tissue are shown in (**M**). * different from Wistar. 1 symbol, $p < 0.05$; 2 symbols, $p < 0.01$.

On the other hand, consumption of sugary solutions either in the same amount of fruit juices or ad libitum resulted in a reduction of adipose tissue weight (Figure 6A–D), a marker of adipose tissue dysfunction, and a further reduction of catalase (Figure 6E–H) and GLO-1 levels (Figure 6I–L) in relation to GK rats maintained with water. Thus, consumption of fruit juices did not change adipose tissue and liver weight, nor changed the lower expression of antioxidant and antiglycant enzymes. Although no differences were observed for AGEs levels in both tissues, the caloric contribution of sugary solutions conduced to liver hypertrophy in diabetic rats, instead of adipose tissue expansion, which was associated with a further downregulation of both antioxidant enzymes.

Diabetic rats had lower heart weight, which was not changed by fruit juices consumption. Instead, the consumption of sugary solutions resulted in an increase of heart weight, being more evident in rats maintained with ad libitum access (Figure 7A–D). In heart, the consumption of sugary solutions led to a compensatory increase of catalase expression, especially when available ad libitum, achieving statistical significance in sugars similar to orange profile (Figure 7E–H). Such increase in catalase levels in rats maintained with *ad libitum* access to sugars may be attributable to the stress caused by the excessive sugar intake. No differences were observed for GLO-1 levels (Figure 7I). The levels of argpyrimidine were not changed by the consumption of fruit juices, but significantly increased in response to sugary solutions, namely with red fruits and pear sugar profile (Figure 7J–M). Similarly, the levels of CML were also increased after consumption of the sugary solutions, namely with red fruits, orange and pear sugars profile, while no major differences were observed after juice consumption (Figure 7N–Q). The heart is particularly susceptible to lipid peroxidation and 8-isoprostane was used as a tissue biomarker of such mechanisms. GK rats have tendentially higher 8-isoprostane levels in the heart, which were in fact reduced by the consumption of fruit juices, especially the peach sample (Figure 7R–U). The rats treated with the sugary solutions revealed 8-isoprostane levels similar to diabetic rats maintained with water.

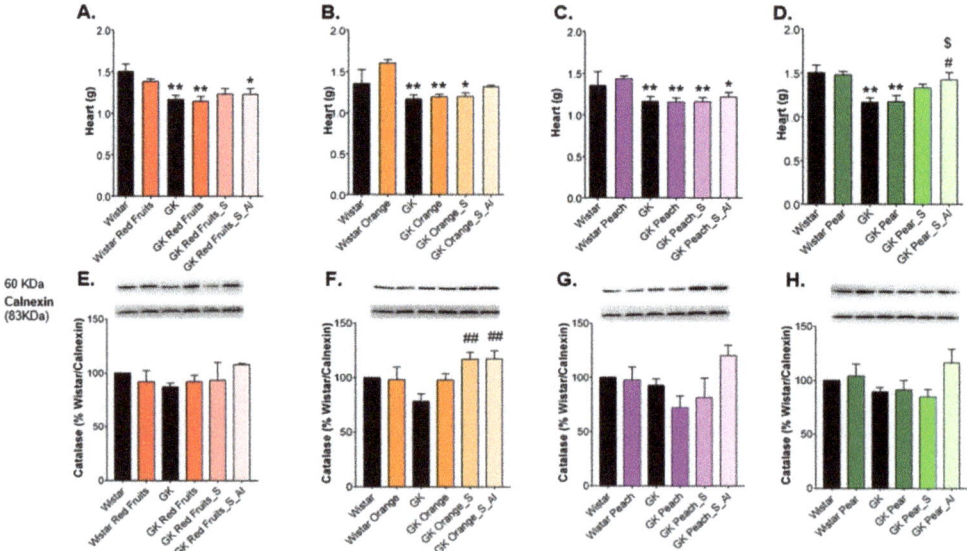

**Figure 7.** *Cont.*

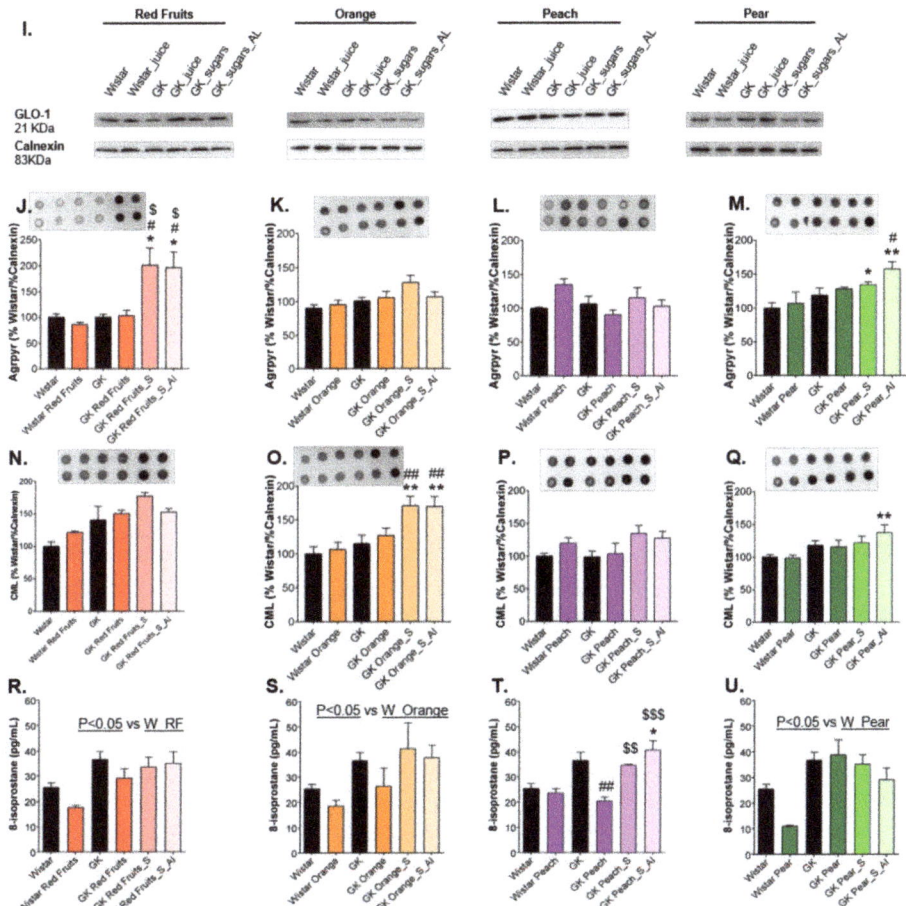

**Figure 7.** Heart weight was recorded (**A–D**) and the levels of catalase were determined by Western blot (**E–H**). Representative western blot membranes of GLO-1 in the heart are shown in (**I**). Heart CML (**J–M**) and argpyrimidine (**N–Q**) were determined by dot blot. 8-Isoprostane levels were determined as a marker of lipid peroxidation (**R–U**). * different from Wistar; # different from GK; $ different from GK_Juice. 1 symbol, $p < 0.05$; 2 symbols, $p < 0.01$.

In kidney, the consumption of fruit juices did not change the weight of the organ in diabetic rats, which was significantly higher in rats maintained with the sugary solutions. Such increase was observed in rats with matched volume of solution but was especially observed in those with ad libitum access (Figure 8A–D). No significant changes were observed in catalase, GLO-1 and CML levels (Figure 8E), while an increase of argpyrimidine levels was observed in rats maintained with the sugary solution similar to pear juice, the one with higher fructose content (Figure 8F–I).

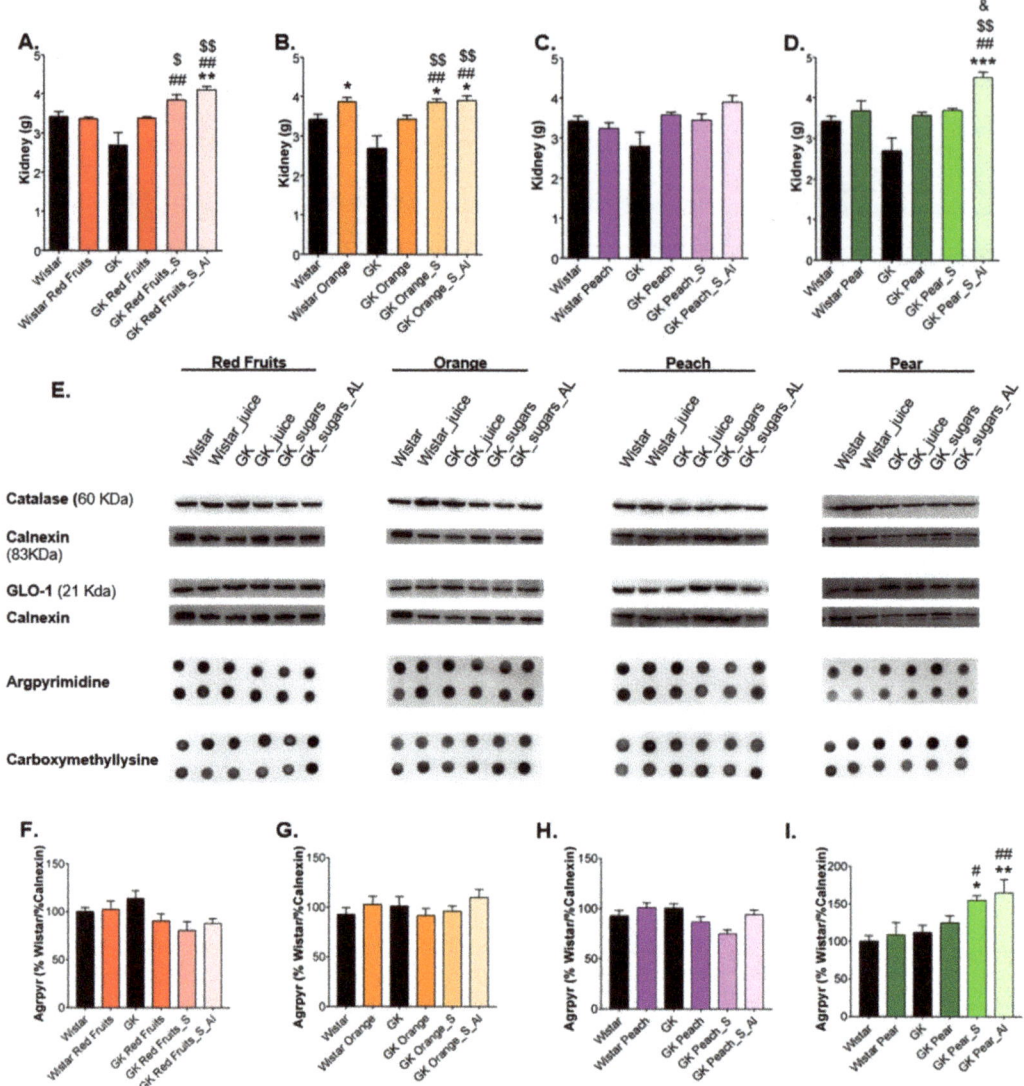

**Figure 8.** Kidney weight was recorded (**A–D**). Representative Western blot membranes of catalase and GLO-1 and dot blot membranes of CML in the kidney are shown in (**E**). Kidney argpyrimidine was determined by dot blot (**F–I**). * different from Wistar; # different from GK; $ different from GK_Juice; & different from GK_S. 1 symbol, $p < 0.05$; 2 symbols, $p < 0.01$.

The existence of oxidative stress particularly in the glomerulus, was assessed through the staining with DHE, a probe for superoxide anion. No changes in DHE reactivity were observed in Wistar rats maintained with fruit juices, in relation to the controls (Figure 9A–C). The diabetic rats maintained with fruit juices revealed a increase of glomerular DHE staining the was only significant for ref fruit sample (Figure 9E,H–K). On the other hand, diabetic rats maintained with the matched volume of the sugary solutions and especially those maintained with ad libitum access to the same solutions revealled a significant increase of DHE staining, being observed in all the samples tested (Figure 9F–K).

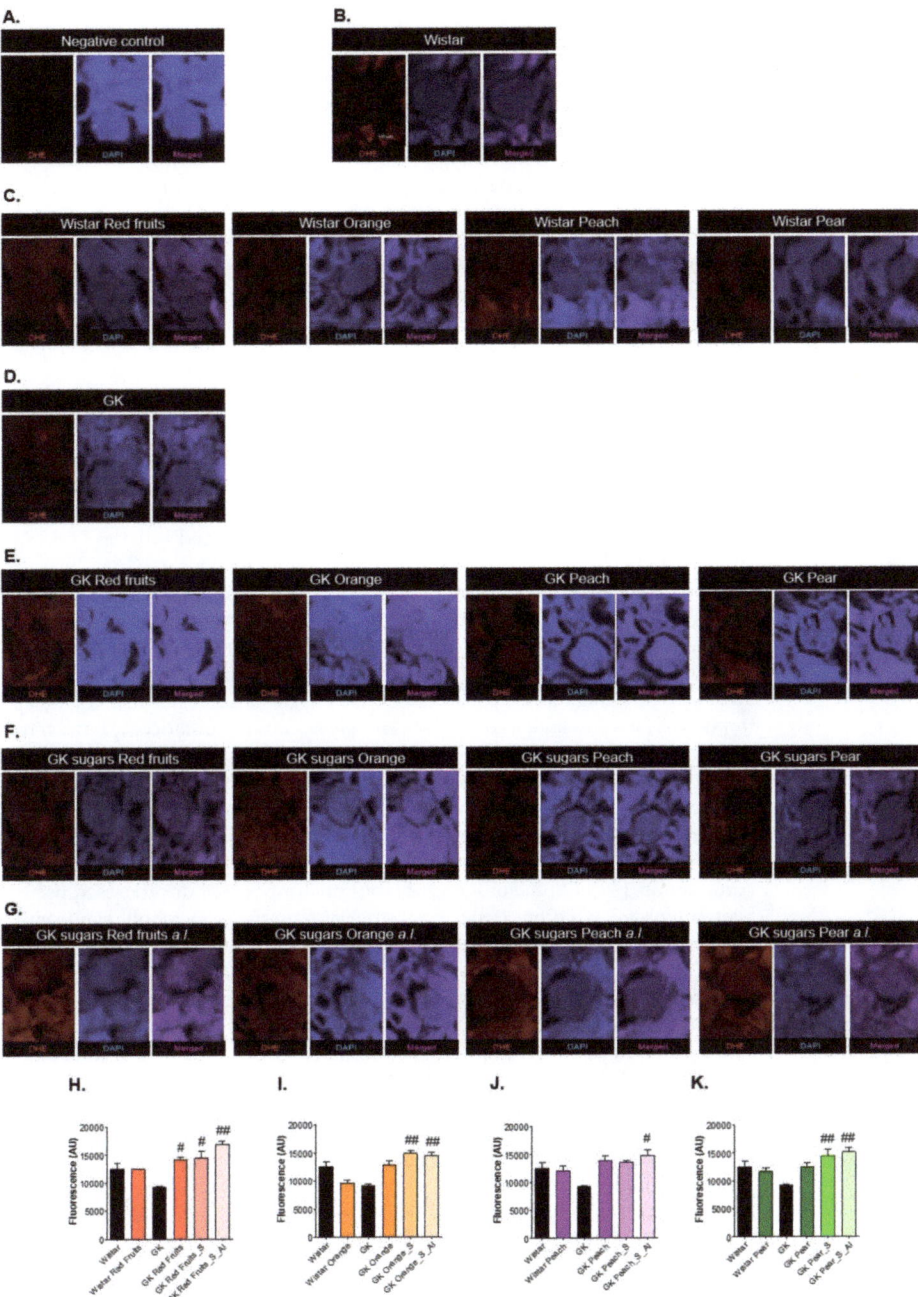

**Figure 9.** Detection of the dihydroethidium (DHE) probe for superoxide anion determination. (**A**) shows the negative control (no probe). Representative images of the glomeruli are shown for control Wistar rats (**B**), Wistar rats maintained with ad libitum access to fruit juices (**C**), control GK rats (**D**), GK rats maintained with ad libitum access to fruit juices (**E**), GK rats treated with respective sugary solutions matched in sugar profile, concentration and quantity (**F**), and GK rats maintained with ad libitum access to the same sugary solutions (**G**). (**H–K**) show the quantification of glomerular DHE staining for the different experimental conditions of each sample tested. # different from GK. 1 symbol, $p < 0.05$; 2 symbols, $p < 0.01$.

## 4. Discussion

In this study, we have demonstrated the distinct role of sugars naturally present in fruit juices and added sugars in impairing oxidative stress, glycation, glucose metabolism and energy balance in an animal model of type 2 diabetes. We have compared sugary solutions with a similar profile of glucose, fructose and sucrose to four different samples of fruit juices. We have shown that sugary solutions induce a higher post-prandial glycaemia and lower total antioxidant capacity of erythrocytes when comparing to the corresponding fruit juices samples. We have also shown that the chronic intake of the same sugary solutions by type 2 diabetic rats, especially when available ad libitum, leads to an imbalance of energy intake regulation, causing increased body weight gain and hyperglycaemia. Such alterations are associated with increased markers of glycation and oxidative stress in several organs. Altogether, heart and kidney appear to be more susceptible to oxidative stress and glycation after an ad libitum consumption of added sugars, while fruit juices were not associated with such alterations.

Consumption of fast-food has been considered in many observational studies as a risk factor for being overweight or obese in both developed and developing regions, even after controlling for energy intake [35]. Higher intake of sugar sweetened drinks was associated with poorer dietary choices and correlated with higher BMI and waist circumference in children [36]. In fact, a recent study by Fox and colleagues has shown increased children's sugar intake from added sources in school breakfasts and lunches [37]. About 63% of children were shown to surpass the limit defined by the Dietary Guidelines for Americans for 24 h intake of added sugars [37]. In adults, increased daily dietary glycemic index was positively associated with higher BMI, with little effect of the percentage of calories from total carbohydrates or total carbohydrate consumption [38]. Increased energy density of foods and macronutrients consumption are usually considered the main determinants for adiposity and metabolic syndrome. However, the source of nutrients are apparently an important factor to take into account, mainly because of other compounds/trace elements that are often present in many foods [39,40]. Such compounds may influence nutrient digestion, absorption, metabolism or biochemical effect, and may be absent in foods or beverages with high amounts of added nutrients (sugars or fat) or may be lost during their industrial processing. The consumption of processed foods with higher sugar and fat content has been suggested as a risk factor for the development of metabolic syndrome components [39]. On the other hand, the consumption of unprocessed natural foods has been suggested as a protective dietary strategy to improve metabolic syndrome components and biochemical markers of disease [39,40].

Consumption of sugar-sweetened beverages (SSB) and fructose-rich fruit juices have been associated with markers of cardiometabolic disease, such as triglycerides (sugars are used for de novo lipogenesis) and HbA1c, as well as with increased risk of arthritis and asthma in pediatric populations, possibly due to increased fructose-induced AGEs formation, RAGE activation and inflammation [41–45]. A recent meta-analysis concluded that increased energy density of meals and food source (processed foods) are key determinants of fructose impact on glycemic control and insulinemia [46]. Data supported that natural sources of fructose-containing sugars or their matched substitution for other macronutrients do not have a negative impact on HbA1c [46]. On the other hand, the addition of the same sugars has harmful effects. The authors disclosed that natural sources like fruit or fruit juices have protective effects on glycemic control, while foods like sweetened milk with added sugars have negative effects [46]. In the present study, fruit juices were supplied ad libitum and no restraint on their consumption was imposed during the treatment period. Remarkably, we show here that ad libitum consumption of fruit juices did not have a negative impact on body weight, glycaemia, glycation and oxidative stress, even in diabetic rats. Such effects were not distinct from those observed in normal rats with ad libitum acess to the same fruit juices. When compared to control Wistar rats, the consumption of fruit juices by Wistar rats did not change any of the parameters studied. Control Wistar rats were also used as normal model to compare the effects of fruit juices and sugary solutions in GK rats. Although 14-weeks-old GK rats are not significantly different from Wistar rats, the consumption of sugary solutions, especially when ad libitum, further increased such differences.

One of the mechanisms for the protective effects of natural sugar sources like fruit juices is the presence of other compounds with the capacity to prevent glycation and oxidative stress. For instance, previous studies have shown that fructose-induced glycation of albumin in vitro was 98% inhibited by pomegranate juice, but less by other fruit juices. Orange, grape or cranberry juice inhibited glycation by 20%, while apple juice didn't confer any protection [47]. Accordingly, citrus juice has been suggested to have beneficial effects on several cardiometabolic markers on patients with type 2 diabetes [48]. On the contrary, beverages or sweetened fruit juices were shown to have higher amounts of AGEs than natural fruit juices [49]. Fruit juices are a natural source of flavonoids and anthocyanins. They have been suggested by several authors as useful in regulating glycaemia and as good supplements or treatment for type 2 diabetes [50–52]. Authors have suggested that such effects may, not only rely in the direct antioxidant properties of the molecules, but also in their ability to modulate mitochondrial function or gut microbiota diversity [53,54].

Another important factor for the protective effects of fruit juices when compared to beverages or sweetened fruit juices is the modulation of satiety mechanisms. Although physical fruit processing for juice preparation has been shown to accelerate gastric emptying and to potentially reduce satiety, the presence of fiber in natural fruit juices was shown to reduce postprandial hyperglycaemia, while increasing the feelings of satiety and fullness [55,56]. Importantly, we here show that fruit juices, besides being a natural source of sugars, have an impact on satiety mechanisms, given that their ad libitum consumption is associated with lower food intake, especially in diabetic rats. Such mechanisms are absent when consuming the corresponding sugary solutions, given that rats fed with matched solutions, not only do not decrease food intake, but actually increase it in most of the samples tested. Remarkably, ad libitum availability of such solutions leads to their significantly higher consumption, also not leading to lower food intake. Altogether, this results in a energy imbalance towards energy intake that leads to weight gain, hyperglycaemia, oxidative stress and glycation. Spetter et al., have shown that fruit juices consumption leads to an inhibition of striatum activation. More, they have shown that activation of anterior cingulate area in the central nervous system predicts subsequent reduction of fruit juices consumption, suggesting a food-specific satiety [57]. Indeed, the role of AGEs and oxidative stress in the hypothalamus must also be considered as a possible mechanisms in the dysregulation of energy imbalance, which needs further investigation. Although little is known regarding the activation of brain areas in response to different sugars composition of foods, it is possible that added sugars, out of a natural matrix with other substances that potentially retard their intestinal absorption and protect from their harmful effects, may cause a distinct impact on such brain areas. Importantly, the pleasantness induced by different sugar content in fruit juices may affect the activation of such areas and can also be modified along the time in order to reduce sugar intake. It was demonstrated that reduction of added sugar to orange juices is well tolerated by the consumers without affecting acceptance [58].

In summary, fruit juices are a natural source of sugars. However, they are ingested in a complex mixture of other nutrients, fibers and other known and unknown compounds that may delay their digestion and absorption, preventing postprandial hyperglycaemia and adverse metabolic effects. Our results show that added sugars have a distinct impact on glycemic control. Matched sugars to four different fruit juices samples do not cause a significative difference on glycaemia, glycation and oxidative stress, even in a diabetic model. Even so, our results show that added sugars have a completely different effect in the modulation of satiety and regulation of energy balance, leading to a poorer glycemic profile and increased levels of glycation and oxidative stress markers, particularly in tissues like the heart and the kidney.

A limitation of our study is the relative short time of juice/sugary solution administration. Future studies could perform administrations for longer periods, in order to undertand the long-term effects of naturally present and added sugars. Longer administrations in more aged diabetic models could reveal more harmful effects of sugars in later stages of disease. Another question that should be answered in the future is the consequences for insulin signalling in liver and epripheral tissues, as well as for insulin secretion and beta-cell viability.

In conclusion, our results reinforce the evidence supporting a noxious role for added sugars in foods, especially when in aqueous solutions, and a harmless effect of fruit sugars without added sugar when consumed moderately, even in diabetic models. We believe that such evidence will help to create the awareness for the need of better food policies and nutritional advices for the general population.

**Author Contributions:** Conceptualization, P.M.; methodology, T.M.-A., B.C., D.A., A.A., C.B., D.S., S.O. and P.M.; software, T.M.-A. and P.M.; validation, T.M.-A. and P.M.; formal analysis, P.M.; investigation, T.M.-A., S.O. and P.M.; resources, R.S. and P.M.; data curation, P.M.; writing—original draft preparation, T.M.-A. and P.M.; writing—review and editing, P.M.; visualization, P.M.; supervision, P.M.; project administration, P.M.; funding acquisition, P.M. All authors have read and agreed to the published version of the manuscript.

**Funding:** This work was supported by the Portuguese Science and Technology Foundation (FCT): Strategic Project UIDB/04539/2020 (CIBB), as well as by COMPETE-FEDER funds (POCI-01-0145-FEDER-007440).

**Institutional Review Board Statement:** The experimental protocol was approved by the local Institutional Animal Care and Use Committee (ORBEA13/18), and all the procedures were performed by licensed users of Federation of Laboratory Animal Science Associations (FELASA) and in accordance with the European Union Directive for Protection of Vertebrates Used for Experimental and Other Scientific Ends (2010/63/EU).

**Informed Consent Statement:** Not applicable.

**Data Availability Statement:** The datasets generated during and/or analyzed during the current study are available from the corresponding author upon reasonable request.

**Acknowledgments:** We thank SUMOL + COMPAL S.A. for providing the juice samples and for financial support.

**Conflicts of Interest:** The study was supported by SUMOL + COMPAL S.A., which is a producer of nectars, soft drinks and 100% fruit juices, having products with only naturally present and with added sugars in their portfolio.

## References

1. Deforche, B.; van Dyck, D.; Deliens, T.; de Bourdeaudhuij, I. Changes in Weight, Physical Activity, Sedentary Behaviour and Dietary Intake during the Transition to Higher Education: A Prospective Study. *Int. J. Behav. Nutr. Phys. Act.* **2015**, *12*, 16. [CrossRef] [PubMed]
2. Bernardo, G.L.; Jomori, M.M.; Fernandes, A.C.; da Costa Proença, R.P. Consumo alimentar de estudantes universitários. *Rev. Nutr.* **2017**, *30*, 847–865. [CrossRef]
3. Vorster, H.H.; Kruger, A.; Wentzel-Viljoen, E.; Kruger, H.S.; Margetts, B.M. Added Sugar Intake in South Africa: Findings from the Adult Prospective Urban and Rural Epidemiology Cohort Study. *Am. J. Clin. Nutr.* **2014**, *99*, 1479–1486. [CrossRef]
4. Sánchez-Pimienta, T.G.; Batis, C.; Lutter, C.K.; Rivera, J.A. Sugar-Sweetened Beverages Are the Main Sources of Added Sugar Intake in the Mexican Population. *J. Nutr.* **2016**, *146*, 1888S–1896S. [CrossRef]
5. Stanhope, K.L. Sugar Consumption, Metabolic Disease and Obesity: The State of the Controversy. *Crit. Rev. Clin. Lab. Sci.* **2016**, *53*, 52–67. [CrossRef]
6. Pereira, M.A. Sugar-Sweetened and Artificially-Sweetened Beverages in Relation to Obesity Risk123. *Adv. Nutr.* **2014**, *5*, 797–808. [CrossRef]
7. Mooradian, A.D.; Smith, M.; Tokuda, M. The Role of Artificial and Natural Sweeteners in Reducing the Consumption of Table Sugar: A Narrative Review. *Clin. Nutr. ESPEN* **2017**, *18*, 1–8. [CrossRef]
8. De Lorgeril, M.; Salen, P. New Insights into the Health Effects of Dietary Saturated and Omega-6 and Omega-3 Polyunsaturated Fatty Acids. *BMC Med.* **2012**, *10*, 50. [CrossRef]

9. Bes-Rastrollo, M.; Sayon-Orea, C.; Ruiz-Canela, M.; Martinez-Gonzalez, M.A. Impact of Sugars and Sugar Taxation on Body Weight Control: A Comprehensive Literature Review. *Obesity* **2016**, *24*, 1410–1426. [CrossRef]
10. Yang, Q.; Zhang, Z.; Gregg, E.W.; Flanders, W.D.; Merritt, R.; Hu, F.B. Added Sugar Intake and Cardiovascular Diseases Mortality among US Adults. *JAMA Intern. Med.* **2014**, *174*, 516–524. [CrossRef]
11. Sluik, D.; van Lee, L.; Engelen, A.I.; Feskens, E.J.M. Total, Free, and Added Sugar Consumption and Adherence to Guidelines: The Dutch National Food Consumption Survey 2007–2010. *Nutrients* **2016**, *8*, 70. [CrossRef]
12. Pfinder, M.; Heise, T.L.; Hilton Boon, M.; Pega, F.; Fenton, C.; Griebler, U.; Gartlehner, G.; Sommer, I.; Katikireddi, S.V.; Lhachimi, S.K. Taxation of Unprocessed Sugar or Sugar-added Foods for Reducing Their Consumption and Preventing Obesity or Other Adverse Health Outcomes. *Cochrane Database Syst. Rev.* **2020**, *4*, CD012333. [CrossRef]
13. World Health Organization. *WHO Guideline: Sugars Intake for Adults and Children*; WHO: Geneva, Switzerland, 2015; Volume 26, pp. 34–36. ISBN 978.92.4.154902 8.
14. Lopes, C.; Torres, D.; Oliveira, A.; Severo, M.; Alarcão, V.; Guiomar, S.; Mota, J. Inquérito Alimentar Nacional e de Atividade Física, IAN-AF 2015–2016: Relatório metodológico. 2017. Available online: https://ian-af.up.pt/sites/default/files/IAN-AF%20Relatorio%20Metodol%C3%B3gico.pdf (accessed on 9 February 2021).
15. Goldfein, K.R.; Slavin, J.L. Why Sugar Is Added to Food: Food Science 101. *Compr. Rev. Food Sci. Food Saf.* **2015**, *14*, 644–656. [CrossRef]
16. McLellan, A.C.; Thornalley, P.J. Glyoxalase Activity in Human Red Blood Cells Fractioned by Age. *Mech. Ageing Dev.* **1989**, *48*, 63–71. [CrossRef]
17. McLellan, A.C.; Thornalley, P.J.; Benn, J.; Sonksen, P.H. Glyoxalase System in Clinical Diabetes Mellitus and Correlation with Diabetic Complications. *Clin. Sci.* **1994**, *87*, 21–29. [CrossRef]
18. Riboulet-Chavey, A.; Pierron, A.; Durand, I.; Murdaca, J.; Giudicelli, J.; van Obberghen, E. Methylglyoxal Impairs the Insulin Signaling Pathways Independently of the Formation of Intracellular Reactive Oxygen Species. *Diabetes* **2006**, *55*, 1289–1299. [CrossRef]
19. Thornalley, P.J. The Glyoxalase System: New Developments towards Functional Characterization of a Metabolic Pathway Fundamental to Biological Life. *Biochem. J.* **1990**, *269*, 1–11. [CrossRef]
20. Thornalley, P.J. Modification of the Glyoxalase System in Human Red Blood Cells by Glucose in Vitro. *Biochem. J.* **1988**, *254*, 751–755. [CrossRef]
21. Delgado-Andrade, C.; Fogliano, V. Dietary Advanced Glycosylation End-Products (dAGEs) and Melanoidins Formed through the Maillard Reaction: Physiological Consequences of their Intake. *Annu. Rev. Food Sci. Technol.* **2018**, *9*, 271–279. [CrossRef]
22. Cuccurullo, C.; Iezzi, A.; Fazia, M.L.; de Cesare, D.; di Francesco, A.; Muraro, R.; Bei, R.; Ucchino, S.; Spigonardo, F.; Chiarelli, F.; et al. Suppression of Rage as a Basis of Simvastatin-Dependent Plaque Stabilization in Type 2 Diabetes. *Arterioscler. Thromb. Vasc. Biol.* **2006**, *26*, 2716–2723. [CrossRef] [PubMed]
23. Hanssen, N.M.J.; Stehouwer, C.D.A.; Schalkwijk, C.G. Methylglyoxal and Glyoxalase I in Atherosclerosis. *Biochem. Soc. Trans.* **2014**, *42*, 443–449. [CrossRef]
24. Lee, H.J.; Howell, S.K.; Sanford, R.J.; Beisswenger, P.J. Methylglyoxal Can Modify GAPDH Activity and Structure. *Ann. N. Y. Acad. Sci.* **2005**, *1043*, 135–145. [CrossRef] [PubMed]
25. Loske, C.; Neumann, A.; Cunningham, A.M.; Nichol, K.; Schinzel, R.; Riederer, P.; Münch, G. Cytotoxicity of Advanced Glycation Endproducts Is Mediated by Oxidative Stress. *J. Neural. Transm.* **1998**, *105*, 1005–1015. [CrossRef]
26. Rosca, M.G.; Mustata, T.G.; Kinter, M.T.; Ozdemir, A.M.; Kern, T.S.; Szweda, L.I.; Brownlee, M.; Monnier, V.M.; Weiss, M.F. Glycation of Mitochondrial Proteins from Diabetic Rat Kidney Is Associated with Excess Superoxide Formation. *Am. J. Physiol. Ren. Physiol.* **2005**, *289*, F420–F430. [CrossRef] [PubMed]
27. Wu, L.; Juurlink, B.H.J. Increased Methylglyoxal and Oxidative Stress in Hypertensive Rat Vascular Smooth Muscle Cells. *Hypertension* **2002**, *39*, 809–814. [CrossRef]
28. Brownlee, M. Biochemistry and Molecular Cell Biology of Diabetic Complications. *Nature* **2001**, *414*, 813–820. [CrossRef]
29. Funk, S.D.; Yurdagul, A.; Orr, A.W. Hyperglycemia and Endothelial Dysfunction in Atherosclerosis: Lessons from Type 1 Diabetes. *Int. J. Vasc. Med.* **2012**, *2012*, 569654. [CrossRef]
30. Sena, C.M.; Matafome, P.; Crisóstomo, J.; Rodrigues, L.; Fernandes, R.; Pereira, P.; Seiça, R.M. Methylglyoxal Promotes Oxidative Stress and Endothelial Dysfunction. *Pharm. Res.* **2012**, *65*, 497–506. [CrossRef]
31. Su, Y.; Lei, X.; Wu, L.; Liu, L. The Role of Endothelial Cell Adhesion Molecules P-Selectin, E-Selectin and Intercellular Adhesion Molecule-1 in Leucocyte Recruitment Induced by Exogenous Methylglyoxal. *Immunology* **2012**, *137*, 65–79. [CrossRef]
32. Rodrigues, T.; Matafome, P.; Santos-Silva, D.; Sena, C.; Seiça, R. Reduction of Methylglyoxal-Induced Glycation by Pyridoxamine Improves Adipose Tissue Microvascular Lesions. Available online: https://www.hindawi.com/journals/jdr/2013/690650/ (accessed on 9 February 2021).
33. Sacramento, J.F.; Martins, F.O.; Rodrigues, T.; Matafome, P.; Ribeiro, M.J.; Olea, E.; Conde, S.V. A2 Adenosine Receptors Mediate Whole-Body Insulin Sensitivity in a Prediabetes Animal Model: Primary Effects on Skeletal Muscle. *Front. Endocrinol.* **2020**, *11*, 262. [CrossRef]
34. Matafome, P.; Santos-Silva, D.; Crisóstomo, J.; Rodrigues, T.; Rodrigues, L.; Sena, C.M.; Pereira, P.; Seiça, R. Methylglyoxal Causes Structural and Functional Alterations in Adipose Tissue Independently of Obesity. *Arch. Physiol. Biochem.* **2012**, *118*, 58–68. [CrossRef] [PubMed]

35. Costa, C.S.; Rauber, F.; Leffa, P.S.; Sangalli, C.N.; Campagnolo, P.D.B.; Vitolo, M.R. Ultra-Processed Food Consumption and Its Effects on Anthropometric and Glucose Profile: A Longitudinal Study during Childhood. *Nutr. Metab. Cardiovasc. Dis.* **2019**, *29*, 177–184. [CrossRef]
36. Collison, K.S.; Zaidi, M.Z.; Subhani, S.N.; Al-Rubeaan, K.; Shoukri, M.; Al-Mohanna, F.A. Sugar-Sweetened Carbonated Beverage Consumption Correlates with BMI, Waist Circumference, and Poor Dietary Choices in School Children. *BMC Public Health* **2010**, *10*, 234. [CrossRef] [PubMed]
37. Fox, M.K.; Gearan, E.C.; Schwartz, C. Added Sugars in School Meals and the Diets of School-Age Children. *Nutrients* **2021**, *13*, 471. [CrossRef] [PubMed]
38. Ma, Y.; Olendzki, B.; Chiriboga, D.; Hebert, J.R.; Li, Y.; Li, W.; Campbell, M.; Gendreau, K.; Ockene, I.S. Association between Dietary Carbohydrates and Body Weight. *Am. J. Epidemiol.* **2005**, *161*, 359–367. [CrossRef] [PubMed]
39. Schröder, H.; Fïto, M.; Covas, M.I. REGICOR investigators Association of Fast Food Consumption with Energy Intake, Diet Quality, Body Mass Index and the Risk of Obesity in a Representative Mediterranean Population. *Br. J. Nutr.* **2007**, *98*, 1274–1280. [CrossRef]
40. Costa, C.S.; del-Ponte, B.; Assunção, M.C.F.; Santos, I.S. Consumption of Ultra-Processed Foods and Body Fat during Childhood and Adolescence: A Systematic Review. *Public Health Nutr.* **2018**, *21*, 148–159. [CrossRef]
41. Yu, Z.; Ley, S.H.; Sun, Q.; Hu, F.B.; Malik, V.S. Cross-Sectional Association between Sugar-Sweetened Beverage Intake and Cardiometabolic Biomarkers in US Women. *Br. J. Nutr.* **2018**, *119*, 570–580. [CrossRef]
42. DeChristopher, L.R.; Uribarri, J.; Tucker, K.L. Intake of High-Fructose Corn Syrup Sweetened Soft Drinks, Fruit Drinks and Apple Juice Is Associated with Prevalent Arthritis in US Adults, Aged 20–30 Years. *Nutr. Diabetes* **2016**, *6*, e199. [CrossRef]
43. DeChristopher, L.R.; Uribarri, J.; Tucker, K.L. Intakes of Apple Juice, Fruit Drinks and Soda Are Associated with Prevalent Asthma in US Children Aged 2–9 Years. *Public Health Nutr.* **2016**, *19*, 123–130. [CrossRef]
44. DeChristopher, L.R.; Tucker, K.L. Excess Free Fructose, High-Fructose Corn Syrup and Adult Asthma: The Framingham Offspring Cohort. *Br. J. Nutr.* **2018**, *119*, 1157–1167. [CrossRef] [PubMed]
45. DeChristopher, L.R.; Tucker, K.L. Excess Free Fructose, Apple Juice, High Fructose Corn Syrup and Childhood Asthma Risk—the National Children's Study. *Nutr. J.* **2020**, *19*. [CrossRef]
46. Choo, V.L.; Viguiliouk, E.; Mejia, S.B.; Cozma, A.I.; Khan, T.A.; Ha, V.; Wolever, T.M.S.; Leiter, L.A.; Vuksan, V.; Kendall, C.W.C.; et al. Food Sources of Fructose-Containing Sugars and Glycaemic Control: Systematic Review and Meta-Analysis of Controlled Intervention Studies. *BMJ* **2018**, *363*, k4644. [CrossRef]
47. Dorsey, P.G.; Greenspan, P. Inhibition of Nonenzymatic Protein Glycation by Pomegranate and Other Fruit Juices. *J. Med. Food* **2014**, *17*, 447–454. [CrossRef] [PubMed]
48. Rampersaud, G.C.; Valim, M.F. 100% Citrus Juice: Nutritional Contribution, Dietary Benefits, and Association with Anthropometric Measures. *Crit. Rev. Food Sci. Nutr.* **2017**, *57*, 129–140. [CrossRef]
49. Takeuchi, M.; Takino, J.; Furuno, S.; Shirai, H.; Kawakami, M.; Muramatsu, M.; Kobayashi, Y.; Yamagishi, S. Assessment of the Concentrations of Various Advanced Glycation End-Products in Beverages and Foods That Are Commonly Consumed in Japan. *PLoS ONE* **2015**, *10*. [CrossRef] [PubMed]
50. AL-Ishaq, R.K.; Abotaleb, M.; Kubatka, P.; Kajo, K.; Büsselberg, D. Flavonoids and Their Anti-Diabetic Effects: Cellular Mechanisms and Effects to Improve Blood Sugar Levels. *Biomolecules* **2019**, *9*, 430. [CrossRef]
51. Wang, Y.; Alkhalidy, H.; Liu, D. The Emerging Role of Polyphenols in the Management of Type 2 Diabetes. *Molecules* **2021**, *26*, 703. [CrossRef] [PubMed]
52. Khoo, H.E.; Azlan, A.; Tang, S.T.; Lim, S.M. Anthocyanidins and Anthocyanins: Colored Pigments as Food, Pharmaceutical Ingredients, and the Potential Health Benefits. *Food Nutr. Res.* **2017**, *61*, 1361779. [CrossRef]
53. Anhê, F.F.; Varin, T.; Barz, M.; Desjardins, Y.; Levy, E.; Roy, D.; Marette, A. Gut Microbiota Dysbiosis in Obesity-Linked Metabolic Diseases and Prebiotic Potential of Polyphenol-Rich Extracts. *Curr. Obes. Rep.* **2015**, *4*, 389–400. [CrossRef]
54. Bendokas, V.; Skemiene, K.; Trumbeckaite, S.; Stanys, V.; Passamonti, S.; Borutaite, V.; Liobikas, J. Anthocyanins: From Plant Pigments to Health Benefits at Mitochondrial Level. *Crit. Rev. Food Sci. Nutr.* **2020**, *60*, 3352–3365. [CrossRef] [PubMed]
55. Krishnasamy, S.; Lomer, M.C.E.; Marciani, L.; Hoad, C.L.; Pritchard, S.E.; Paul, J.; Gowland, P.A.; Spiller, R.C. Processing Apples to Puree or Juice Speeds Gastric Emptying and Reduces Postprandial Intestinal Volumes and Satiety in Healthy Adults. *J. Nutr.* **2020**, *150*, 2890–2899. [CrossRef] [PubMed]
56. Bosch-Sierra, N.; Marqués-Cardete, R.; Gurrea-Martínez, A.; Grau-Del Valle, C.; Morillas, C.; Hernández-Mijares, A.; Bañuls, C. Effect of Fibre-Enriched Orange Juice on Postprandial Glycaemic Response and Satiety in Healthy Individuals: An Acute, Randomised, Placebo-Controlled, Double-Blind, Crossover Study. *Nutrients* **2019**, *11*, 3014. [CrossRef] [PubMed]
57. Spetter, M.S.; de Graaf, C.; Viergever, M.A.; Smeets, P.A.M. Anterior Cingulate Taste Activation Predicts Ad Libitum Intake of Sweet and Savory Drinks in Healthy, Normal-Weight Men. *J. Nutr.* **2012**, *142*, 795–802. [CrossRef] [PubMed]
58. De Oliveira Pineli, L.D.L.; de Aguiar, L.A.; Fiusa, A.; de Assunção Botelho, R.B.; Zandonadi, R.P.; Melo, L. Sensory Impact of Lowering Sugar Content in Orange Nectars to Design Healthier, Low-Sugar Industrialized Beverages. *Appetite* **2016**, *96*, 239–244. [CrossRef]

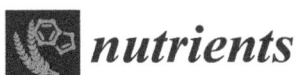

Article

# The Effect of Probiotics (MCP® BCMC® Strains) on Hepatic Steatosis, Small Intestinal Mucosal Immune Function, and Intestinal Barrier in Patients with Non-Alcoholic Fatty Liver Disease

Mohamad Hizami Mohamad Nor [1,†], Nurainina Ayob [2,†], Norfilza M. Mokhtar [2,3], Raja Affendi Raja Ali [1,3], Geok Chin Tan [3,4], Zhiqin Wong [1,3], Nor Hamizah Shafiee [5], Yin Ping Wong [4], Muaatamarulain Mustangin [4] and Khairul Najmi Muhammad Nawawi [1,3,*]

[1] Gastroenterology and Hepatology Unit, Department of Medicine, Faculty of Medicine, Universiti Kebangsaan Malaysia, Kuala Lumpur 56000, Malaysia; hizami84@gmail.com (M.H.M.N.); draffendi@ppukm.ukm.edu.my (R.A.R.A.); wzhiqin@ppukm.ukm.edu.my (Z.W.)
[2] Department of Physiology, Faculty of Medicine, Universiti Kebangsaan Malaysia, Kuala Lumpur 56000, Malaysia; ainina.ayob@yahoo.com (N.A.); norfilza@ppukm.ukm.edu.my (N.M.M.)
[3] GUT Research Group, Faculty of Medicine, Universiti Kebangsaan Malaysia, Kuala Lumpur 56000, Malaysia; tangc@ppukm.ukm.edu.my
[4] Department of Pathology, Faculty of Medicine, Universiti Kebangsaan Malaysia, Kuala Lumpur 56000, Malaysia; ypwong@ppukm.ukm.edu.my (Y.P.W.); amar@ppukm.ukm.edu.my (M.M.)
[5] Dietetics Programme, Faculty of Health Sciences, Universiti Kebangsaan Malaysia, Kuala Lumpur 56000, Malaysia; mizahnur91@gmail.com
* Correspondence: knajmi@ukm.edu.my
† These authors contributed equally to this work.

**Abstract:** Treatment for non-alcoholic fatty liver disease (NAFLD) currently consists of lifestyle modifications such as a low-fat diet, weight loss, and exercise. The gut microbiota forms part of the gut–liver axis and serves as a potential target for NAFLD treatment. We investigated the effect of probiotics on hepatic steatosis, fibrosis, and biochemical blood tests in patients with NAFLD. At the small intestinal mucosal level, we examined the effect of probiotics on the expression of CD4+ and CD8+ T lymphocytes, as well as the tight junction protein zona occluden-1 (ZO-1). This was a randomized, double-blind, placebo-controlled trial involving ultrasound-diagnosed NAFLD patients ($n$ = 39) who were supplemented with either a probiotics sachet (MCP® BCMC® strains) or a placebo for a total of 6 months. Multi-strain probiotics (MCP® BCMC® strains) containing six different *Lactobacillus* and *Bifidobacterium* species at a concentration of 30 billion CFU were used. There were no significant changes at the end of the study in terms of hepatic steatosis (probiotics: $-21.70 \pm 42.6$ dB/m, $p = 0.052$ vs. placebo: $-10.72 \pm 46.6$ dB/m, $p = 0.29$) and fibrosis levels (probiotics: $-0.25 \pm 1.77$ kPa, $p = 0.55$ vs. placebo: $-0.62 \pm 2.37$ kPa, $p = 0.23$) as measured by transient elastography. Likewise, no significant changes were found for both groups for the following parameters: LiverFAST analysis (steatosis, fibrosis and inflammation scores), alanine aminotransferase, total cholesterol, triglycerides, and fasting glucose. In the immunohistochemistry (IHC) analysis, no significant expression changes were seen for CD4+ T lymphocytes in either group (probiotics: $-0.33 \pm 1.67$, $p = 0.35$ vs. placebo: $0.35 \pm 3.25$, $p = 0.63$). However, significant reductions in the expression of CD8+ T lymphocytes ($-7.0 \pm 13.73$, $p = 0.04$) and ZO-1 (Z-score = $-2.86$, $p = 0.04$) were found in the placebo group, but no significant changes in the probiotics group. In this pilot study, the use of probiotics did not result in any significant clinical improvement in NAFLD patients. However, at the microenvironment level (i.e., the small intestinal mucosa), probiotics seemed to be able to stabilize the mucosal immune function and to protect NAFLD patients against increased intestinal permeability. Therefore, probiotics might have a complementary role in treating NAFLD. Further studies with larger sample sizes, a longer duration, and different probiotic strains are needed to evaluate the real benefit of probiotics in NAFLD.

Citation: Mohamad Nor, M.H.; Ayob, N.; Mokhtar, N.M.; Raja Ali, R.A.; Tan, G.C.; Wong, Z.; Shafiee, N.H.; Wong, Y.P.; Mustangin, M.; Nawawi, K.N.M. The Effect of Probiotics (MCP® BCMC® Strains) on Hepatic Steatosis, Small Intestinal Mucosal Immune Function, and Intestinal Barrier in Patients with Non-Alcoholic Fatty Liver Disease. *Nutrients* 2021, 13, 3192. https://doi.org/10.3390/nu13093192

Academic Editors: Silvia V. Conde and Fatima O. Martins

Received: 19 August 2021
Accepted: 9 September 2021
Published: 14 September 2021

**Publisher's Note:** MDPI stays neutral with regard to jurisdictional claims in published maps and institutional affiliations.

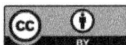

Copyright: © 2021 by the authors. Licensee MDPI, Basel, Switzerland. This article is an open access article distributed under the terms and conditions of the Creative Commons Attribution (CC BY) license (https://creativecommons.org/licenses/by/4.0/).

**Keywords:** NAFLD; probiotics; gut microbiota; mucosal immune function; intestinal permeability

## 1. Introduction

Non-alcoholic fatty liver disease (NAFLD) refers to the presence of hepatic steatosis in the absence of other causes of heavy hepatic fat accumulation, such as heavy alcohol intake. It is one of the most common causes of chronic liver disease nowadays. It has an estimated global prevalence of 25%, with the highest prevalence in the Middle East and South America (31.8% and 30.5% respectively) [1]. A recent meta-analysis on the prevalence of NAFLD in Asian countries ($n$ = 237 studies with 13,044,518 individuals as pooled participants), revealed an overall NALFD prevalence of 29.6%, with an increasing prevalence trend over time (1999–2005: 25.3%; 2006–2011: 28.5%; 2012–2017: 33.9%) [2]. This has given rise to a new epidemic in chronic liver disease and increased disease burden.

Treatment options for the NAFLD are limited and mainly revolve around lifestyle interventions such as weight loss via dietary therapy and exercise [3]. It has to be treated early owing to its tendency to progress to end-stage liver cirrhosis and the possible subsequent complication of hepatocellular carcinoma. As our understanding of the pathogenesis of NAFLD has evolved, it has been suggested that disturbances in the gut microbiota composition, leading to gut dysbiosis that can lead to gut–liver axis derangement, is one of the possible factors that triggers local inflammatory cascades [4,5]. Gut dysbiosis theoretically disrupts the arrangement of the adjacent intestinal epithelial cells by loosening tight junctions, which subsequently triggers the response of adaptive immunity. Tight junction proteins such as zona occludens-1 (ZO-1), which is considered to be one of the more important components in junctional complexes, plays a significant role in maintaining the monolayer integrity of epithelial cells through cell–cell communication [6]. The translocation of microbial endotoxins, such as lipopolysaccharides, have been shown to induce steatosis, inflammation, and fibrosis, as well as elevated inflammatory cytokines, such as TNF-alpha (TNF-$\alpha$) [7]. Therefore, probiotics present a possible target of treatment by manipulating the gut microbiota and modulating intestinal permeability and local mucosal inflammation.

Several methods are available for manipulating the microbiota and its influence on the gut–liver axis, such as the use of prebiotics, probiotics, synbiotics, or faecal microbiota transplants. Probiotics are live microorganisms that, when administered in adequate amounts, confer a health benefit on the host [8]. Prebiotics are selectively indigestible fermented compounds that can induce the growth or activity of beneficial microorganisms [9]. Synbiotics, on the other hand, are a combination of both prebiotics and probiotics. A number of studies involving animals and humans have demonstrated the benefits of pro/synbiotics in NAFLD, such as improving the hepatic steatosis level, reducing hepatic inflammation, and improving biochemical parameters such as alanine aminotransferase (ALT), fasting glucose, and lipid profiles [10–12].

In other diseases, gut microbiota manipulation has been shown to improve outcomes. In an animal study, the use of resistant starch to alter the gut microbiota by shifting the composition of the gut microbiota towards butyrate-producing bacteria, was shown to slow the progress of chronic kidney disease in a mouse model of 5/6 nephrectomy [13]. The use of *L. mucosae A1* has been shown to reduce severe lipid accumulation in the serum, liver, and aortic sinus of ApoE-/-mice on a Western diet, while also reducing the serum lipopolysaccharide-binding protein content of mice, reflecting improved metabolic endotoxemia [14]. In humans, the use of *Lactobacillus rhamnosus GG*-supplemented formula was shown to increase tolerance of infants to cow's milk allergy by expanding the butyrate-producing bacterial strains in the gut [15]. A larger meta-analysis of supplementation with the same strain was shown to reduce antibiotic-associated diarrhea for any reason [16]. Furthermore, 6 months of supplementation with probiotics (MCP® BCMC® strains) containing six viable microorganisms of *Lactobacillus* and *Bifidobacterium* strains in post-surgical colorectal cancer patients was shown to reduce the level of pro-inflammatory cytokines (TNF-α, IL-6, IL10, IL-12, IL-17A, IL-17C, and IL-22) compared with the pre-treatment level [17].

Hence, we conducted a randomized, double-blind, placebo-controlled trial to assess whether probiotic supplementation can improve hepatic steatosis, fibrosis, and other clinical biomarkers in NAFLD patients. Since the small intestine is responsible for most nutrient absorption and digestion, it is prudent to explore the role of the small intestine in the development of NAFLD. Therefore, we also determined the effect of probiotics on changes in the expression of CD4+ and CD8+ T lymphocytes (mucosal immune function) as well as ZO-1 (small intestinal barrier).

## 2. Methodology

### 2.1. Study Design

A randomized, double-blind, placebo-controlled pilot study involving patients from the Universiti Kebangsaan Malaysia Medical Centre (UKMMC) was conducted, and the protocol was approved by the institutional ethics committee (UKM PPI/111/8/JEP-2019-456). The trial was registered at the US National Institutes of Health website (http://www.clinical-trials.gov) #NCT04074889.

### 2.2. Patient Recruitment

The inclusion criteria were: patients aged 18 years old and above with an ultrasound diagnosis of fatty liver, a baseline-controlled attenuation parameter (CAP) score measured by FibroScan of $\geq$263 dB/m, and a baseline ALT of more than 35 IU/L for males and 25 IU/L for females. Patients with evidence of other chronic liver diseases, such as concomitant hepatitis B or C infections, and autoimmune hepatitis disorder or alcoholic liver disease, were excluded from this study. Other exclusion criteria consisted of evidence of acute disorders affecting the liver such as drug-induced liver injury, the presence of hepatocellular carcinoma (or liver metastases), any biliary diseases (which would explain the raised ALT, such as gallstones), or evidence of liver cirrhosis. Patients were advised to stop taking any nutritional supplements and to temporarily discontinue any lipid-lowering drugs, beginning at least 4 weeks prior to the study. The recruitment period lasted for a period of 6 months (September 2019 to February 2020).

### 2.3. Clinical Assessment and Intervention

At baseline measurement, patients' comorbidities (diabetes mellitus, hypertension and dyslipidemia) were recorded. Body mass index (BMI) classifications were performed as per Malaysian clinical practice guidelines [18]. Therefore, underweight refers to a BMI of <18.5 kg/m$^2$, normal weight a BMI of 18.5–22.9 kg/m$^2$, pre-obesity a BMI of 23.0–27.4 kg/m$^2$, and obesity a BMI of >27.5 kg/m$^2$. Blood samples were investigated and a transient elastography was also performed. These tests will be elaborated in the next section.

The baseline dietary pattern was assessed using a Food Frequency Questionnaire (FFQ), a semiquantitative tool for assessing the dietary patterns of patients (adjusted for the Malaysian diet) at the baseline and after the intervention [19]. The FFQ was analyzed to ensure there were no significant differences in the nutritional intake between the two groups, before and after the intervention. All patients were instructed to maintain their current diet and lifestyles. The patients were also instructed to not embark on any weight loss or diet program.

The random allocation sequence was generated by a computer model using Microsoft Excel to create blocks of four in order to allow even numbers in each interventional arm. The randomization was performed by the principal investigators, who held the allocation sequence. After the baseline measurement had been completed, sachets containing the probiotics or a placebo were given to the participants according to their assigned group.

Both the investigators and the patients were blinded to the content of the sachets, and an independent investigator held the code, which was revealed at the end of the study.

### 2.4. Laboratory Investigations

A set of blood investigations was carried out before and after the intervention that included triglycerides (TG), alpha-2-macroglobulin, total cholesterol (TC), gamma-glutamyl transferase (GGT), ALT, aspartate transaminase (AST), total bilirubin, fasting glucose, haptoglobin, and apolipoprotein A1. These measurements were then inputted into an algorithm developed by Fibronostics (LiverFAST) to estimate the level of steatosis, fibrosis, and inflammation based on the blood results. This algorithm has been shown to have a prediction outcome in terms of steatosis and fibrosis that is comparable with liver stiffness measurements measured by transient elastography and liver biopsy, as it can objectively estimate the level of steatosis, fibrosis, and inflammation to be not significant, minimal, moderate, significant, or severe [20,21].

### 2.5. Immunohistochemistry Analysis

Duodenal samples (the second part of the duodenum) from the NAFLD patients were obtained by performing oesophagogastroduodenoscopy (OGD) before and after the intervention. Immunohistochemistry was performed on serial 3 mm sections of the formalin-fixed paraffin-embedded duodenum biopsy samples. The slides were treated with rabbit monoclonal CD4 antibody (Cell Marque, Sigma Aldrich, Burlington, VT, USA) at a dilution of 1:100, mouse monoclonal CD8 antibody (Dako, Agilent Technologies, Santa Clara, CA, US), and rabbit monoclonal to ZO-1 tight junction antibody (Abcam, Cambridge, UK) at a dilution of 1:300. The slides were incubated for 30 min at room temperature, followed by treatment with secondary antibodies and horseradish peroxidase (HRP) for another 30 min. The slides were finally visualized with diaminobenzidine, counterstained with hematoxylin, dehydrated, and mounted. Brown staining of CD4+, CD8+ and ZO-1 on the cell cytoplasm and membrane was classified as positive staining. External positive controls were always included in the batch of slides (CD4+ and CD8+: tonsil; ZO-1: kidney).

The immunostaining was reviewed and scored independently by two histopathologists. We counted the average number of CD4+ or CD8+ T lymphocytes in at least three selected villi, which was later analyzed as the mean number of labelled nuclei over a total of 100 enterocytes. In the lamina propria, the staining was examined semi-quantitatively in the cytoplasmic area and scored as follows: 0: no staining; +: focal staining; ++: regional staining; and +++: no loss. For ZO-1, the results were expressed semi-quantitatively, as previously reported [22]; in brief, cytoplasmic labelling intensity was scored as follows: 0: complete loss; +: moderate loss; ++: focal loss; +++: very focal loss; and ++++: no loss. The staining index score for CD4+, CD8+, and ZO-1 was based on the immunopositive area.

### 2.6. Transient Elastography

A FibroScan 502, manufactured by Echosens (Paris, France) was used in the study to obtain the liver stiffness measurement (LSM, kPa) and the controlled attenuation parameter (CAP, dB/m). A CAP score of $\geq 263$ was taken as the cut-off value to indicate the presence of hepatic steatosis [23]. The measurement was considered reliable if there were at least 10 valid readings, a success reading rate of at least 70%, and an interquartile range/median (IQR/M) of less than 20%. The same equipment was used throughout the study, and all the measurements were performed only by the trained principal investigator of this study in order to eliminate inter-operator variability.

### 2.7. Probiotics and Compliance

The probiotics used were Microbial Cell Preparation (MCP) (Hexbio®; comprising MCP® BCMC® strains) from B-Crobes Laboratory Sdn. Bhd. Their specifications are listed in Table 1. Patients were instructed to consume the product twice a day (in the morning and evening, either with or without meals). The product can be mixed with one glass of water (approximately 250 mL) before consumption, or consumed directly. On the other hand, the placebo contained the same excipients but without the live bacteria. The content of both the probiotics and placebo were packed in a similar-looking sachet and were indistinguishable from each other both in terms of colour, taste, and smell, and were labelled as A or B. Sachets were kept in a dry place below 25 °C and away from direct sunlight. The subjects of the study were also told to do the same. The shelf life of the sachets was 2 years, and the sachets were delivered to the study site at 3-month intervals.

**Table 1.** Contents of the probiotics used in the study.

| Form | White Granules, Packed in a Sachet Form |
|---|---|
| Concentration | 30 billion colony-forming units (CFU) |
| Strains | MCP® BCMC® strains consisting of *Lactobacillus acidophilus* BCMC 12,130 (107 mg), *Lactobacillus casei* subsp. BCMC 12,313 (107 mg), *Lactobacillus lactis* BCMC 12,451 (107 mg), *Bifidobacterium bifidum* BCMC 02290 (107 mg), *Bifidobacterium infantis* BCMC 02129 (107 mg) and *Bifidobacterium longum* BCMC 02120 (107 mg) |
| Product weight | 3 g |
| Manufacturer | B-Crobes Laboratory Sdn. Bhd., GMP, manufactured in Malaysia |

Compliance was checked via the sachet count method during the 3-month appointment with the subjects and another count at the end of the study. A periodic check was also carried out via phone calls and text messages. We accepted compliance rates between 85% and 100% [24].

*2.8. Statistical Analysis*

Descriptive statistics were computed and are presented as means ± standard deviation, as the data were normally distributed. All statistical analyses were performed using SPSS software version 20.0 (SPSS Inc. Chicago, IL, USA) for Windows. Demographic data are presented as means and standard deviations for the normally distributed data. The data were analyzed with a paired sample t-test to account for reductions within the group (probiotics or placebo). An independent sample t-test was used to compare the mean reduction between the groups. For non-normally distributed data, the values are presented as medians (IQR) and the mean differences were calculated using Wilcoxon signed-rank tests. For the IHC analysis, paired sample t-tests were performed to determine changes in the number of CD4+ and CD8+ T lymphocytes in the villi, while the Wilcoxon signed-rank test was used for cytoplasmic staining of CD4+, CD8+, and ZO-1 in the lamina propria, villi, and crypts. A $p$-value of $\leq 0.05$ was considered to be statistically significant.

*2.9. Primary and Secondary Outcomes*

The primary outcome was the mean difference in hepatic steatosis, as measured by CAP in dB/m by FibroScan after probiotics/placebo supplementation. Secondary outcomes included the mean difference in fibrosis score (as measured by FibroScan), the mean difference in selected liver enzymes and lipid profiles (which includes serum total cholesterol, triglycerides, ALT, AST, GGT and fasting blood glucose), and the computed scores (LiverFAST), such as the steatosis, fibrosis, and activity (correlating to hepatic inflammation) scores. The other secondary outcomes were the mean differences in CD4+ and CD8+ T lymphocyte counts observed in the villi, the percentage of proteins in areas of the lamina propria, as well as in the villi and crypts for the tight junction protein ZO-1.

## 3. Results

*3.1. Baseline Characteristics*

Eighty-five percent of the total patients enrolled in the study completed the intervention, with 15 patients in the probiotics group and 17 patients in the placebo group, as shown in Figure 1. The baseline demographics data are summarized in Table 2. The reasons for dropout included an inability to come to the follow-up appointments due to work commitments, getting pregnant during the trial, and logistics issues of the patients. None of the studied patients had any compliance issues related to intolerance or side-effects of the probiotics/placebo. The majority of the participants were in the obese category. No statistically significant difference existed between the two groups regarding their baseline anthropometric measurements, transient elastography, or biochemical blood tests. Data were analyzed per-protocol.

**Table 2.** Baseline characteristics of the studied patients. Values are presented as means (SD) for normally distributed data.

|  | Total (n = 39) | Probiotics (n = 17) | Placebo (n = 22) | p-Value |
|---|---|---|---|---|
| Age | 53.44 (14.13) | 54.70 (10.19) | 52.47 (16.73) | 0.63 |
| Gender |  |  |  |  |
| Male | 28 | 11 | 17 |  |
| Female | 11 | 6 | 5 |  |
| Diabetes mellitus |  |  |  |  |
| Yes | 19 | 9 | 10 |  |
| No | 20 | 8 | 12 |  |
| Hypertension |  |  |  |  |
| Yes | 21 | 11 | 10 |  |
| No | 18 | 6 | 12 |  |
| Metabolic characteristics |  |  |  |  |
| Height, m | 1.64 (0.08) | 1.62 (0.09) | 1.65 (0.07) | 0.21 |
| Weight, kg | 76.70 (13.45) | 75.00 (14.80) | 78.03 (12.51) | 0.49 |
| BMI, kg/m$^2$ | 29.62 (8.46) | 31.33 (12.02) | 28.30 (3.90) | 0.63 |
| Nutritional intake |  |  |  |  |
| Average kcal | 1731.82 (348.62) | 1759.94 (408.39) | 1710.09 (302.85) | 0.66 |
| Carbohydrate, g | 202.79 (40.86) | 194.39 (46.82) | 209.29 (35.35) | 0.26 |
| % of total kcal | 46% | 44% | 48% |  |
| Total fat, g | 67.23 (20.78) | 67.46 (21.81) | 61.31 (19.84) | 0.34 |
| % of total kcal | 33% | 34% | 32% |  |
| Protein, g | 85.16 (23.93) | 91.64 (26.34) | 80.16 (21.16) | 0.14 |
| % of total kcal | 19% | 20% | 18% |  |
| Serum biochemistry |  |  |  |  |
| ALT, IU/L | 72.02 (34.77) | 70.29 (28.21) | 73.36 (39.71) | 0.78 |
| AST, IU/L | 46.92 (18.27) | 44.35 (12.67) | 48.90 (21.74) | 0.44 |
| GGT, IU/L | 70.10 (54.41) | 65.94 (34.07) | 73.31 (66.69) | 0.68 |
| Triglycerides, mmol/L | 2.06 (0.79) | 2.04 (0.79) | 2.09 (0.81) | 0.84 |
| Total Cholesterol, mmol/L | 5.79 (0.89) | 5.93 (0.90) | 5.68 (0.88) | 0.38 |
| Fasting glucose, mmol/L | 5.34 (1.31) | 5.13 (0.96) | 5.50 (1.53) | 0.38 |
| Serum LiverFAST |  |  |  |  |
| Steatosis score | 0.64 (0.15) | 0.67 (0.16) | 0.62 (0.14) | 0.41 |
| Fibrosis score | 0.30 (0.20) | 0.28 (0.17) | 0.33 (0.22) | 0.46 |
| Activity score | 0.42 (0.23) | 0.42 (0.21) | 0.43 (0.24) | 0.85 |
| Transient elastography |  |  |  |  |
| Liver stiffness, kPa | 7.44 (2.76) | 7.25 (2.76) | 7.58 (2.82) | 0.37 |
| Controlled attenuated parameter, dB/m | 333.51 (34.35) | 339.11 (34.39) | 329.18 (35.15) | 0.71 |

ALT, alanine aminotransferase; AST, aspartate aminotransferase; BMI, body mass index; GGT, gamma-glutamyl transferase.

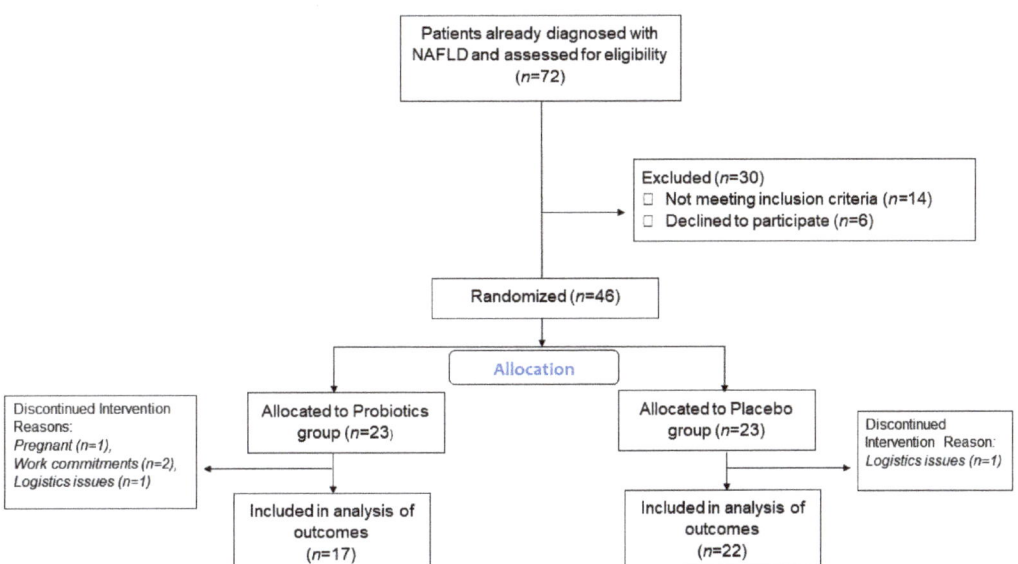

**Figure 1.** Consolidated Standards of Reporting Trials flow diagram of the study participants. NAFLD, non-alcoholic fatty liver disease.

### 3.2. Hepatic Steatosis, Fibrosis and Activity Scores

The post-intervention hepatic steatosis scores in the probiotics group showed a greater reduction in the mean CAP score, from 339.17 ± 33.58 dB/m to 317.41 ± 40.37 dB/m (a mean reduction of −21.70 dB/m, $p = 0.052$) compared with that of the placebo group, which was from 329.18 ± 35.15 dB/m to 318.45 ± 45.37 dB/m (a mean reduction of −10.72 dB/m; $p = 0.29$). However, the improvement in CAP scores in the probiotics group was not statistically significant. For the hepatic fibrosis score measured using FibroScan, there was no statistically significant difference within the probiotics (from 7.25 ± 2.76 kPa to 6.99 ± 2.74 kPa; $p = 0.55$) and placebo (from 7.58 ± 2.82 kPa to 6.95 ± 2.19 kPa; $p = 0.23$) groups.

LiverFAST was also used to evaluate the hepatic steatosis, fibrosis, and inflammatory activity scores in NAFLD patients. For the probiotics group after supplementation with probiotics, we did not elicit any improvement in the scores for all three parameters (steatosis score: $p = 0.06$; fibrosis score: $p = 0.88$; activity score: $p = 0.78$). Likewise, no improvement in the score was seen in the placebo group (steatosis score: $p = 0.053$; activity score: $p = 0.57$). In fact, the median fibrosis score showed a significant increase after the 6-month study period from 0.27 (0.15–0.45) to 0.33 (0.15–0.36) ($p = 0.022$; Tables 3 and 4).

Table 3. Clinical parameters at baseline and the end of the study by intervention group.

|  | Probiotics (n = 17) | | | Placebo (n = 22) | | |
|---|---|---|---|---|---|---|
|  | Baseline | End of Study | p-Value | Baseline | End of Study | p-Value |
| Steatosis (CAP), dB/m | 339.17 (33.58) | 317.41 (40.37) | 0.05 | 329.18 (35.15) | 318.45 (45.37) | 0.29 |
| Liver stiffness, kPa | 7.25 (2.76) | 6.99 (2.74) | 0.55 | 7.58 (2.82) | 6.95 (2.19) | 0.23 |
| ALT, IU/L | 70.29 (28.21) | 84.29 (70.55) | 0.26 | 73.36 (39.71) | 74.50 (38.73) | 0.84 |
| AST, IU/L | 44.35 (12.67) | 46.35 (23.19) | 0.64 | 48.90 (21.74) | 45.50 (25.80) | 0.36 |
| GGT, IU/L | 65.94 (34.07) | 72.17 (56.90) | 0.45 | 73.31 (66.69) | 74.63 (81.94) | 0.81 |
| * Steatosis score | 0.72 (0.53–0.80) | 0.76 (0.64–0.85) | 0.06 | 0.67 (0.52–0.74) | 0.73 (0.51–0.79) | 0.053 |
| * Fibrosis score | 0.26 (0.15–0.40) | 0.22 (0.18–0.36) | 0.88 | 0.27 (0.15–0.45) | 0.33 (0.15–0.36) | 0.022 |
| Activity score | 0.42 (0.21) | 0.41 (0.24) | 0.78 | 0.43 (0.24) | 0.44 (0.25) | 0.57 |
| * Body mass index, kg/m$^2$ | 28.50 (25.0–31.60) | 30.0 (26.20–32.90) | 0.048 | 28.50 (25.05–31.15) | 29.60 (25.85–32.03) | 0.002 |
| Triglycerides, mg/dL | 2.04 (0.79) | 1.94 (0.75) | 0.55 | 2.09 (0.81) | 2.01 (1.01) | 0.66 |
| Total cholesterol, mg/dL | 5.93 (0.90) | 6.17 (1.38) | 0.31 | 5.68 (0.88) | 5.74 (1.46) | 0.79 |
| Fasting glucose, mg/dL | 5.13 (0.96) | 5.6 (1.09) | 0.06 | 5.50 (1.53) | 5.14 (0.68) | 0.28 |

ALT, alanine aminotransferase; AST, aspartate aminotransferase; CAP, controlled attenuated parameter; GGT, gamma-glutamyl transferase. Values are presented as the mean (standard deviation), unless stated otherwise. * Values are presented as the median (interquartile range). Analysis was performed by Wilcoxon signed-rank tests due to a non-normal distribution.

Table 4. Mean changes in the study parameters between the groups from baseline to the end of the study.

|  | Probiotics (n = 17) | | Placebo (n = 22) | | |
|---|---|---|---|---|---|
|  | Mean | SD | Mean | SD | p-Value |
| Steatosis, dB/m | −21.7 | 42.60 | −10.72 | 46.64 | 0.45 |
| Liver stiffness, kPa | −0.25 | 1.77 | −0.62 | 2.37 | 0.59 |
| ALT, IU/L | 14.0 | 50.04 | 1.13 | 26.39 | 0.30 |
| AST, IU/L | 2.00 | 17.31 | −3.40 | 17.09 | 0.33 |
| GGT, IU/L | 6.2 | 33 | 1.35 | 28.38 | 0.60 |
| Steatosis score | 0.049 | 0.09 | 0.042 | 0.11 | 0.83 |
| Fibrosis score | 0.01 | 0.10 | 0.06 | 0.09 | 0.18 |
| Activity score | −0.12 | 0.15 | 0.015 | 0.13 | 0.56 |
| Body mass index, kg/m$^2$ | 0.7 | 1.46 | 0.82 | 1.06 | 0.81 |
| Triglycerides, mg/dL | −0.10 | 0.68 | −0.07 | 0.77 | 0.90 |
| Total cholesterol, mg/dL | 0.23 | 0.93 | 0.05 | 1.07 | 0.59 |
| Fasting glucose, mg/dL | 0.46 | 0.94 | −0.44 | 1.31 | 0.03 |

ALT, alanine aminotransferase; AST, aspartate aminotransferase; GGT, gamma-glutamyl transferase. Values are presented as the mean (standard deviation). (−) denotes a reduction in the measurement at the end of the study compared with the baseline.

### 3.3. Biochemical Blood Tests

Other biochemical parameters such as ALT, AST, GGT, total cholesterol, triglycerides, and fasting glucose did not show any significant differences within both groups after the intervention (Tables 3 and 4).

### 3.4. Immunohistochemistry Analysis

#### 3.4.1. Expression of CD4+ T Lymphocytes

Quantitatively, there was no significant difference in the mean post-intervention CD4+ T lymphocyte count in the small intestinal villi for both the probiotics (from $2.30 \pm 1.83$ to $1.97 \pm 1.50$; $p = 0.35$) and placebo (from $2.03 \pm 1.68$ to $2.38 \pm 4.82$; $p = 0.63$) groups. Similarly, the cytoplasmic staining of the small intestinal lamina propria did not show any significant change in expression for both groups (probiotics: Z-score = 0.00, $p = 1.00$; placebo: Z-score= −0.302, $p = 0.76$) (Figures 2 and 3).

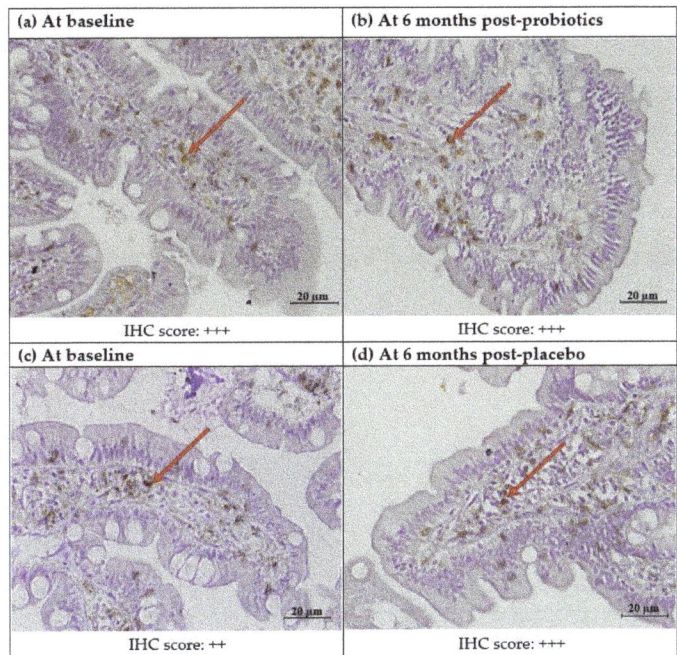

**Figure 2.** Immunohistochemicalstaining of CD4+ protein in the duodenal mucosa (CD4+, 400X). (**a**) Duodenal mucosa of a patient with NAFLD at baseline. (**b**) Duodenal mucosa of a patient with NAFLD after 6 months of probiotics. (**c**) Duodenal mucosa of a patient with NAFLD at baseline. (**d**) Duodenal mucosa of a patient with NAFLD after 6 months of the placebo. The arrows show brownish staining of the CD4+ T lymphocytes in the lamina propria. Semi-quantitatively, both the probiotics and placebo groups did not show any difference in the percentage of staining before and after the intervention. Staining score: 0: no staining; +: focal staining; ++: regional staining; and +++: no loss.

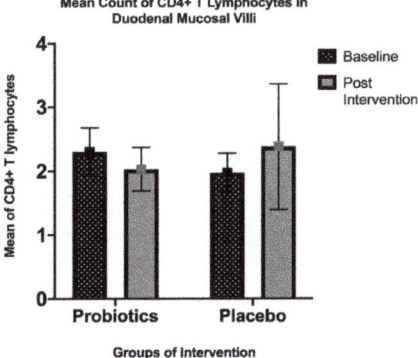

**Figure 3.** Immunohistochemical staining analysis of CD4+ T lymphocytes in the villi of the duodenal mucosa in NAFLD patients. There was a slight decrease in the mean count of intraepithelial CD4+ T lymphocytes observed in the probiotics group after 6 months of the intervention (from $2.30 \pm 1.83$ to $1.97 \pm 1.50$; $p = 0.35$), while the placebo group showed a slight increase in the mean intraepithelial CD4+ T lymphocyte count (from $2.03 \pm 1.68$ to $2.38 \pm 4.82$; $p = 0.63$). Both groups did not show any significant changes.

### 3.4.2. Expression of CD8+ T Lymphocytes

The quantitative analysis in the small intestinal villi showed that there was a significant decrease in the CD8+ T lymphocyte count for the placebo group (from 30.51 ± 16.85 to 23.51 ± 10.61; $p = 0.04$), but not for the probiotics group (from 25.40 ± 17.81 to 20.58 ± 8.72; $p = 0.21$). However, the same trend was not seen in the semi-quantitative analysis for cytoplasmic staining in the lamina propria (Figures 4 and 5).

### 3.4.3. Expression of ZO-1

There was no significant change in ZO-1 expression after the intervention for both groups, when analyzed semi-quantitatively in the small intestinal villi (probiotics: Z-score = −0.97, $p = 0.33$; placebo: Z-score = −0.73, $p = 0.47$). On the other hand, semi-quantitative analysis in the crypt area showed a significant reduction in ZO-1 expression for the placebo group (Z-score = −2.86, $p = 0.04$) but no significant change for the probiotics group (Z-score = −0.93, $p = 0.35$) (Figure 6).

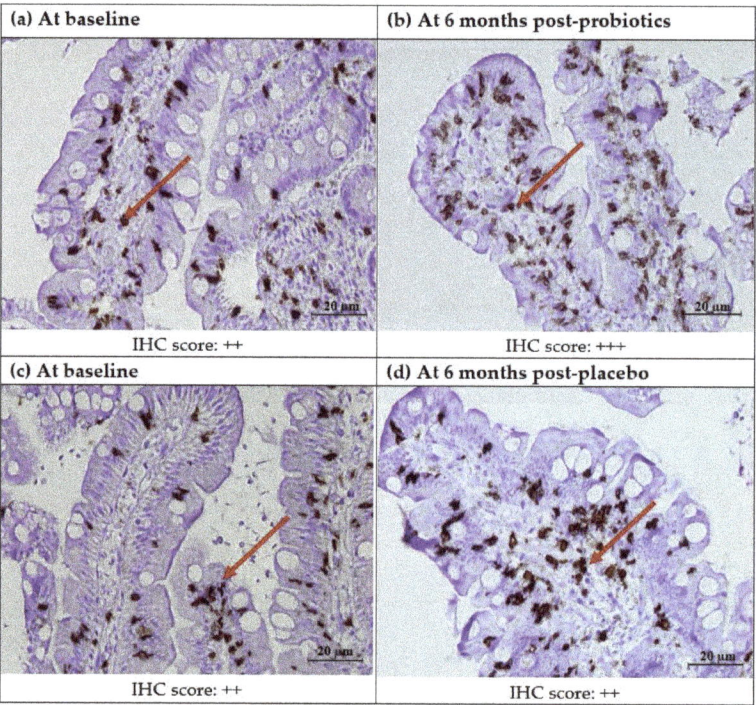

**Figure 4.** Immunohistochemical staining of CD8+ protein in the duodenal mucosa (CD8+,400X). (**a**) Duodenal mucosa of a patient with NAFLD at baseline. (**b**) Duodenal mucosa of a patient with NAFLD after 6 months of probiotics. (**c**) Duodenal mucosa of a patient with NAFLD at baseline. (**d**) Duodenal mucosa of a patient with NAFLD after 6 months of the placebo. Red arrows show brownish CD8+ T lymphocytes in the lamina propria. Semi-quantitatively, no significant post-intervention difference was seen in either the probiotics of placebo groups. Staining score: 0: no staining; +: focal staining; ++: regional staining; and +++: no loss.

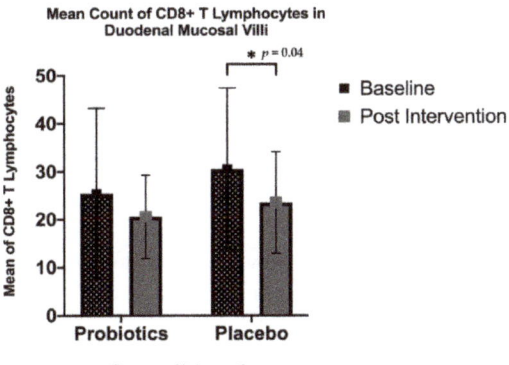

**Figure 5.** Immunohistochemical staining analysis of CD8+ T lymphocytes in the villi of the duodenal mucosa in NAFLD patients. There was a significant decrease in the mean count of intraepithelial CD8+T lymphocytes observed in the placebo group after 6 months of the intervention (from 30.51 ± 16.85 to 23.51 ± 10.61, * $p = 0.04$), while the probiotics group showed a slight decrease in the mean intraepithelial CD8+T lymphocyte count; however, this was not statistically significant ($p = 0.211$).

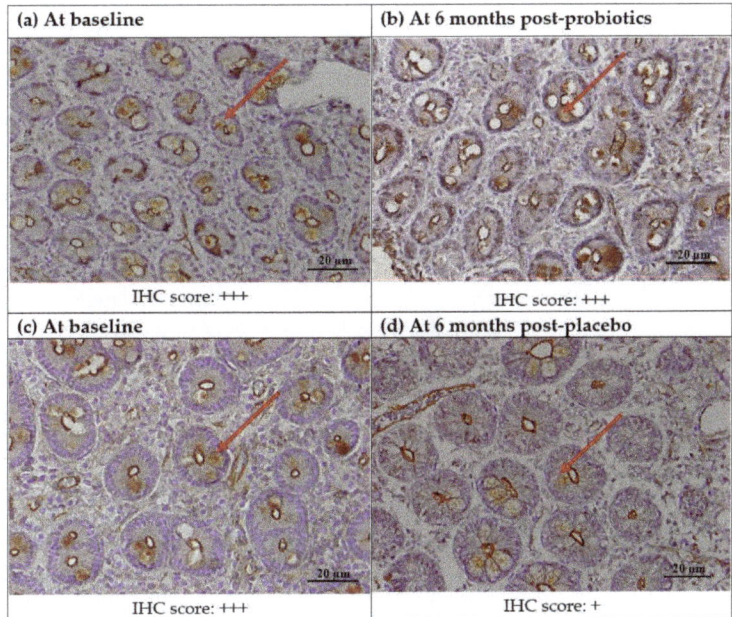

**Figure 6.** Immunohistochemical staining of tight junction zonula occluden-1 (ZO-1) protein in the duodenal mucosa (ZO-1400X). (**a**) Duodenal mucosa of a patient with NAFLD at baseline. (**b**) Duodenal mucosa of a patient with NAFLD after 6 months of probiotics. (**c**) Duodenal mucosa of a patient with NAFLD at baseline. (**d**) Duodenal mucosa of a patient with NAFLD after 6 months of the placebo. Brownish ZO-1 IHC staining was observed in the intestinal crypts (red arrows). There was a significant reduction in ZO-1 expression in the post-intervention placebo group (Z-score = −2.86, $p = 0.04$) but not in the probiotics group (Z-score = −0.93, $p = 0.35$). Staining score: 0: complete loss; +: moderate loss; ++: focal loss; +++: very focal loss; and ++++: no loss.

## 3.5. Nutritional Analysis

Based on the FFQ, there was a significant decrease in the daily total fat intake in the probiotics group after the intervention compared with the placebo group ($-10.63 \pm 18.56$ g, $p < 0.05$ vs. $-2.53 \pm 21.32$ g, $p = 0.58$). Other macronutrients showed no significant difference in either of the two groups, as shown in Table 5.

Table 5. Dietary intake from baseline to the end of the study within the groups.

|  | Probiotics (n = 17) | | | Placebo (n = 22) | | |
| --- | --- | --- | --- | --- | --- | --- |
|  | Baseline | End of Study | p-Value | Baseline | End of Study | p-Value |
| Calories, kcal | 1759.94 (408) | 1645.03 (565) | 0.39 | 1636.04 (457) | 1637.11 (485) | 0.98 |
| Carbohydrates, g | 194.39 (46.82) | 215.31 (63.87) | 0.26 | 209.29 (35.35) | 213.24 (46.46) | 0.70 |
| Protein, g | 91.64(26.34) | 83.23 (23.77) | 0.14 | 80.16 (21.16) | 86.97 (21.75) | 0.13 |
| Total fat, g | 67.46 (21.81) | 56.82 (18.60) | <0.05 | 61.31 (19.84) | 58.77 (16.96) | 0.58 |

Value presented in Mean (standard deviation).

LiverFAST categories:

(I) Fibrosis score: 0–0.27, no fibrosis, F0; 0.28–0.48, minimal, F1; 0.49–0.58, moderate, F2; 0.59–0.74, significant, F3; 0.75–1.00, severe, F4

(II) Steatosis score: 0.69–1.0, no steatosis, S0; 0.38–0.56, minimal, S1; 0.57–0.68, moderate, S2; 0.69–1.00, severe, S3

(III) Activity score: 0–0.29, no activity, A0; 0.3–0.52, minimal, A1; 0.53–0.62, moderate, A2; 0.63–0.72, significant, A3; 0.73–1.00, severe, A4

## 4. Discussion

There was no specific gut microbiota associated with NAFLD. However, multiple studies have shown how a dysbiotic environment exists in NAFLD and non-alcoholic steatohepatitis (NASH) patients. Michail et al. (2015) compared three groups, which were lean healthy children, obese children without NAFLD, and obese children with NAFLD. Using faecal samples, they found that children with NAFLD had more *Gammaproteobacteria* and *Epsilonproteobacteria* (at class level) and *Prevotella* (at genus level) compared with healthy controls [25]. Zhu et al. (2012) found a higher prevalence of *Proteobacteria* (phylum level), *Enterobacteriaceace* (family level), and *Escherichia* (genus level) in children with NASH [26]. In contrast to the study by Zhu et al., Mouzaki et al. (2013) found a lower percentage of *Bacteroidetes* in NASH patients compared with healthy controls, independent of their diet or body mass index [27]. On the other hand, Wong et al. (2015) did not find any change in *Bacteroidetes* levels between the NASH patients and healthy controls [28]. Instead, the abundance of *Firmicutes* decreased in the NASH patients compared with healthy controls. These inconsistencies may be due to various factors, such as the different geographical locations, diets, ages, and the population studied [29].

There have been multiple studies concerning the manipulation of the gut microbiota in order to achieve a clinical improvement in hepatic steatosis and inflammation, together with other measured laboratory parameters, using either prebiotics, probiotics or synbiotics. Mofidi et al. (2017), in a randomized placebo-controlled trial involving 50 patients, were able to demonstrate a greater reduction in hepatic steatosis and fibrosis measured by transient elastography. The researchers used synbiotics consisting of multiple strains of *Lactobacillus* sp. and *Bifidobacterium* sp. compared with a placebo group over 28 weeks [10]. Similarly, Eslamparast et al. (2014), in a study involving 52 patients, were also able to demonstrate a greater reduction in ALT, GGT, and high sensitivity C-reactive protein in the synbiotics group compared with the placebo group [30]. A meta-analysis in 2013 of four other randomized controlled trials also showed the positive effect of probiotics in reducing ALT and total cholesterol [31]. Duseja et al. (2019) demonstrated an improvement in the liver histology of patients with NAFLD after taking probiotics compared with the usual care group [32]. However, most recently in 2020, Scorletti et al., in one of the largest studies, which involved 104 patients for a duration of 10 to 14 months, revealed no significant difference in liver steatosis in both the synbiotics and placebo groups [33].

Probiotics have been shown to affect the mucosal immune function, as well as the intestinal barrier in fatty liver subjects or models. Jiang et al. (2015) revealed a decreased number of duodenal CD4+ and CD8+ T lymphocytes in a NAFLD group compared with healthy controls [34]. This finding was in agreement with other recent studies by Zhao et al. (2021) and Ma et al. (2016), which also found a selective loss of intrahepatic CD4+ T lymphocytes in both human and animal models due to lipid metabolism dysregulation [35,36]. Another new published study by Antonucci et al. (2020) showed the suppression of circulating CD4+ and CD8+ T lymphocytes activation due to infiltration of polymorphonuclear neutrophils (PMNs), which were elevated in NAFLD and NASH patients [37]. However, a few studies that used liver tissues instead of duodenal tissues displayed contrasting results. A study by Her et al. (2020) conducted on a humanized mouse model with an induced high-fat high-calorie diet (HFHD), which showed an increasing trend of effector memory T cells and human CD4+ after 20 weeks of observation [38]. This can also be seen in another study by Hu et al. (2016), which concluded that a high activation of hepatic CD4+ and CD8+ T lymphocytes was due to gut-derived lymphocytes that migrated to the liver [39]. The study indicated that immune cells with different localizations might exhibit different immune responses.

Zonula occluden proteins, which comprise ZO-1, ZO-2, and ZO-3, are tight junction proteins that are responsible for controlling the paracellular pathway of solutes between the linings of adjacent epithelial cells [40]. Miele et al. (2009) found a disruption of intestinal tight junction ZO-1 with evidence of a small increase in intestinal bacteria overgrowth in biopsy-proven NAFLD patients [22]. An animal study by Feng et al. (2019) manipulated ApoE$^{-/+}$ mice with a standard and high-fat diet (HFD) supplemented with curcumin for 16 weeks [41]. The expression of ZO-1 was upregulated in HFD mice supplemented with curcumin, in concordance with reduced circulating lipopolysaccharide levels. An animal study by Kim et al. (2019) reported upregulation of ZO-1, Claudin-3, and Mucin-4 in a dextran sodium sulphate-induced model after *Lactobacillus paracasei* treatment for 8 days [42].

In our study, we did not find a statistically significant reduction in the level of hepatic steatosis for the probiotics group. Additionally, no improvement was seen in other biochemical blood parameters. To our knowledge, our study is currently the first to be conducted in the local Malaysian setting. Malaysia, compared with other countries, has a more diversified dietary intake, due to the multiethnic population in the country. So far, data on gut microbiota prevalence in Malaysia are still limited. Chong et al. (2015) revealed that the northern Malaysian population has high levels of *Bacteroidetes* and *Firmicutes* (phyla). In their sub-analysis of Aboriginal children, an abundant amount of *Aeromonadales* (order) was seen in comparison with the more dominant presence of *Bacteroidetes* and *Firmicutes* [43]. Neoh et al. (2018), in a study of 15 patients living in urban areas, showed three prevalent gut phyla: *Bacteroidetes, Firmicutes,* and *Fusobacterium* [44]. In addition, Lee et al. (2014), in a sub-analysis, revealed how the Malaysian gut microbiota was much more diverse compared with that of people who live in New York [45]. The differing local gut microbiota may have affected the results of this study. Further data on the local gut microbiota may be needed, and a larger sample size may be suggested if similar studies are repeated in a local population at a later time.

Our study's findings are comparable with some previous studies, in which the placebo group showed a significant reduction in expression of CD8+ T lymphocytes and ZO-1 after 6 months. Although we failed to demonstrate a significant improvement in the expression of CD8+ T lymphocytes and ZO-1 for the probiotics group, we revealed no significant reduction in their expression, unlike in the placebo group. Therefore, this study gives an insight into the thought that probiotics might play a role in stabilizing mucosal immune function, as well as preventing intestinal permeability in NAFLD patients.

There are several limitations of the study that need to be mentioned. The sample size for the study was relatively small and may have led to a high probability of Type I statistical errors and a higher chance of confounding factors affecting the results. Participants were also instructed not to significantly change their diet during the study, but we found a significant decrease in total fat intake in the probiotics group, which may also have affected the final results. However, the anorexigenic effect of probiotics has been studied in several animal models and human studies; for example, Bjerg et al. (2014) showed that intraluminal infusion of *Lactobacillus casei W8* into an ex vivo porcine ileum resulted in increased *GLP-1* secretion, which can potentially suppress the appetite acutely. Ingestion of a high concentration of *Lactobacillus casei W8* prior to ad libitum lunch also resulted in a lower energy intake compared with those who consumed the placebo [46]. Although the fat intake was reduced in our probiotics group, it is worth mentioning that it still remains within the range recommended by the Malaysian nutritional committee and the joint FAO/WHO recommendations [47,48] However, our baseline characteristics indicated a diet rich in protein, as the total intake exceeded the recommended nutritional guidelines (61 g/day for men and 52 g/day for women). The total fat intake seems to be within the recommended intake (61 to 73 g for men and 53 to 63 g for women). The carbohydrate intake was also within the recommended level, not exceeding 50% of the daily total energy intake. This trend of higher dietary protein intake compared with carbohydrates and other macronutrients has been shown in several studies looking at the average dietary trends of various cohorts of the Malaysian population, either in central urban populations or in suburban East Malaysian populations [49,50]. This trend, however, has been observed globally and is predominant in countries with emerging economies where the improving economic status enables its population to consume more foods of animal origin; hence, we did not expect significant changes in our population's diet compared with many developing and developed countries [51]. Although FibroScan has been proven to have a good correlation with liver histology in NAFLD, liver biopsy still remains the gold standard of liver histology assessments, something that was not performed in this study due to the invasive nature of the test. Another study limitation was that we did not collect stool samples for gut microbiota analyses.

The strength of this study was that it quantified the dietary composition of the patients in an objective manner. Using the FFQ, the investigators were able to compute the dietary pattern of the participants at baseline, and the analysis could easily be repeated at the end of the study, which allowed us to identify the reduction in total fat intake in the probiotics group. The use of serum-based LiverFAST also eliminated operator-dependent variability in assessing hepatic steatosis. We used multiple strains of *Lactobacillus and Bifidobacterium* at a high concentration in order to restore gut dysbiosis, while other studies used either single or multiple strains of a similar genus at a much lower concentration [10,29–33].

## 5. Conclusions

In this pilot study, the use of probiotics for a 6-month duration did not show any significant clinical improvement in NAFLD patients, namely hepatic steatosis, fibrosis, and activity scores, as well as biochemical blood tests. However, in the microenvironment of the small intestine, probiotics seemed to be able to stabilize the mucosal immune function, as shown by the reduced expression of CD8+ T lymphocytes in the placebo group, but not in the probiotics group. Additionally, probiotics were able to protect NAFLD patients against increased intestinal permeability, which was seen in the placebo group. Therefore, probiotics might play a complementary role in treating NAFLD. Further studies with larger sample sizes, a longer duration, and different probiotic strains are needed in order to evaluate the real benefit of probiotics in the management of NAFLD.

**Author Contributions:** Conceptualization, K.N.M.N., R.A.R.A., N.M.M. and Z.W.; methodology and participants recruitment, K.N.M.N., M.H.M.N., N.A., N.M.M., G.C.T., N.H.S., Y.P.W. and M.M.; data analysis, K.N.M.N., M.H.M.N., N.A., G.C.T., N.H.S., Y.P.W. and M.M.; writing—original draft preparation, M.H.M.N. and N.A.; writing—review and editing, K.N.M.N., R.A.R.A., N.M.M. and Z.W.; supervision, K.N.M.N., R.A.R.A., N.M.M., Z.W. and G.C.T. All authors have read, critically appraised and agreed to the published version of the manuscript.

**Funding:** This study was funded by the Fundamental Research Grant Scheme of the Ministry of Higher Education (Project Code: FRGS/1/2018/SKK02/UKM/03/2) and by the Young Lecturers' Incentive Grant (GGPM) of the National University of Malaysia (GGPM-2019-036). We would like to acknowledge B-Crobes Laboratory Sdn. Bhd. for their industrial support.

**Institutional Review Board Statement:** The study was conducted according to the guidelines of the Declaration of Helsinki, and was approved by the UKM ethics committee (UKM PPI/111/8/JEP-2019-456).

**Informed Consent Statement:** Written informed consent was obtained from all subjects involved in the study.

**Data Availability Statement:** The raw data of the clinical outcomes and IHC results are available from the corresponding author on reasonable request.

**Conflicts of Interest:** The authors hereby declare no conflict of interest.

## References

1. Younossi, Z.M.; Koenig, A.B.; Abdelatif, D.; Fazel, Y.; Henry, L.; Wymer, M. Global epidemiology of nonalcoholic fatty liver disease—Meta-analytic assessment of prevalence, incidence, and outcomes. *Hepatology* **2016**, *64*, 73–84. [CrossRef]
2. Li, J.; Zou, B.; Yeo, Y.H.; Feng, Y.; Xie, X.; Lee, D.H.; Fujii, H.; Wu, Y.; Kam, L.Y.; Ji, F.; et al. Prevalence, incidence, and outcome of non-alcoholic fatty liver disease in Asia, 1999–2019: A systematic review and meta-analysis. *Lancet Gastroenterol. Hepatol.* **2019**, *4*, 389–398. [CrossRef]
3. Jennison, E.; Patel, J.; Scorletti, E.; Byrne, C.D. Diagnosis and management of non-alcoholic fatty liver disease. *Postgrad. Med. J.* **2019**, *95*, 314–322. [CrossRef] [PubMed]
4. Buzzetti, E.; Pinzani, M.; Tsochatzis, E.A. The multiple-hit pathogenesis of non-alcoholic fatty liver disease (NAFLD). *Metabolism* **2016**, *65*, 1038–1048. [CrossRef] [PubMed]
5. Bashiardes, S.; Shapiro, H.; Rozin, S.; Shibolet, O.; Elinav, E. Non-alcoholic fatty liver and the gut microbiota. *Mol. Metab.* **2016**, *5*, 782–794. [CrossRef] [PubMed]
6. Jadhav, K.; Cohen, T.S. Can you trust your gut? Implicating a disrupted intestinal microbiome in the progression of NAFLD/NASH. *Front. Endocrinol.* **2020**, *11*, 592157. [CrossRef] [PubMed]
7. MacIejewska, D.; Łukomska, A.; Dec, K.; Skonieczna-Zydecka, K.; Gutowska, I.; Skórka-Majewicz, M.; Styburski, D.; Misiakiewicz-Has, K.; Pilutin, A.; Palma, J. Diet-induced rat model of gradual development of non-alcoholic fatty liver dis-ease (NAFLD) with lipopolysaccharides (LPS) secretion. *Diagnostics* **2019**, *9*, 205. [CrossRef]
8. Sander, M.E. Probiotics: Definition, sources, selection, and uses. *Clin. Infect. Dis.* **2008**, *46*, S58–S61. [CrossRef]
9. Lim, C.C.; Ferguson, L.R.; Tannock, G.W. Dietary fibres as "prebiotics": Implications for colorectal cancer. *Mol. Nutr. Food Res.* **2005**, *49*, 609–619. [CrossRef]
10. Mofidi, F.; Poustchi, H.; Yari, Z.; Nourinayyer, B.; Merat, S.; Sharafkhah, M.; Malekzadeh, R.; Hekmatdoost, A. Synbiotic supplementation in lean patients with non-alcoholic fatty liver disease: A pilot, randomised, double-blind, placebo-controlled, clinical trial. *Br. J. Nutr.* **2017**, *117*, 662–668. [CrossRef]
11. Loguercio, C.; De Simone, T.; Federico, A.; Terracciano, F.; Tuccillo, C.; Di Chicco, M.; Cartenì, M.; Del Vecchio Blanco, C. Gut-liver axis: A new point of attack to treat chronic liver damage? *Am. J. Gastroenterol.* **2002**, *97*, 2144–2146. [CrossRef] [PubMed]
12. Li, Z.; Yang, S.; Lin, H.; Huang, J.; Watkins, P.A.; Moser, A.B.; DeSimone, C.; Song, X.Y.; Diehl, A.M. Probiotics and antibodies to TNF inhibit inflammatory activity and improve non-alcoholic fatty liver disease. *Hepatology* **2003**, *37*, 343–350. [CrossRef] [PubMed]
13. Karaduta, O.; Glazko, G.; Dvanajscak, Z.; Arthur, J.; Mackintosh, S.; Orr, L.; Rahmatallah, Y.; Yeruva, L.; Tackett, A.; Zybailov, B. Resistant starch slows the progression of CKD in the 5/6 nephrectomy mouse model. *Physiol. Rep.* **2020**, *8*, e14610. [CrossRef] [PubMed]
14. Jiang, T.; Wu, H.; Yang, X.; Li, Y.; Zhang, Z.; Chen, F.; Zhao, L.; Zhang, C. *Lactobacillus mucosae* strain promoted by a high-fiber diet in genetic obese child alleviates lipid metabolism and modifies gut microbiota in apoe-/- mice on a western diet. *Microorganisms* **2020**, *8*, 1225. [CrossRef]
15. 15. Canani, R.B.; Sangwan, N.; Stefka, A.; Nocerino, R.; Paparo, L.; Aitoro, R.; Calignano, A.; Khan, A.A.; Gilbert, J.A.; Nagler, C.R. Lactobacillus rhamnosus GG-supplemented formula expands butyrate-producing bacterial strains in food allergic infants. *ISME J.* **2015**, *10*, 742–750. [CrossRef] [PubMed]

16. Szajewska, H.; Kołodziej, M. Systematic review with meta-analysis: *Lactobacillus rhamnosus* GG in the prevention of antibiotic-associated diarrhea in children and adults. *Aliment. Pharmacol. Ther.* **2015**, *42*, 1149–1157. [CrossRef]
17. Zaharuddin, L.; Mokhtar, N.M.; Nawawi, K.N.M.; Ali, R.A.R. A randomized double-blind placebo-controlled trial of probiotics in post-surgical colorectal cancer. *BMC Gastroenterol.* **2019**, *19*, 131. [CrossRef] [PubMed]
18. Ismail, I.S.; Bebakar, W.; Kamaruddin, N. Clinical Practice Guidelines on management of obesity 2004. Putrajaya: Ministry of Health Malaysia, Academy of Medicine of Malaysia, Malaysian Association for the Study of Obesity, Malaysian Endocrine and Metabolic Society. 2004. Available online: https://www.moh.gov.my/moh/resources/Penerbitan/CPG/Endocrine/5a.pdf (accessed on 5 September 2021).
19. Nurul-fadhilah, A.; Teo, P.S.; Foo, L.H. Validity and reproducibility of a food frequency questionnaire (FFQ) for dietary as-sessment in Malay adolescents in Malaysia. *Asia Pac. J. Clin. Nutr.* **2012**, *21*, 97–103.
20. Poynard, T.; Ratziu, V.; Naveau, S.; Thabut, D.; Charlotte, F.; Messous, D.; Capron, D.; Abella, A.; Massard, J.; Ngo, Y.; et al. The diagnostic value of biomarkers (SteatoTest) for the prediction of liver steatosis. *Comp. Hepatol.* **2005**, *4*, 10. [CrossRef]
21. Munteanu, M.; Tiniakos, D.; Anstee, Q.; Charlotte, F.; Marchesini, G.; Bugianesi, E.; Trauner, M.; Romero, G.M.; Oliveira, C.; Day, C. Diagnostic performance of FibroTest, SteatoTest and ActiTest in patients with NAFLD using the SAF score as histological reference. *Aliment. Pharmacol Ther.* **2016**, *44*, 877–889. [CrossRef]
22. Miele, L.; Valenza, V.; La Torre, G.; Montalto, M.; Cammarota, G.; Ricci, R.; Mascianà, R.; Forgione, A.; Gabrieli, M.L.; Perotti, G.; et al. Increased intestinal permeability and tight junction alterations in nonalcoholic fatty liver disease. *Hepatology* **2009**, *49*, 1877–1887. [CrossRef]
23. Chan, W.-K.; Mustapha, N.R.N.; Mahadeva, S. Controlled attenuation parameter for the detection and quantification of hepatic steatosis in nonalcoholic fatty liver disease. *J. Gastroenterol. Hepatol.* **2014**, *29*, 1470–1476. [CrossRef]
24. Krueger, K.P.; Felkey, B.G.; Berger, B.A. Improving adherence persistence: A review assessment of interventions description of steps toward a national adherence initiative. *J. Am. Pharm. Assoc.* **2003**, *43*, 668–679. [CrossRef]
25. Michail, S.; Lin, M.; Frey, M.R.; Fanter, R.; Paliy, O.; Hilbush, B.; Reo, N.V. Altered gut microbial energy and metabolism in children with non-alcoholic fatty liver disease. *FEMS Microbiol. Ecol.* **2014**, *91*, 1–9. [CrossRef] [PubMed]
26. Zhu, L.; Baker, S.S.; Gill, C.; Liu, W.; Alkhouri, R.; Baker, R.D.; Gill, S.R. Characterization of gut microbiomes in nonalcoholic steatohepatitis (NASH) patients: A connection between endogenous alcohol and NASH. *Hepatology* **2012**, *57*, 601–609. [CrossRef] [PubMed]
27. Mouzaki, M.; Comelli, E.M.; Arendt, B.M.; Bonengel, J.; Fung, S.K.; Fischer, S.; McGilvray, I.D.; Allard, J.P. Intestinal microbiota in patients with non-alcoholic fatty liver disease. *Hepatology* **2013**, *58*, 120–127. [CrossRef]
28. Wong, V.W.-S.; Wong, G.L.-H.; Chan, H.L.-Y.; Yeung, D.K.W.; Chan, R.; Chim, A.M.-L.; Chan, C.K.M.; Tse, Y.K.; Woo, J.; Chu, W.C.W. Bacterial endotoxin and non-alcoholic fatty liver disease in the general population: A prospective cohort study. *Aliment. Pharmacol. Ther.* **2015**, *42*, 731–740. [CrossRef]
29. Delzenne, N.M.; Knudsen, C.; Beaumont, M.; Rodriguez, J.; Neyrinck, A.; Bindels, L.B. Contribution of the gut microbiota to the regulation of host metabolism and energy balance: A focus on the gut–liver axis. *Proc. Nutr. Soc.* **2019**, *78*, 319–328. [CrossRef]
30. Eslamparast, T.; Poustchi, H.; Zamani, F.; Sharafkhah, M.; Malekzadeh, R.; Hekmatdoost, A. Synbiotic supplementation in nonalcoholic fatty liver disease: A randomized, double-blind, placebo-controlled pilot study. *Am. J. Clin. Nutr.* **2014**, *99*, 535–542. [CrossRef] [PubMed]
31. Ma, Y.Y.; Li, L.; Yu, C.H.; Shen, Z.; Chen, L.H.; Li, Y.M. Effects of probiotics on nonalcoholic fatty liver disease: A meta-analysis. *World J. Gastroenterol.* **2013**, *19*, 6911–6918. [CrossRef]
32. Duseja, A.; Acharya, S.K.; Mehta, M.; Chhabra, S.; Rana, S.; Das, A.; Dattagupta, S.; Dhiman, R.K.; Chawla, Y.K. High potency multistrain probiotic improves liver histology in non-alcoholic fatty liver disease (NAFLD): A randomised, double-blind, proof of concept study. *BMJ Open Gastroenterol.* **2019**, *6*, e000315. [CrossRef] [PubMed]
33. Scorletti, E.; Afolabi, P.R.; Miles, E.A.; Smith, D.E.; Almehmadi, A.; Alshathry, A.; Childs, C.E.; Del Fabbro, S.; Bilson, J.; Moyses, H.E. Synbiotics alter fecal microbiomes, but not liver fat or fibrosis, in a randomized trial of patients with non-alcoholic fatty liver disease. *Gastroenterology* **2020**, *158*, 1597–1610.e7. [CrossRef] [PubMed]
34. Jiang, W.; Wu, N.; Wang, X.; Chi, Y.; Zhang, Y.; Qiu, X.; Hu, Y.; Li, J.; Liu, Y. Dysbiosis gut microbiota associated with in-flammation and impaired mucosal immune function in intestine of humans with non-alcoholic fatty liver disease. *Sci. Rep.* **2015**, *5*, 8096. [CrossRef] [PubMed]
35. Zhao, C.; Lou, F.; Li, X.; Ma, J.; Zhu, Z.; Li, H.; Zhai, Y.; Chen, H.; Zhang, Q.; Liu, Z.; et al. Correlation of CD3+/CD4+, and serum CK-18 fragment levels with glucose and lipid metabolism in elderly type 2 diabetes patients with nonalcoholic fat-ty liver disease. *Am. J. Transl. Res.* **2021**, *13*, 2546–2554.
36. Ma, C.; Kesarwala, A.; Eggert, T.; Medina-Echeverz, J.; Kleiner, D.E.; Jin, P.; Stroncek, P.J.D.F.; Terabe, M.; Kapoor, V.; Elgindi, M.; et al. NAFLD causes selective CD4+ T lymphocyte loss and promotes hepatocarcinogenesis. *Nature* **2016**, *531*, 253–257. [CrossRef] [PubMed]
37. Antonucci, L.; Porcu, C.; Timperi, E.; Santini, S.J.; Iannucci, G.; Balsano, C. circulating neutrophils of nonalcoholic steatohepatitis patients show an activated phenotype and suppress T lymphocytes activity. *J. Immunol. Res.* **2020**, *2020*, 4570219. [CrossRef]
38. Her, Z.; Tan, J.H.L.; Lim, Y.-S.; Tan, S.Y.; Chan, X.Y.; Tan, W.W.S.; Liu, M.; Yong, K.S.M.; Lai, F.; Ceccarello, E.; et al. CD4+ T cells mediate the development of liver fibrosis in high fat diet-induced NAFLD in humanized mice. *Front. Immunol.* **2020**, *11*, 580968. [CrossRef]

39. Hu, Y.; Zhang, H.; Li, J.; Cong, X.; Chen, Y.; He, G.; Chi, Y.; Liu, Y. Gut-derived lymphocyte recruitment to liver and induce liver injury in non-alcoholic fatty liver disease mouse model. *J. Gastroenterol. Hepatol.* **2016**, *31*, 676–684. [CrossRef]
40. Bauer, H.C.; Zweimueller-Mayer, J.; Steinbacher, P.; Lametschwandtner, A. The dual role of zonula occludens (ZO) proteins. *J. Biomed. Biotechnol.* **2010**, *2010*, 402593. [CrossRef]
41. Feng, D.; Zou, J.; Su, D.; Mai, H.; Zhang, S.; Li, P.; Zheng, X. Curcumin prevents high-fat diet-induced hepatic steatosis in ApoE−/− mice by improving intestinal barrier function and reducing endotoxin and liver TLR4/NF-κB inflammation. *Nutr. Metabol.* **2019**, *16*, 79. [CrossRef]
42. Kim, W.-K.; Jang, Y.J.; Seo, B.; Han, D.H.; Park, S.; Ko, G. Administration of *Lactobacillus paracasei* strains improves immunomodulation and changes the composition of gut microbiota leading to improvement of colitis in mice. *J. Funct. Foods* **2018**, *52*, 565–575. [CrossRef]
43. Chong, C.W.; Ahmad, A.F.; Lim, Y.A.L.; Teh, C.S.J.; Yap, I.K.S.; Lee, S.C.; Chin, Y.T.; Loke, P.; Chua, K.H. Effect of ethnicity and socioeconomic variation to the gut microbiota composition among pre-adolescent in Malaysia. *Sci. Rep.* **2015**, *5*, srep13338. [CrossRef] [PubMed]
44. Neoh, H.-M.; Osman, M.A.; Ab Mutalib, N.S.; Chin, S.F.; Ang, M.Y.; Mazlan, L.; Ngiu, C.S.; Jamal, R. IDDF2018-ABS-0199 Gut microbiome profiling of malaysians: A snapshot. *BMJ* **2018**, *67*, A13. [CrossRef]
45. Lee, S.C.; Tang, M.S.; Lim, Y.A.L.; Choy, S.H.; Kurtz, Z.D.; Cox, L.M.; Gundra, U.M.; Cho, I.; Bonneau, R.; Blaser, M.J.; et al. Helminth colonization is associated with increased diversity of the gut microbiota. *PLoS Negl. Trop. Dis.* **2014**, *8*, e2880. [CrossRef] [PubMed]
46. Bjerg, A.T.; Kristensen, M.; Ritz, C.; Holst, J.J.; Rasmussen, C.; Leser, T.D.; Wellejus, A.; Astrup, A. *Lactobacillus paracasei* subsp paracasei L. *casei* W8 suppresses energy intake acutely. *Appetite* **2014**, *82*, 111–118. [CrossRef]
47. Nishida, C.; Martinez, N.F. FAO/WHO scientific update on carbohydrates in human nutrition: Introduction. *Eur. J. Clin. Nutr.* **2007**, *61*, S1–S4. [CrossRef]
48. Ministry of Health Malaysia. *Recommended Nutrient Intakes for Malaysia*; Ministry of Health Malaysia: Putrajaya, Malaysia, 2005.
49. Lee, Y.Y.; Muda, W.A.M.W. Dietary intakes and obesity of Malaysian adults. *Nutr. Res. Pr.* **2019**, *13*, 159–168. [CrossRef]
50. Ismail, S.; Shamsuddin, K.; Latiff, K.; Saad, H. Food consumption among overweight and obese working Malay women in urban settings. *Int. J. Community Med. Public Health* **2016**, *3*, 658–662. [CrossRef]
51. FAO. *The State of Food and Agriculture Leveraging Food Systems for Inclusive Rural Transformation*; FAO: Rome, Italy, 2017.

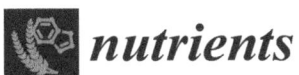

Article

# A High Protein Diet Is More Effective in Improving Insulin Resistance and Glycemic Variability Compared to a Mediterranean Diet—A Cross-Over Controlled Inpatient Dietary Study

Francesca Tettamanzi [1,†], Vincenzo Bagnardi [2,†], Panayiotis Louca [3], Ana Nogal [3], Gianna Serafina Monti [4], Sara P. Mambrini [5,6], Elisa Lucchetti [7], Sabrina Maestrini [7], Silvia Mazza [5], Ana Rodriguez-Mateos [8], Massimo Scacchi [5,9], Ana M. Valdes [10,‡], Cecilia Invitti [11,‡] and Cristina Menni [3,*,‡]

1. Department of Biomedical Sciences, Humanitas University, 20072 Pieve Emanuele, Italy; francesca.tettamanzi@st.hunimed.eu
2. Department of Statistics and Quantitative Methods, University of Milan-Bicocca, 20126 Milan, Italy; vincenzo.bagnardi@unimib.it
3. Department of Twin Research, King's College London, St Thomas' Hospital Campus, London SE1 7EH, UK; panayiotis.louca@kcl.ac.uk (P.L.); ana.nogal_macho@kcl.ac.uk (A.N.)
4. Department of Economics Management and Statistics, University of Milan-Bicocca, 20126 Milan, Italy; gianna.monti@unimib.it
5. Laboratory of Metabolic Research, Istituto Auxologico Italiano, IRCCS, S. Giuseppe Hospital, 28824 Piancavallo, Italy; s.mambrini@auxologico.it (S.P.M.); s.mazza@auxologico.it (S.M.); massimo.scacchi@unimi.it (M.S.)
6. International Center for the Assessment of Nutritional Status (ICANS), Department of Food, Environmental and Nutritional Sciences (DeFENS), University of Milan, 20100 Milan, Italy
7. Istituto Auxologico Italiano, IRCCS, S. Giuseppe Hospital, 28824 Piancavallo, Italy; e.lucchetti@auxologico.it (E.L.); s.maestrini@auxologico.it (S.M.)
8. Department of Nutritional Sciences, King's College London, Franklin Wilkins Building, London SE1 9NH, UK; ana.rodriguez-mateos@kcl.ac.uk
9. Department of Clinical Sciences and Community Health, University of Milan, 20122 Milan, Italy
10. Inflammation, Injury and Recovery Sciences, School of Medicine, University of Nottingham, Nottingham NG5 1PB, UK; ana.valdes@nottigham.ac.uk
11. Laboratory of Research in Preventive Medicine, IRCCS Istituto Auxologico Italiano, 20100 Milan, Italy; invitti@auxologico.it
* Correspondence: cristina.menni@kcl.ac.uk
† These two authors contributed equally to this paper.
‡ These three authors contributed equally to this paper.

**Abstract:** The optimal dietary pattern to improve metabolic function remains elusive. In a 21-day randomized controlled inpatient crossover feeding trial of 20 insulin-resistant obese women, we assessed the extent to which two isocaloric dietary interventions—Mediterranean (M) and high protein (HP)—improved metabolic parameters. Obese women were assigned to one of the following dietary sequences: M–HP or HP–M. Cardiometabolic parameters, body weight, glucose monitoring and gut microbiome composition were assessed. Sixteen women completed the study. Compared to the M diet, the HP diet was more effective in (i) reducing insulin resistance (insulin: Beta (95% CI) = $-6.98$ ($-12.30$, $-1.65$) µIU/mL, $p = 0.01$; HOMA-IR: $-1.78$ (95% CI: $-3.03$, $-0.52$), $p = 9 \times 10^{-3}$); and (ii) improving glycemic variability ($-3.13$ ($-4.60$, $-1.67$) mg/dL, $p = 4 \times 10^{-4}$), a risk factor for T2D development. We then identified a panel of 10 microbial genera predictive of the difference in glycemic variability between the two diets. These include the genera *Coprococcus* and *Lachnoclostridium*, previously associated with glucose homeostasis and insulin resistance. Our results suggest that morbidly obese women with insulin resistance can achieve better control of insulin resistance and glycemic variability on a high HP diet compared to an M diet.

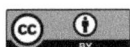

**Keywords:** high protein diet; Mediterranean diet; insulin resistance; glycemic variability; obesity; gut microbiome; dietary intervention

## 1. Introduction

An obesity pandemic is gripping the globe, with higher demand and availability for energy-dense foods, accompanied by increasingly sedentary lifestyles [1–3]. This is a major public health concern, as obesity often confers an increased risk of developing a wide range of complex and life-changing diseases, including cardiovascular and cerebrovascular disease, type II diabetes and cancers [4–7]. Therefore, the development and implementation of effective and affordable measures to combat obesity is of utmost importance. As well as encouraging increased physical activity, many efforts to reduce obesity and its associated disorders have focused on the impact of diet and nutrition [8]. In particular, the Mediterranean (M) diet, a diet characterized by high levels of polyphenols, mono- and polyunsaturated fatty acids (MUFAs and PUFAs), antioxidants, and fiber, as well as low levels of salt, sugar and saturated fatty acids [9], has been associated with improved health outcomes [9]. Greater adherence to the M diet has been associated with reduced risk of cardiovascular disease [9,10], which also supports weight loss [11]. A high-protein (HP) diet, comprising low carbohydrate, high fat and high protein intake, has also been suggested as a potential dietary intervention for obesity prevention [12] with HP diets corresponding to greater weight loss compared to similar isocaloric diets with standard protein content [13]. A HP diet has also been shown to lead to a greater weight loss compared to a high-carbohydrate diet, along with an improvement in insulin parameters, highlighting its power to lower the risk of type 2 diabetes and cardiovascular diseases [14,15]. Over the short term, a HP diet has been suggested to more effectively aid weight loss in contrast to a low-fat diet, and has been shown to change body composition in overweight or obese men [14]. The mechanisms supporting the HP diets' effects on weight loss efficacy is theorized to be related to increased satiety [16] and it has been suggested that this enhances an individual's metabolic rate [17]. Recent evidence suggests that the benefits of any dietary intervention are intrinsically linked to an individual's metabolic profile [18]. The exact role of the gut microbiome in nutrient metabolism is still unclear, but various studies have linked microbial diversity and specific bacteria to a propensity for obesity, as well as to the metabolism of dietary compounds found in the M diet, including omega-3 fatty acids and polyphenols [19,20]. Here, we aimed to explore the differential effects on metabolic parameters elicited by the M and HP diets. As these effects are reported to be exacerbated in obese individuals with impaired metabolic response, we conducted a 21-day randomized crossover controlled dietary trial in 20 insulin-resistant women with obesity.

## 2. Materials and Methods

A flowchart of the study design is presented in Figure 1.

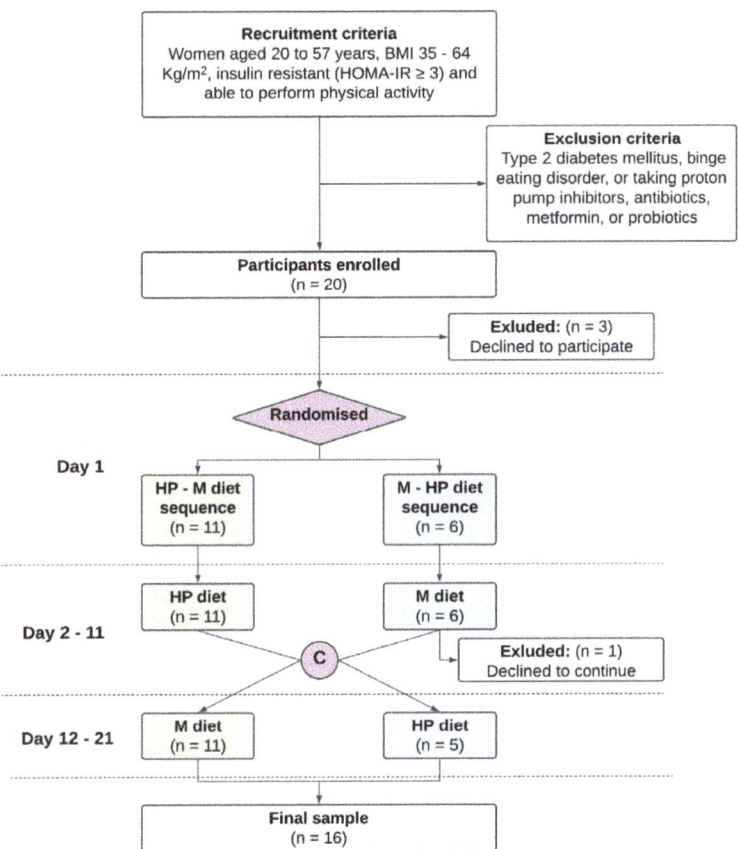

**Figure 1.** Study flowchart.

*2.1. Study Design and Participants*

This is an open-label, single-center randomized crossover controlled dietary trial in an inpatient setting. Participants were assigned to receive, in a 1:1 ratio, one of the two following dietary sequences: hypocaloric M diet followed by hypocaloric HP diet (sequence M–HP) or vice versa (sequence HP–M). Each period of intervention lasted 10 days with no washout before the switch from the first to the second diet. Participants were at San Giuseppe Hospital, Piancavallo of the IRCCS Istituto Auxologico Italiano, where they were hospitalized throughout the duration of the trial. Patients eligible for the study were women aged 20 to 57 years with BMI 35–64 kg/m$^2$, insulin resistant (HOMA-IR $\geq$ 3) and able to perform physical activity. Exclusion criteria included individuals suffering from type 2 diabetes mellitus (defined by the presence of occasional plasma glucose value of $\geq$200 mg/dL or a fasting plasma glucose of $\geq$126 mg/dl or an HbA1c $\geq$ 6.5% ($\geq$48 mmol/mol Hb)), binge eating disorder, taking proton pump inhibitors, antibiotics, metformin or probiotics. Moreover, women included in the study were not following any specific dietary patterns in the 6 months preceding study enrolment, and were characterized by prandial hyperphagia, excessive carbohydrates, lipid and sodium consumption, poor fiber intake and insufficient hydration.

The study protocol was approved by the Institutional Ethical Committee (2018_01_30_02) and all participants provided written informed consent before the trial.

## 2.2. Study Procedures

Eligible patients were randomly allocated into two groups on day 1: sequence M–HP or sequence HP–M. The M diet was composed of approximately 55% carbohydrates (whole wheat), 25% fat (PUFA from olive oil, almonds and pistachios) and 20% protein (fish, goat cheese and legumes). The HP diet was composed of approximately 40% carbohydrate, 30% fat and 30% protein. Both diets had the same caloric intake, which was 500 Kcal less than the individual daily caloric requirement, and a similar equally moderate glycemic load ranging between 11 and 19. Moreover, for both the M and HP diets, the energy derived from the consumption of simple carbohydrates (represented mainly by fruits and dairy products) was lower than 15% of the total energy. Animal and vegetable proteins were provided in both diets. In the M diet, protein consumption was in line with the relevant Food Guide Pyramid. Second courses included mainly white meat, bluefish, goat cheese and legumes. In the HP diet, proteins sources were mainly white meat, fish and eggs (Table S1).

On day 1, baseline measurements of clinical variables were obtained for each participant, including height, weight, waist and hip circumference, blood pressure, heart rate and body composition as measured by phase-sensitive, single-frequency bioimpedance analyzer (BIA 101, Akern, Pisa, Italy). Resting energy expenditure (REE) was assessed with indirect computerized calorimetry (Vmax 29, Sensor Medics, Yorba Linda, CA, USA), and the total energy expenditure (TEE) was estimated by multiplying the REE by Physical Activity Level (PAL), which was 1.2 for all, i.e., $TEE = REE \times 1.2$. 500 kcal were subtracted from the individual TEE to determine the diet hypocaloric target. Additionally, fasting blood samples for insulin and lipids (total, LDL and HDL cholesterol, triglycerides) measurement and stool samples were collected. Fecal samples were immediately frozen at −20 °C. For the gut microbiota analysis, samples were stored at −80 °C directly until processing following 3–5 h refrigeration.

Measurements and sample collections were repeated during clinical visits on days 6, 11, 16, and 21. Adherence to the diet was closely monitored by the nurses. Throughout the study, glucose levels were monitored by flash continuous glucose monitoring (FSL-FGM; Free-Style Libre™; Abbott, Witney, Oxfordshire, UK).

## 2.3. 16S rRNA Gut Microbiome

Microbial 16S rRNA gene was extracted from fecal samples and sequenced using the Illumina MiSeq platform at the Genetic Laboratory, Erasmus Medical Centre in Rotterdam, the Netherlands. The Microbiota pipeline 25 was used to filter and cluster reads into Operational Taxonomic Units (OTU) based on 97% similarity against the SILVA database v132 [20,21]. Microbial diversity indices were calculated using the platform QIIME 2 (v2018.11) as the average value after rarefying the OTU table to 13678 reads. Shannon and Simpson indices were calculated to describe the alpha diversity (i.e., microbial diversity within individual samples) [22,23]:

$Shannon\ Index = -\sum_{i=1}^{s}(p_i log_2 p_i)$, where $s$ is the number of OTUs and $p_i$ the proportion of the community represented by OTU $i$.

$Simpson\ Index = 1 - \sum p_i^2$, where $p_i$ is the proportion of the community represented by OTU $i$.

## 2.4. Study Outcomes

The primary study outcomes were insulin and HOMA-IR measured as the change from baseline concentration during each diet (i.e., the difference between insulin, HOMA-IR from day 11 to day 1 for the first diet in the sequence, and between day 21 and day 11 for the second diet in the sequence) and glycemic variability. Individual HOMA-IR was computed as $HOMA\text{-}IR = (fasting\ insulin \times fasting\ glucose)/405$ with glucose measured in mg/dl and insulin in μU/L.

Individual glycemic variability was measured for each diet as daily mean standard deviation (SD) of glucose concentration during continuous monitoring, that is, for each individual the mean standard deviation was calculated as $SD = 1/dx \sum SD_d$, where $SD_d$ is standard deviation of each day's glucose measurements in HP or M diet. For overall evaluation of CGM data, we also computed (i) the difference between diets in mean blood glucose concentration and (ii) the percentage of time of sensor glucose concentration within target range (within 70–180 mg/dL), in hypoglycemic (below 70 mg/dL) and hyperglycemic (above 180 mg/dl) conditions. All CGM metrics were calculated using the R package iglu [24]. Secondary study outcomes included change from baseline in weight waist to hip ratio, fat to lean mass ratio, lipids, blood pressure, heart rate and microbial diversity metrics.

*2.5. Statistical Analysis*

The analysis dataset included all participants who completed the dietary sequence and had measurement of the main study outcomes at least at the beginning and at the end of each intervention period (i.e., day 1, 11 and 21) (Figure 1). According to the intention-to-treat principle, patients were analyzed in the dietary sequence assigned. Baseline characteristics of the study population were described as mean values along with their standard deviations (SD). To adjust for treatment period and sequence, a linear mixed effect regression model was fitted, which included as fixed predictors treatment type (HP over M), treatment period (P1 over 2) and sequence (HP–M over M–HP). The effect of the type of diet on glycemic variability was evaluated by calculating the difference in SD of glucose concentration between HP and M diets, and applying linear mixed effect regression model as described above. Additional study outcomes, including clinical, microbial and other glucose-related variables, were similarly analyzed. Estimates of unadjusted and adjusted mean values along with their 95% Confidence Intervals (CI) were calculated for each outcome. Mean differences and CI were standardized to obtain comparable effect sizes for considered variables, and were represented in forest plots.

Exploratory sub-analyses were performed to evaluate the association of baseline microbial taxa with the difference between HP and M diet in individual glucose variability ($SD_{HP} - SD_M$, with SD as defined above), by using a Lasso regression model with zero sum constraint to account for the compositional nature of microbial data [25]. Relative abundances (RA) of OTU agglomerated to genus level were calculated, filtered if sparse in less than 80% of the samples, and log transformed before the analysis. For variable selection, 5-fold cross-validation was applied to tune the regularization term lambda. Associations were expressed as beta regression coefficients.

Statistical analyses were performed using the statistical software SAS 9.4 (SAS Institute, Cary, NC, USA) and R version 3.6.2. A *p*-value less than 0.05 was considered statistically significant.

## 3. Results

Between April and December 2018, 20 patients were enrolled in the study at the Piancavallo Hospital, Italy. Of them, three patients decided not to take part in the study before randomization, and one patient assigned to sequence M–HP discontinued the study after the first diet; 16 participants completed the dietary sequence assigned and represented the analysis set (Figure 1). As depicted in Figure 1, participants were enrolled in the study and randomly allocated on day 1 to one of two dietary sequences: the HP–M indicates high protein diet followed by Mediterranean diet, and the M–HP indicates the Mediterranean diet followed by high protein diet. Crossover (C) to the second diet occurred on day 12.

The characteristics of the participants at study entry are presented in Table 1. On average, women were slightly younger, had a lower BMI, fasting glucose, insulin and HOMA-IR in the HP–M group compared to the M–HP group. However, differences were not statistically significant.

Table 1. Clinical and biochemical characteristics of obese women at baseline.

| Phenotype | HP–M | M–HP |
|---|---|---|
| N | 11 | 5 |
| Sex, n (%) | 11 (100%) | 5 (100%) |
| Impaired Fasting Glucose, n (%) | 3 (27.3%) | 1 (20%) |
| Age, years | 36.18 (12.55) | 42.40 (15.32) |
| Weight, Kg | 118.94 (17.98) | 130.86 (38.84) |
| BMI, Kg/m$^2$ | 44.56 (4.61) | 50.40 (10.79) |
| Waist to hip ratio | 0.86 (0.07) | 0.91 (0.12) |
| Fat to lean mass ratio * | 1.06 (0.16) | 1.28 (0.25) |
| SBP, mmHg | 127.27 (11.04) | 129.00 (11.40) |
| DBP, mmHg | 79.09 (8.61) | 79.00 (8.94) |
| Heart Rate, bpm | 82.55 (11.71) | 78.40 (15.47) |
| Triglycerides, mmol/L | 1.27 (0.34) | 1.58 (0.56) |
| Total cholesterol, mmol/L | 4.12 (0.78) | 4.65 (0.86) |
| LDL cholesterol, mmol/L | 1.61 (0.43) | 1.94 (0.45) |
| HDL cholesterol *, mmol/L | 1.17 (0.11) | 1.00 (0.08) |
| Glucose, mg/dL | 93.27 (8.13) | 94.80 (6.53) |
| Insulin, µIU/mL | 19.98 (8.28) | 24.42 (11.52) |
| HOMA-IR | 4.60 (2.05) | 5.61 (2.43) |
| HbA1c, % | 5.55 (0.25) | 5.68 (0.44) |
| Shannon Index | 5.76 (0.42) | 5.58 (0.37) |
| Simpson Index | 0.96 (0.01) | 0.96 (0.01) |

Mean (SD). HP: high protein diet; M: Mediterranean diet; BMI: body mass index; SBP: systolic blood pressure, DBP: diastolic blood pressure, LDL: low-density lipoprotein; HDL: high-density lipoprotein; HOMA-IR: homeostasis model assessment of insulin resistance; HbA1c: hemoglobin A1c; * Statistically significant difference between two sequence groups according to *t*-test (fat to lean mass ratio: $p$ = 0.05; HDL cholesterol: $p$ = 0.01).

The HP and M diets led to a similar loss of body weight, with a mean change from baseline of −2.71 (95% CI: −3.59, −1.82) kg and −2.09 (95% CI: −2.71, −1.46) kg, respectively (Figure S1). Moreover, reduction in body weight was greater during the first period and diminished in the second part of the study, regardless of the dietary sequence (Figure S1). Changes in other biometric measures such as BMI, waist to hip ratio and fat to lean mass ratio lipids, blood pressure and in gut microbiome composition (Shannon and Simpson indexes) were also similar after the two diets (Figure S1).

### 3.1. Improvement in Insulin Resistance and HOMA-IR

In order to investigate whether an improvement in insulin resistance could be achieved after the two diets, we compared elicited effects on insulin and HOMA-IR variation using linear mixed effect regression models, with adjustment for treatment period and intervention sequence.

As shown in Figure 2A, the HP diet was more effective in reducing insulin levels, leading to a mean change from baseline of −3.50 (95% CI: −8.22, 1.21) µIU/mL, while higher levels were registered after the M diet with a value of 1.55 (95% CI: −1.08, 4.18) µIU/mL. Similarly, the HP diet led to a greater reduction in HOMA-IR with respect to the M diet with mean change from baseline of −0.996 (95% CI: −2.11, 0.12) and 0.32 (95% CI: −0.32, 0.96). Differences in the two outcomes between diets were statistically significant ($p$ = 0.01, $p$ = 9 × 10$^{-3}$). Reduction in glucose concentration was slightly greater in HP diet (−2.44 (95% CI: −6.02, 1.14) mg/dL) with respect to M diet (−1.88b (95% CI: −491, 1.16) mg/dL), however the difference between the two interventions was not statistically significant ($p$ = 0.55).

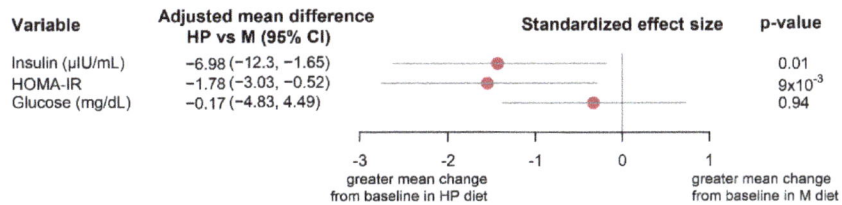
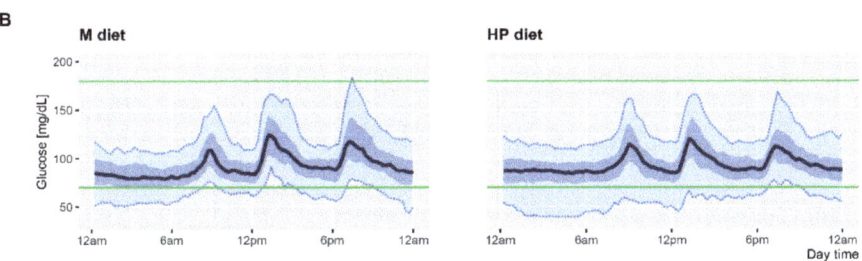
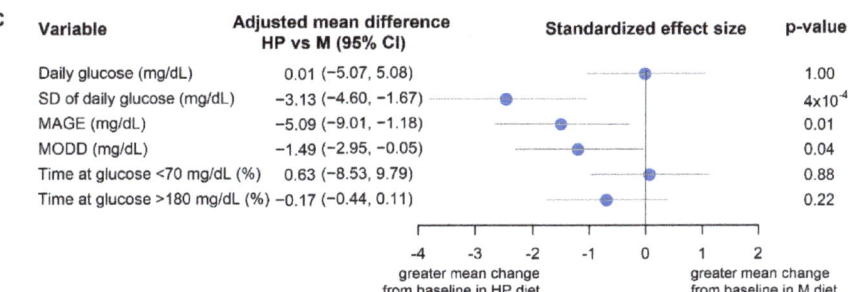

**Figure 2.** (**A**) Effect of diet on the mean change from baseline of insulin, HOMA-IR and glucose. Mean differences between high protein and Mediterranean diet in change from baseline of considered variables along with related standardized effect size and *p*-values are shown. Estimates were calculated using a mixed effect regression model, after adjusting for dietary sequence and treatment period. (**B**) Summary sensor glucose profiles for 24 h during (i) Mediterranean) and (ii) high protein diet. The solid blue line represents the median, the dark-blue shaded areas the interquartile range, while the light-blue shaded areas the 5th–95th percentile range. Green lines represent the normal range of glucose concentration, 70–180 mg/dL. (**C**) Effect of diet on glucose-related outcomes. Mean difference in glucose-related indices between high protein and Mediterranean diets along with related standardized effect size and *p*-values are shown. Estimates were calculated using a mixed effect regression model, after adjusting for dietary sequence and treatment period. HP: high protein diet, M: Mediterranean diet; HOMA-IR: homeostasis model assessment of insulin resistance CI: confidence interval; SD: standard deviation; MAGE: mean amplitude of glycemic excursions; MODD: mean of daily differences; ($N$ = 16).

### 3.2. Effect of HP and M Diets on Glycemic Variability

To further investigate the possible differential effect of the two dietary regimens on glucose variability, continuous monitoring data on glucose concentration were analyzed. Figure 2B shows 24 h sensor glucose profiles for each diet (individual patients' profiles are reported in Figure S2). Mean differences between interventions in SD of glucose concentration and other glucose summary outcomes, after adjustment for dietary sequence and treatment period, are presented in Figure 2C along with related standardized effect size and *p*-values (means of glucose outcomes in the two groups are reported in Table S2).

Patients while on HP diet improved glycemic variability, showing a significant reduction in SD of glucose concentration (Figure 2C), with a mean of 14.79 (95% CI: 12.83, 16.75) mg/dL compared to 17.92 (95% CI: 15.96, 19.89) mg/dL observed during M diet ($p = 4 \times 10^{-4}$ for the difference) as reported in Table S2. Consistent results were also observed for both mean amplitude of glycemic excursions (MAGE) and the mean of daily differences (MODD) [26], Figure 2C. CGM data supported the previous indication that glucose levels were not affected by the type of diet, as the mean daily concentration of blood glucose was comparable in the two groups (Figure 2C).

Patients spent similar sensor time at glucose levels below 70 mg/dL during HP diet and M diet. Time spent in hyperglycemic conditions at glucose levels above 180 mg/dL was limited and comparable for the two diets. No differences were detected between diets in indices of low and high blood glucose risks (data not shown).

### 3.3. Association of Baseline Gut Microbial Composition at Genus Level with Glucose Variability

We further investigated whether the patients' gut microbiome composition could be related to the difference in glycemic variability observed in the two diets. After aggregating OTUs into 148 genera, with the use of a zero sum constraint regression model, we identified a panel of 10 microbial genera (Figure 3).

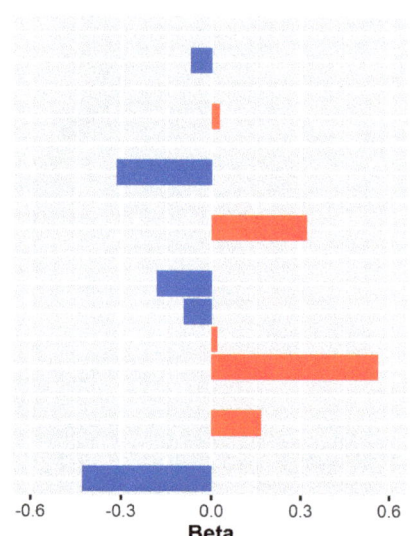

**Figure 3.** Microbial genera associated with the difference in glucose standard deviation between diets. Association between baseline microbial composition and mean difference of glucose index between HP and M diets was evaluated using zero sum constraint regression model. Results are reported in terms of beta regression coefficients, where the increase in the relative abundance of the selected genus at baseline is associated with an increased difference (red bars) or a decreased difference (blue bars) in SD of glucose concentration between HP and M diets. OTUs at baseline were first agglomerated to genus level. Relative abundances were filtered for sparsity and log transformed before the analysis. SD: standard deviation; (*N* = 16).

Of the 10 identified microbial taxa, 4 genera were annotated to the family of *Lachnospiraceae* (with opposite directions), one genus to *Ruminococcaceae* (with negative direction), *Peptostreptococcaceae* (with positive direction), *Acidaminococcaceae* (with negative direction), *Clostridiaceae* (with positive direction), *Coriobacteriaceae* (with negative direction) and *Desulfovibrionaceae* (with positive direction) families.

## 4. Discussion

In this 21-day randomized crossover controlled inpatient feeding trial, we found the HP diet to be more effective in reducing insulin resistance and in improving glycemic variability, compared to the M diet in 16 morbidly obese women with pre-diabetes. Moreover, we identified a panel of 10 microbial genera underlying the difference in glycemic variability between the two diets. These include microbes previously associated with the regulation of glucose homeostasis and insulin resistance [25,27].

We have also reported that both diets are equally effective in reducing weight (Figure S1) with participants consistently losing more weight during the first half of the study, compared to the second half. The lack of difference observed in weight, waist to hip ratio and BMI between the M and HP diets suggests that the weight loss observed may be primarily due to the isocaloric nature of the two diets, rather than specific dietary components. Moreover, participants may have benefitted overall from improved nutrition (increased fiber, PUFA, etc.) compared to their previous dietary habits; however, this information was unavailable for study.

Beneficial effects on health outcomes and metabolic functions have been reported in individuals adhering to both HP and M diets [28,29]. A HP diet has been linked with greater improvements in metabolic health and insulin sensitivity in individuals, mainly obese, overweight or insulin-resistant, when compared to alternate diets if weight loss is achieved [30,31]. Indeed, a greater decrease in HOMA-IR/insulin was reported in (i) obese women on an 8-week HP compared to those on a low protein diet [32]; (ii) in obese women on a 9-month isocaloric HP-low carbohydrate diet compared to those adhering to a standard isocaloric diet [33]; (iii) in overweight and obese women with the highest protein uptake in a 6-month calorie reduced diet with increasing protein content (20%, 27% or 35%) [33,34], among others. Our results are consistent and support, in this study group, a greater improvement in insulin resistance and related parameters after following an HP diet.

In our study, HP and M diets did not elicit an effect on the mean glucose level, both during clinical visits and when using 24 h glucose monitoring data. This observation is in line with several studies that reported no effect on the mean glucose levels after high protein intake in T2D patients [35]. However, we found a lower glycemic variability in morbidly obese women following the HP diet. Glucose variability is a risk factor for T2D development and complications [36], and increases in variability may be considered an additional parameter in the assessment of glucose homeostasis at the early stages of glucose dysregulation [37,38]. Reducing glucose variability by diet in non-diabetic patients may be clinically relevant because at early stages of dysglycemia; there is a decline of the cardiac autonomic function that is related to glucose variability and HOMA-IR [39]. In addition, glucose variability is associated with in-hospital complications and longer hospitalization following surgery [40–42] and with mortality in critically ill subjects [43].

Several studies have linked glycemic control to gut microbiome composition [36,44,45]. When we investigated the role of gut microbiome composition in our study, we found that *Eubacterium xylanophilum*, *Desulfovibrio*, *Terrisporobacter*, *Clostridium sensu stricto* and *Coprococcus* presented a positive effect on glycemic variability following the HP diet. This suggests that these genera might play an important role in improving host glucose homeostasis. For instance, *Coprococcus* might exert such a positive effect by its production of short-chain fatty acids (SCFA) [46]. Several studies have reported the benefits of SCFA in glucose homeostasis by regulating the blood glucose levels and glucose uptake [46]. Likewise, *Coprococcus* spp. might be able to metabolize the vitamins folate and biotin, which have been associated with lower plasma glucose levels [27]. On the other hand, a negative association was found with *Ruminococcus*, *Eggerthelia*, *Eubacterium hallii*, *Lachnoclostridium* and *Phascolarctobacterium*, suggesting that they might negatively impact glucose metabolism, and thus, type-2 diabetes. We have previously investigated the functional capabilities of *Lachnoclostridium spp.* and reported that *Lachnoclostridium* might metabolize both choline and phosphatidylethanolamine [27], which are precursors of trimethylamine

(TMA) and TMA-N-oxide (TMAO), thereby negatively regulating glucose metabolism and insulin sensitivity [37].

Our study benefits from a highly controlled nature; we can be confident in participants' adherence to the diet and its effect on the observed changes. However, we cannot infer any information about the long-term effects of either diet, as this study was only 21 days long, with participants spending 10 days on each diet. A study over a longer time course may reveal differences between the M and HP diets.

We also note some limitations. Our study has a small sample size with only 20 participants and a drop-out rate of 20%. Second, there was no wash-out period between the two diets. Third, study participants did not do an oral glucose tolerance test. Although the OGTT provides useful information about glucose tolerance, it does not infer on insulin sensitivity/resistance per se [47]. Moreover, under fasting conditions, basal insulin secretion determines a relatively constant level of insulinemia that will be lower or higher in accordance with insulin sensitivity such that hepatic glucose production matches whole body glucose disposal under fasting conditions. Thus, surrogate indexes based on fasting glucose and insulin concentrations, such as HOMA-IR, provide a greater reflection of primarily hepatic insulin sensitivity/resistance. Finally, only 11 participants provided stool samples for the entire duration of the study. Further work to investigate the role of gut microbiome composition and diversity in individual response to dietary intervention would be of considerable interest. Moreover, the study design lacked a wash-out period between dietary crossovers, as dietary effects may be brought about over a longer duration, some crossover effects of the previous diets may have been observed.

## 5. Conclusions

In conclusion, we find that the HP diet is more effective in reducing insulin resistance and in improving glycemic variability in morbidly obese women with pre-diabetes and have identified a panel of 10 microbes underlying the difference in glycemic variability between the two diets. Further investigation is required to elucidate the links between dietary interventions, the microbiome and clinical outcomes, as well as to identify measures that are predictive of individual response to intervention. Continued investigation of these interactions will contribute to the development of stratified intervention and prevention strategies for obesity and its associated health problems.

**Supplementary Materials:** The following are available online at https://www.mdpi.com/article/10.3390/nu13124380/s1, Table S1. Details on food provided with the two diets. Table S2. Difference between the two diets in glycemic exposure, control and variability. Figure S1. Effect of diet on the mean change from baseline of anthropometric measures, blood pressure, heart rate and lipids. Figure S2. Individual 24 h median sensor glucose profiles according to the type of diet.

**Author Contributions:** Conceptualization: A.M.V., C.I. and C.M. Project administration/recruitment: S.P.M., S.M. (Sabrina Maestrini), S.M. (Silvia Mazza), E.L. and M.S. Formal analysis: F.T. and V.B. Study coordination/supervision: M.S., C.I. and C.M. Resources: G.S.M. and A.R.-M. Writing—original draft preparation: F.T., V.B., P.L., A.N., A.M.V. and C.M.; writing—review and editing: all. All authors have read and agreed to the published version of the manuscript.

**Funding:** This work is funded by the NIHR Nottingham BRC. C.M., A.N. and P.L. are funded by the Chronic Disease Research Foundation. AMV is supported by the National Institute for Health Research Nottingham Biomedical Research Centre.

**Institutional Review Board Statement:** The study was conducted according to the guidelines of the Declaration of Helsinki, and approved by the Institutional Review Board of Instituto Auxologico Italiano.

**Informed Consent Statement:** Informed consent was obtained from all subjects involved in the study.

**Data Availability Statement:** Data for this study is deposited on Mendeley (Mendeley Data, V1, doi:10.17632/nsnm9tjrnt.1).

**Acknowledgments:** We thank all the participants for contributing and supporting our research.

**Conflicts of Interest:** AMV is a consultant for Zoe Global Ltd. (London, UK). All other authors declare no competing financial interests.

## References

1. Kim, R.; Lee, D.H.; Subramanian, S.V. Understanding the Obesity Epidemic. *BMJ* **2019**, *366*, l4409. [CrossRef] [PubMed]
2. D'Innocenzo, S.; Biagi, C.; Lanari, M. Obesity and the Mediterranean Diet: A Review of Evidence of the Role and Sustainability of the Mediterranean Diet. *Nutrients* **2019**, *11*, 1306. [CrossRef]
3. Seidell, J.C.; Halberstadt, J. The Global Burden of Obesity and the Challenges of Prevention. *Ann. Nutr. Metab.* **2015**, *66*, 7–12. [CrossRef] [PubMed]
4. Guh, D.P.; Zhang, W.; Bansback, N.; Amarsi, Z.; Birmingham, C.L.; Anis, A.H. The Incidence of Co-Morbidities Related to Obesity and Overweight: A Systematic Review and Meta-Analysis. *BMC Public Health* **2009**, *9*, 88. [CrossRef] [PubMed]
5. Poirier, P.; Giles, T.D.; Bray, G.A.; Hong, Y.; Stern, J.S.; Xavier Pi-Sunyer, F.; Eckel, R.H. Obesity and Cardiovascular Disease: Pathophysiology, Evaluation, and Effect of Weight Loss. *Circulation* **2006**, *113*, 898–918. [CrossRef]
6. Drozdz, D.; Alvarez-Pitti, J.; Wójcik, M.; Borghi, C.; Gabbianelli, R.; Mazur, A.; Herceg-Čavrak, V.; Lopez-Valcarcel, B.G.; Brzeziński, M.; Lurbe, E.; et al. Obesity and Cardiometabolic Risk Factors: From Childhood to Adulthood. *Nutrients* **2021**, *13*, 4176. [CrossRef]
7. Pergola, G.D.; De Pergola, G.; Silvestris, F. Obesity as a Major Risk Factor for Cancer. *J. Obes.* **2013**, *2013*, 291546. [CrossRef]
8. Ba, S.; Swinburn, B.A.; Caterson, I.; Seidell, J.C.; James, W.P.T. Diet, Nutrition and the Prevention of Excess Weight Gain and Obesity. *Public Health Nutr.* **2004**, *7*, 123–146. [CrossRef]
9. Widmer, R.J.; Jay Widmer, R.; Flammer, A.J.; Lerman, L.O.; Lerman, A. The Mediterranean Diet, Its Components, and Cardiovascular Disease. *Am. J. Med.* **2015**, *128*, 229–238. [CrossRef]
10. Martinez-Lacoba, R.; Pardo-Garcia, I.; Amo-Saus, E.; Escribano-Sotos, F. Mediterranean Diet and Health Outcomes: A Systematic Meta-Review. *Eur. J. Public Health* **2018**, *28*, 955–961. [CrossRef]
11. Shai, I.; Schwarzfuchs, D.; Henkin, Y.; Shahar, D.R.; Witkow, S.; Greenberg, I.; Golan, R.; Fraser, D.; Bolotin, A.; Vardi, H.; et al. Weight Loss with a Low-Carbohydrate, Mediterranean, or Low-Fat Diet. *N. Engl. J. Med.* **2008**, *359*, 229–241. [CrossRef]
12. Astrup, A.; Raben, A.; Geiker, N. The Role of Higher Protein Diets in Weight Control and Obesity-Related Comorbidities. *Int. J. Obes.* **2015**, *39*, 721–726. [CrossRef]
13. Campos-Nonato, I.; Hernandez, L.; Barquera, S. Effect of a High-Protein Diet versus Standard-Protein Diet on Weight Loss and Biomarkers of Metabolic Syndrome: A Randomized Clinical Trial. *Obes. Facts* **2017**, *10*, 238–251. [CrossRef]
14. McAuley, K.A.; Hopkins, C.M.; Smith, K.J.; McLay, R.T.; Williams, S.M.; Taylor, R.W.; Mann, J.I. Comparison of High-Fat and High-Protein Diets with a High-Carbohydrate Diet in Insulin-Resistant Obese Women. *Diabetologia* **2005**, *48*, 8–16. [CrossRef]
15. Kitabchi, A.E.; McDaniel, K.A.; Wan, J.Y.; Tylavsky, F.A.; Jacovino, C.A.; Sands, C.W.; Nyenwe, E.A.; Stentz, F.B. Effects of High-Protein Versus High-Carbohydrate Diets on Markers of -Cell Function, Oxidative Stress, Lipid Peroxidation, Proinflammatory Cytokines, and Adipokines in Obese, Premenopausal Women Without Diabetes: A Randomized Controlled Trial. *Diabetes Care* **2013**, *36*, 1919–1925. [CrossRef]
16. Moon, J.; Koh, G. Clinical Evidence and Mechanisms of High-Protein Diet-Induced Weight Loss. *J. Obes. Metab. Syndr.* **2020**, *29*, 166–173. [CrossRef]
17. Yamaoka, I.; Hagi, M.; Doi, M. Circadian Changes in Core Body Temperature, Metabolic Rate and Locomotor Activity in Rats on a High-Protein, Carbohydrate-Free Diet. *J. Nutr. Sci. Vitaminol.* **2009**, *55*, 511–517. [CrossRef]
18. Manach, C.; Milenkovic, D.; Van de Wiele, T.; Rodriguez-Mateos, A.; de Roos, B.; Garcia-Conesa, M.T.; Landberg, R.; Gibney, E.R.; Heinonen, M.; Tomás-Barberán, F.; et al. Addressing the Inter-Individual Variation in Response to Consumption of Plant Food Bioactives: Towards a Better Understanding of Their Role in Healthy Aging and Cardiometabolic Risk Reduction. *Mol. Nutr. Food Res.* **2017**, *61*, 1600557. [CrossRef]
19. Menni, C.; Zierer, J.; Pallister, T.; Jackson, M.A.; Long, T.; Mohney, R.P.; Steves, C.J.; Spector, T.D.; Valdes, A.M. Omega-3 Fatty Acids Correlate with Gut Microbiome Diversity and Production of N-Carbamylglutamate in Middle Aged and Elderly Women. *Sci. Rep.* **2017**, *7*, 11079. [CrossRef]
20. Mompeo, O.; Spector, T.D.; Matey Hernandez, M.; Le Roy, C.; Istas, G.; Le Sayec, M.; Mangino, M.; Jennings, A.; Rodriguez-Mateos, A.; Valdes, A.M.; et al. Consumption of Stilbenes and Flavonoids Is Linked to Reduced Risk of Obesity Independently of Fiber Intake. *Nutrients* **2020**, *12*, 1871. [CrossRef]
21. Boers, S.A.; Hiltemann, S.D.; Stubbs, A.P.; Jansen, R.; Hays, J.P. Development and Evaluation of a Culture-Free Microbiota Profiling Platform (MYcrobiota) for Clinical Diagnostics. *Eur. J. Clin. Microbiol. Infect. Dis.* **2018**, *37*, 1081–1089. [CrossRef]
22. Shannon, C.E.; Weaver, W. *The Mathematical Theory of Communication*; University of Illinois Press: Champaign, IL, USA, 1998; ISBN 9780252098031.
23. Hurlbert, S.H. The Nonconcept of Species Diversity: A Critique and Alternative Parameters. *Ecology* **1971**, *52*, 577–586. [CrossRef]
24. Broll, S.; Urbanek, J.; Buchanan, D.; Chun, E.; Muschelli, J.; Punjabi, N.; Gaynanova, I. Interpreting Blood GLUcose Data with R Package Iglu. *PLoS ONE* **2021**, *16*, e0248360. [CrossRef]
25. Lin, W.; Shi, P.; Feng, R.; Li, H. Variable Selection in Regression with Compositional Covariates. *Biometrika* **2014**, *101*, 785–797. [CrossRef]
26. Service, F.J.; Nelson, R.L. Characteristics of Glycemic Stability. *Diabetes Care* **1980**, *3*, 58–62. [CrossRef]

27. Nogal, A.; Louca, P.; Zhang, X.; Wells, P.M.; Steves, C.J.; Spector, T.D.; Falchi, M.; Valdes, A.M.; Menni, C. Circulating Levels of the Short-Chain Fatty Acid Acetate Mediate the Effect of the Gut Microbiome on Visceral Fat. *Front. Microbiol.* **2021**, *12*, 711359. [CrossRef]
28. Mirabelli, M.; Chiefari, E.; Arcidiacono, B.; Corigliano, D.M.; Brunetti, F.S.; Maggisano, V.; Russo, D.; Foti, D.P.; Brunetti, A. Mediterranean Diet Nutrients to Turn the Tide against Insulin Resistance and Related Diseases. *Nutrients* **2020**, *12*, 1066. [CrossRef]
29. Feidantsis, K.; Methenitis, S.; Ketselidi, K.; Vagianou, K.; Skepastianos, P.; Hatzitolios, A.; Mourouglakis, A.; Kaprara, A.; Hassapidou, M.; Nomikos, T.; et al. Comparison of Short-Term Hypocaloric High-Protein Diets with a Hypocaloric Mediterranean Diet: Effect on Body Composition and Health-Related Blood Markers in Overweight and Sedentary Young Participants. *Nutrition* **2021**, *91–92*, 111365. [CrossRef] [PubMed]
30. Tricò, D.; Moriconi, D.; Berta, R.; Baldi, S.; Quinones-Galvan, A.; Guiducci, L.; Taddei, S.; Mari, A.; Nannipieri, M. Effects of Low-Carbohydrate versus Mediterranean Diets on Weight Loss, Glucose Metabolism, Insulin Kinetics and β-Cell Function in Morbidly Obese Individuals. *Nutrients* **2021**, *13*, 1345. [CrossRef]
31. Rietman, A.; Schwarz, J.; Tomé, D.; Kok, F.J.; Mensink, M. High Dietary Protein Intake, Reducing or Eliciting Insulin Resistance? *Eur. J. Clin. Nutr.* **2014**, *68*, 973–979. [CrossRef]
32. Yılmaz, S.K.; Eskici, G.; Mertoğlu, C.; Ayaz, A. Effect of Different Protein Diets on Weight Loss, Inflammatory Markers, and Cardiometabolic Risk Factors in Obese Women. *J. Res. Med. Sci.* **2021**, *26*, 28. [PubMed]
33. Luis, D.A.; de Luis, D.A.; Izaola, O.; Aller, R.; de la Fuente, B.; Bachiller, R.; Romero, E. Effects of a High-Protein/low Carbohydrate versus a Standard Hypocaloric Diet on Adipocytokine Levels and Insulin Resistance in Obese Patients along 9 months. *J. Diabetes Its Complicat.* **2015**, *29*, 950–954. [CrossRef] [PubMed]
34. Mateo-Gallego, R.; Marco-Benedí, V.; Perez-Calahorra, S.; Bea, A.M.; Baila-Rueda, L.; Lamiquiz-Moneo, I.; de Castro-Orós, I.; Cenarro, A.; Civeira, F. Energy-Restricted, High-Protein Diets More Effectively Impact Cardiometabolic Profile in Overweight and Obese Women than Lower-Protein Diets. *Clin. Nutr.* **2017**, *36*, 371–379. [CrossRef] [PubMed]
35. Yu, Z.; Nan, F.; Wang, L.Y.; Jiang, H.; Chen, W.; Jiang, Y. Effects of High-Protein Diet on Glycemic Control, Insulin Resistance and Blood Pressure in Type 2 Diabetes: A Systematic Review and Meta-Analysis of Randomized Controlled Trials. *Clin. Nutr.* **2020**, *39*, 1724–1734. [CrossRef]
36. Stolar, M. Glycemic Control and Complications in Type 2 Diabetes Mellitus. *Am. J. Med.* **2010**, *123*, S3–S11. [CrossRef]
37. Subramaniam, S.; Fletcher, C. Trimethylamine N-Oxide: Breathe New Life. *Br. J. Pharmacol.* **2018**, *175*, 1344–1353. [CrossRef]
38. Chakarova, N.; Dimova, R.; Grozeva, G.; Tankova, T. Assessment of Glucose Variability in Subjects with Prediabetes. *Diabetes Res. Clin. Pract.* **2019**, *151*, 56–64. [CrossRef]
39. Dimova, R.; Chakarova, N.; Grozeva, G.; Tankova, T. Evaluation of the Relationship between Cardiac Autonomic Function and Glucose Variability and HOMA-IR in Prediabetes. *Diabetes Vasc. Dis. Res.* **2020**, *17*, 147916412095861. [CrossRef]
40. Akirov, A.; Diker-Cohen, T.; Masri-Iraqi, H.; Shimon, I. High Glucose Variability Increases Mortality Risk in Hospitalized Patients. *J. Clin. Endocrinol. Metab.* **2017**, *102*, 2230–2241. [CrossRef]
41. Shohat, N.; Foltz, C.; Restrepo, C.; Goswami, K.; Tan, T.; Parvizi, J. Increased Postoperative Glucose Variability Is Associated with Adverse Outcomes Following Orthopaedic Surgery. *Bone Jt. J.* **2018**, *100-B*, 1125–1132. [CrossRef]
42. Li, X.; Zhou, X.; Wei, J.; Mo, H.; Lou, H.; Gong, N.; Zhang, M. Effects of Glucose Variability on Short-Term Outcomes in Non-Diabetic Patients After Coronary Artery Bypass Grafting: A Retrospective Observational Study. *Heart Lung Circ.* **2019**, *28*, 1580–1586. [CrossRef]
43. Siegelaar, S.E.; Holleman, F.; Hoekstra, J.B.L.; DeVries, J.H. Glucose Variability; Does It Matter? *Endocr. Rev.* **2010**, *31*, 171–182. [CrossRef]
44. Zeevi, D.; Korem, T.; Zmora, N.; Israeli, D.; Rothschild, D.; Weinberger, A.; Ben-Yacov, O.; Lador, D.; Avnit-Sagi, T.; Lotan-Pompan, M.; et al. Personalized Nutrition by Prediction of Glycemic Responses. *Cell* **2015**, *163*, 1079–1094. [CrossRef]
45. Berry, S.E.; Valdes, A.M.; Drew, D.A.; Asnicar, F.; Mazidi, M.; Wolf, J.; Capdevila, J.; Hadjigeorgiou, G.; Davies, R.; Al Khatib, H.; et al. Human Postprandial Responses to Food and Potential for Precision Nutrition. *Nat. Med.* **2020**, *26*, 964–973. [CrossRef]
46. Nogal, A.; Valdes, A.M.; Menni, C. The Role of Short-Chain Fatty Acids in the Interplay between Gut Microbiota and Diet in Cardio-Metabolic Health. *Gut Microbes* **2021**, *13*, 1897212. [CrossRef]
47. Souto, D.L.; Dantas, J.R.; Oliveira, M.M.D.S.; Rosado, E.L.; Luiz, R.R.; Zajdenverg, L.; Rodacki, M. Does Sucrose Affect the Glucose Variability in Patients with Type 1 Diabetes? A Pilot Crossover Clinical Study. *Nutrition* **2018**, *55–56*, 179–184. [CrossRef]

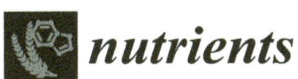

Article

# The Relationship between Macronutrient Distribution and Type 2 Diabetes in Asian Indians

Amisha Pandya *, Mira Mehta and Kavitha Sankavaram

Department of Nutrition and Food Science, University of Maryland, College Park, MD 20742, USA; mmehta@umd.edu (M.M.); kavitha@umd.edu (K.S.)
* Correspondence: apdiabetesstudy@verizon.net; Tel.: +1-240-676-6594

**Abstract:** Asian Indians (AIs) are at increased risk for type 2 diabetes mellitus than other ethnic groups. AIs also have lower body mass index (BMI) values than other populations, so can benefit from strategies other than weight reduction. Macronutrient distributions are associated with improved glycemic control; however, no specific distribution is generally recommended. This study looks at whether a macronutrient distribution of 50:30:20 (percent of total calories from carbohydrates, fats, and protein) is related to diabetes status in AIs. Diet and Hemoglobin A1c (HbA1c) were assessed from convenience sample of AI adults in Maryland. A ratio of actual to needed calories using the 50:30:20 macronutrient distribution was then tested against diabetes status to identify associations. All groups except non-diabetic females, were in negative energy balance. The non-diabetic group consumed larger actual to needed ratios of protein than pre-diabetics and diabetics. However, all groups consumed protein at the lower end of the Acceptable Macronutrient Distribution Range (AMDR), and the quality of all macronutrients consumed was low. Therefore, weight loss may not be the recommendation for diabetes management for AIs. Increasing protein and insoluble fiber consumption, could play a critical role.

**Keywords:** macronutrient distribution; type 2 diabetes mellitus management; type 2 diabetes in Asian Indians immigrants to the US

**Citation:** Pandya, A.; Mehta, M.; Sankavaram, K. The Relationship between Macronutrient Distribution and Type 2 Diabetes in Asian Indians. *Nutrients* **2021**, *13*, 4406. https://doi.org/10.3390/nu13124406

Academic Editors: Silvia V. Conde and Fatima O. Martins

Received: 12 November 2021
Accepted: 7 December 2021
Published: 9 December 2021

**Publisher's Note:** MDPI stays neutral with regard to jurisdictional claims in published maps and institutional affiliations.

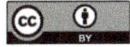

**Copyright:** © 2021 by the authors. Licensee MDPI, Basel, Switzerland. This article is an open access article distributed under the terms and conditions of the Creative Commons Attribution (CC BY) license (https://creativecommons.org/licenses/by/4.0/).

## 1. Introduction

Asian Indians (AIs) in India as well as those who have emigrated to the United States and other western nations are seeing an increase in incidence and prevalence of type 2 diabetes mellitus (T2DM) [1]. Prevalence of T2DM among AIs is estimated at 9.3% across India [2], and 18% in the US [3]. In one Indian State, Gujarat, estimates are 7–14% [4]. Rates of undiagnosed T2DM in AIs in India as well as in other countries is estimated to be approximately 50% [5].

There are complex and poorly understood reasons for the increasing incidence and prevalence of T2DM in AIs, including pathophysiological and sociocultural characteristics specific to this population. AIs have unique physical attributes and cultural attitudes that increase their risk for T2DM compared to other ethnic groups [6]. For example, two commonly cited factors for insulin resistance (IR), a precursor to the development of T2DM, are obesity, as measured by body mass index (BMI), and adverse fat distribution, neither of which seem to be associated with high basal insulin levels in this population [7]. AIs have younger onset for T2DM, and lower BMI values as compared with other populations [1,8–11]. The age of onset for T2DM in AIs is estimated to occur 10 years earlier than in Europeans, and AIs require lower BMI cut-offs for effective identification of T2DM risk [5]. Additionally, AIs may be predisposed to IR and T2DM because AI children are born smaller, have more fat, and less lean muscle [6]. Reduced lean muscle mass at birth is significant because lean muscle mass contains more mitochondria than fat tissue and so is more metabolically efficient. However, because the secretion of insulin is triggered by adipose tissue upon consumption of food, individuals with higher adipose to lean muscle mass ratios may have increased blood insulin levels, which can trigger a negative feedback response resulting in insulin receptor dysfunction leading to IR and T2DM.

The Asian Indian diet is also high in carbohydrates, and with urbanization and migration, there has been a growing tendency towards processed, refined and higher fat convenience foods, coupled with decreases in physical activity seen both in AIs living in India and abroad [12,13].

The purpose of this study is two-fold: (1) to describe the dietary intake of Asian Indian adults with and without T2DM, and (2) to determine whether there is an association between diabetes status and diet indicative of T2DM. Dietary intake was examined as both dietary quantity as well as dietary quality. Dietary quantity was measured by macronutrients (carbohydrates, fat, and protein) as a proportion of total kilocalories. Dietary quality was indicated by consumption of soluble and insoluble fiber, cholesterol, saturated fat, trans fat, and sugar; both were assessed relative to diabetes status.

## 2. Materials and Methods

### 2.1. Study Population

A convenience sample of 59 AI adults from Mangal Mandir, a Hindu temple in the Baltimore/Washington Metropolitan Area, was taken over a period of three months. Subjects included AI adults $\geq$ 18 years of age, literate in English, and residents of the US for >5 years. Participants' demographic information such as age, gender, education, income and number of years in US were collected.

### 2.2. Data Collection

Diabetes status was assessed by hemoglobin A1c readings obtained via physician ordered lab results during a health fair, run by community physicians, and held at the Mangal Mandir temple; an event used to initiate the study. For study participants with no physician's diagnosis of diabetes or with pre-diabetes, physician ordered labs for fasting blood glucose and hemoglobin A1c were not warranted and therefore were not available. Glucose and HbA1c point of care (POC) monitors were used for those that did not have fasting blood glucose and HbA1c readings from their physicians to confirm diabetes status. Cut-offs used for no-diabetes, pre-diabetes and diabetes are those widely accepted by the American Diabetes Association (ADA), the World Health Organization (WHO), and the International Diabetes Federation (IDF); >5.7% = no diabetes, $\geq$5.7% but <6.5% = pre-diabetes, and $\geq$6.5% = diabetes. Hemoglobin A1c level was chosen as the exclusive diagnostic variable because it was the most reliable measure of diabetes status. The collection of fasting blood glucose after 8 h of fasting was found not to be feasible and could not always be obtained from participant physician ordered lab results (about 13% of participants were missing this data point). Therefore, fasting blood glucose was dropped as a diagnostic variable. The accuracy of Bayer's A1cNow+ monitor was confirmed for non-clinical diagnoses of diabetes with up to 98% agreement, or non-significant difference, between the device and laboratory results [14–18]. Participants also provided self-report of their diabetes status which was compared to their HbA1c to determine the rate of undiagnosed diabetes in this population.

All participants completed a 163-item food frequency questionnaire (FFQ) validated with AIs that gave a one-year retrospective to their dietary intake [19,20]. Diet quantity was measured by the proportion of total kilocalories consumed daily in the form of the three energy producing macronutrients, carbohydrates, fats, and proteins contributing to metabolic efficiency and examined by diabetes status. Diet quality was assessed by the consumption of harmful fats such as saturated and trans-fat, dietary cholesterol, and fiber content of carbohydrates as seen in consumption of insoluble and soluble fiber. Basal metabolic rate (BMR) calculations were performed using five different methods, all varied slightly but they each generally followed the same trend by diabetes status.

The initial selection of BMR equations was based on methods used in various studies. There was consideration given to equations applied to Asian Indians in India, however, their use over other methods was not validated in the literature [21–23]. There are four equations commonly cited in the literature. They are the Owen, Mifflin-St. Jeor, Harris Benedict, and the WHO/FAO/UNU; there is varying agreement as to which method is the most reliable [24–27]. The BMR provided by the Tanita Scale (BC-558 Ironman Segmental Body Composition Monitor) used to capture bioelectrical impedance measures was added to previously mentioned four methods. Each method has its predictive variability, and none can be validated as the most accurate predictor in Asian Indian populations. Thus, all were considered in the analysis and correlational analysis confirmed that all five methods were significantly correlated with one another ($p < 0.0001$). For simplicity, the Owen method was selected for the remainder of the analyses. BMR establishes the minimum caloric intake needed to meet energy requirement assuming no physical activity. Energy requirements for each participant were calculated (BMR + kilocalories burned through physical activity).

*2.3. Macronutrient Distribution*

Although the United States Institute of Medicine's (IOM's) Acceptable Macronutrient Distribution Ranges (AMDR) offers recommended ranges of macronutrient intake, no specific recommendations exist to achieve optimal metabolic efficiency, however, there is some evidence that suggests that a macronutrient distribution of 50:30:20 (percent of total calories from carbohydrates, fats, and protein) can be metabolically favorable [28–31]. To establish a reference value for macronutrient distribution, total caloric energy requirement as determined from BMR + kilocalories burned through physical activity, was multiplied by a standard recommended proportion of total kilocalories for each macronutrient (50 percent of total kilocalories from carbohydrates, 30 percent of total kilocalories from fat, and 20 percent of total kilocalories from protein) to obtain the daily required grams of each macronutrient. A ratio of actual to needed kilocalories from each macronutrient was then calculated by dividing daily intake of macronutrients (carbohydrate, fat, and protein) by the daily required grams of each macronutrient. These ratios of actual to needed carbohydrates, fats and proteins were then tested against diabetes status to identify associations.

*2.4. Statistical Analysis*

Descriptive statistics such as mean, standard deviations and correlational analyses were used to describe the data and establish covariance for any variables. Univariate analyses of variance, including *t*-tests, ANOVAs, and linear and logistic regression models were used to determine the association of diet across diabetes status groups. Multiple linear logistic regression was used to determine the relationship between diet and diabetes status. Those participating as married couples, warranted the data being examined to determine any effect this may have had on variable confounding. A correlational analysis was performed between males and females of participant couples.

## 3. Results
*3.1. Participant Demographics*

Fifty-nine individuals initially expressed interest in participating in the study, and 39 participants completed the study (power = 0.76). Study participants were about equally divided by gender (49% male and 51% female) with an average age of 65.2 years (67.4 years for males and 63.0 years for females). About 72% of participants were married. Participants were predominantly Gujarati immigrants (95%) who had lived an average of 37 years in the United States (39 years for males and 35 years for females). Ninety-seven percent of all participants were born in India or Africa, and 3% were born in the United States. Almost two thirds (61.5%) of participants had earned a bachelor's degree or less and 38.5% had earned post graduate or professional degrees. Participants were almost equally split in terms of household income, with 56.4% earning less than or equal to USD 100,000 annually and 43.6% earning more than USD 100,000 annually. Almost three quarters of participants were vegetarian (58% of males and 90% of females, $p < 0.0310$). About 90% of participants, both male and female, consumed alcohol occasionally (1–2 times/month) or never, and most participants did not have a history of smoking (92% overall, 100% for females, and 84% for males). About 53% of males and 70% of females reported primarily being responsible for grocery shopping in their households, whereas most females were predominantly responsible for cooking (0% of males, and 90% of females, $p < 0.0001$).

*3.2. Diabetes Status*

Participant self-report was compared to HbA1c groupings for both diabetes and pre-diabetes to determine the rate of undiagnosed diabetes in this population. Although, 71% of participants correctly self-reported having diabetes and 88% self-reported having pre-diabetes, there were 12% undiagnosed for diabetes and 39% undiagnosed for pre-diabetes. Overall, there were 39% undiagnosed for diabetes and prediabetes, by gender that broke down to be 26% of males and 50% of females.

Participants were 18% non-diabetic (10% male and 8% female), 49% were pre-diabetic (13% male and 36% females), and 33% were diabetic (26% male and 8% female); the difference by gender across these three diabetes status groups is significant ($F = 0.0017$, $p = 0.0197$). Figure 1 shows the breakout of diabetes status group by gender.

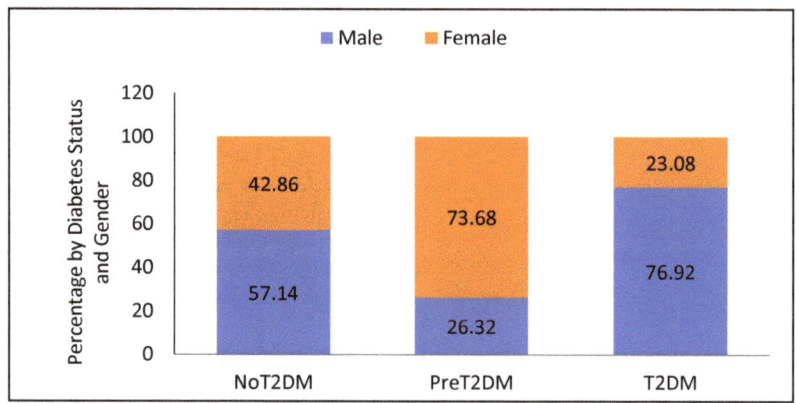

**Figure 1.** Participants by diabetes status and gender (T2DM = Type 2 Diabetes Mellitus).

*3.3. Participant Diets*

Participants consumed an average of 1463.7 kilocalories per day (1600.9 for males and 1333.3 for females, $p = 0.01$). Figure 2 shows the macronutrient intake per day (in grams) for all participants as well as for males and females separately. Daily consumption of protein averaged 51.4 g across all participants (46.8 g for females and 56.4 g for males), carbohydrates averaged 201.3 g across all participants (181.3 g for females and 222.4 g for males), and fats averaged 49.5 g across all participants (46.4 g for females and 52.9 g for males).

Among married participants, couples consumed similar diets, however, participants were not significantly correlated on diabetes status. Therefore, comparisons by diabetes status or gender would still reveal real differences between Asian Indian male and female non-diabetics, pre-diabetics and diabetics.

Although males and females consumed significantly different amounts of total kilocalories per day, they did not differ significantly when each macronutrient was examined as the percent of total kilocalories, or when macronutrient components were examined as proportion of their respective macronutrient. Protein, as a percent of total kilocalories, was about 14% for both males and females, carbohydrates, as a percent of total kilocalories, was 56% for males and 55% for females, and fat, as a percent of total kilocalories, was 29% for males and 31% for females.

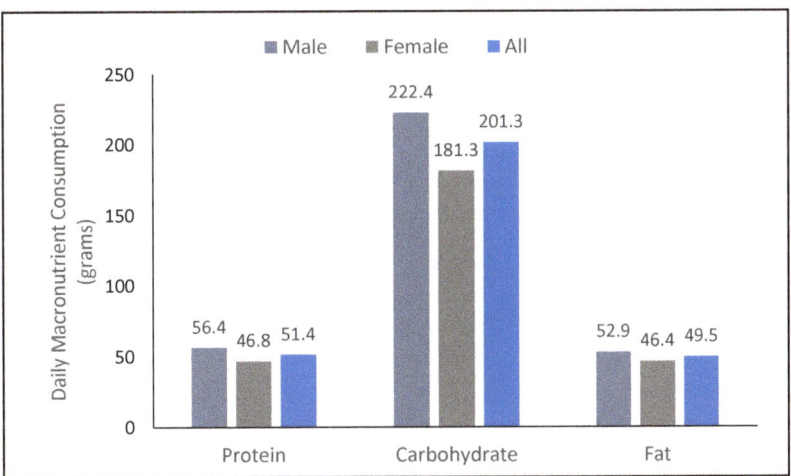

**Figure 2.** Daily macronutrient consumption.

Although the percentages of total kilocalories from protein, carbohydrates, and fats for both males and females fell within acceptable macronutrient distribution ranges for daily consumption by adults in the US as recommended by the Food and Nutrition Board, Institute of Medicine, National Academies [32], protein as percent of total kilocalories was at the lower recommended ranges for daily consumption. Table 1 provides a comparison of the IOM's AMDR with participant daily intakes. Participants had lower than recommended daily ranges for total fiber consumption (16.10 g for females and 19.00 g for males, IOM recommendations ranged 21–25% for females and 30–38% for males) and dramatically less than the maximum allowances for sugar (<1% for both males and females; IOM maximum allowance is 25%). No recommendations were given by the IOM for monounsaturated fatty acids and the nutrient data for this study did not break out polyunsaturated fatty acids into n-6 (linoleic acid) and n-3 (α-linolenic acid), so those comparisons were not possible. Saturated fat and trans fatty acids were consumed in small quantities by participants (<1% and <<1% respectively), and cholesterol was consumed in relatively small quantities as well (5.35% of total kilocalories for females, and 6.63% for males).

Looking at these dietary components by diabetes status reveals that there was a significant difference between the proportion of trans fat consumed of total fat across groups. Non-diabetics consumed the largest proportion (1%), pre-diabetics consumed a smaller proportion (0.2%), and diabetics consumed the smallest proportion of all (0.08%), $p = 0.036$*. There was a difference in the consumption of cholesterol as a proportion of total fat, but it was not significant ($p = 0.2225$). Non-diabetics again consumed the largest proportions (2.67) followed by diabetic (1.85), and then pre-diabetic (1.41), $p = 0.0636$. These differences were not seen when looking at males alone, but were when looking at females alone, albeit not significantly. Non-diabetic females consumed 1% of total fat from trans-fat, whereas pre-diabetic consumed 0.1%, and diabetic consumed 0.03%, $p = 0.0522$. For proportion of cholesterol, non-diabetic females consumed the most (3.03), followed by pre-diabetic females (1.40), and then diabetic females (0.74), $p = 0.0867$.

**Table 1.** Dietary Components as Compared to IOM's Acceptable Macronutrient Distribution Ranges (AMDR).

| Variable | IOM Males | IOM Females | Female (n = 20) | Male (n = 19) |
|---|---|---|---|---|
| Protein as Percent of Total Kilocalories | 10–35% | 10–35% | 14.1% | 14.0% |
| Carbohydrates as Percent of Total Kilocalories | 45–65% | 45–65% | 54.5% | 56.0% |
| Fat as Percent of Total Kilocalories | 20–35% | 20–35% | 31.0% | 29.3% |
| Total Fiber | 30–38 g | 21–25 g | 16.1 g | 19.0 g |
| Soluble Fiber | NA | NA | 7.3g | 8.6g |
| Insoluble Fiber | NA | NA | 7.4g | 9.5g |
| Sugar | 25% | 25% | 0.76% | 0.87% |
| Monounsaturated Fat | NA | NA | 1.4% | 1.3% |
| Polyunsaturated Fat | NA | NA | 0.77% | 0.69% |
| n-6 (linoleic acid) | 5–10% | 5–10% | NA | NA |
| n-3 (α-linolenic acid) | 0.6–1.2% | 0.6–1.2% | NA | NA |
| Saturated Fat | Minimal | Minimal | 12.7g (0.94%) | 14.8g (0.91%) |
| Trans Fat | Minimal | Minimal | 0.20g (0.01%) | 0.19g (0.01%) |
| Cholesterol | Minimal | Minimal | 68.9g (5.35%) | 106.4g (6.63%) |

IOM: Institute of Medicine.

### 3.4. BMR by Diabetes Status

Table 2 provides the mean BMR by gender and diabetes status. BMR establishes the minimum caloric intake needed to meet energy requirement assuming no physical activity. Energy requirements for each participant were calculated (BMR + kilocalories burned through physical activity).

**Table 2.** Basal Metabolic Rate (BMR) Calculated Using Five Different Methods by Gender and Diabetes Status.

| BMR Method | No-Diabetes | Pre-Diabetes | Diabetes |
|---|---|---|---|
| All | (n = 7) | (n = 19) | (n = 13) |
|  | Mean (SD) | Mean (SD) | Mean (SD) |
| Owen | 1435.73 (280.7) | 1335.14 (176.8) | 1545.64 (208.2) |
| Harris-Benedict | 1359.18 (300.2) | 1291.30 (140.0) | 1411.39 (186.9) |
| Mifflin St. Jeor | 1286.67 (307.4) | 1192.23 (193.9) | 1381.08 (203.2) |
| WHO | 1253.27 (177.0) | 1276.27 (106.9) | 1362.19 (116.2) |
| Tanita Scale | 1347.50 (303.0) | 1252.87 (183.2) | 1455.81 (234.7) |
| Females | (n = 3) | (n = 14) | (n = 3) |
| Owen | 1161.72 (53.5) | 1238.49 (52.3) | 1209.09 (72.5) |
| Harris-Benedict | 1188.51 (157.0) | 1238.88 (96.7) | 1198.90 (107.4) |
| Mifflin St. Jeor | 1049.64 (193.2) | 1103.50 (126.8) | 1086.58 (129.0) |
| WHO | 1147.99 (110.2) | 1248.83 (99.2) | 1247.90 (136.7) |
| Tanita Scale | 1101.83 (111.8) | 1164.61 (94.3) | 1094.50 (119.0) |
| Males | (n = 4) | (n = 5) | (n = 10) |
| Owen | 1641.23 (155.7) | 1605.76 (86.8) | 1646.60 (86.9) |
| Harris-Benedict | 1487.18 (.335.9) | 1438.10 (145.7) | 1475.14 (156.3) |
| Mifflin St. Jeor | 1464.45 (256.6) | 1440.68 (110.2) | 1469.43 (117.5) |
| WHO | 1332.23 (187.5) | 1353.08 (96.8) | 1396.47 (90.4) |
| Tanita Scale | 1531.75 (263.9) | 1500.00 (136.1) | 1564.20 (117.1) |

Figures 3–5 show the average BMR, average caloric intake needed to meet energy requirements and average caloric intake by diabetes status and gender. Correlational analysis shows that BMR is significantly correlated with total caloric intake for all par-

ticipants (0.4251, $p$ = 0.0070), but not for males only (0.0334, $p$ = 0.8920), or females only (0.1088, $p$ = 0.6478). However, BMR was significantly correlated with total caloric intake needed to meet energy requirements for all participants, males only and females only (0.7799, $p$ < 0.0001; 0.6738, $p$ = 0.0016; 0.6865, $p$ = 0.0008, respectively). Total caloric intake to meet energy needs significantly exceeds total kilocalories consumed for all participants as well as for males only and females only (0.3015, $p$ = 0.0625; 0.0444, $p$ = 0.8569; 0.2550, $p$ = 0.2779, respectively), except for female non-diabetics, whose caloric intake exceeds total kilocalories needed for energy needs.

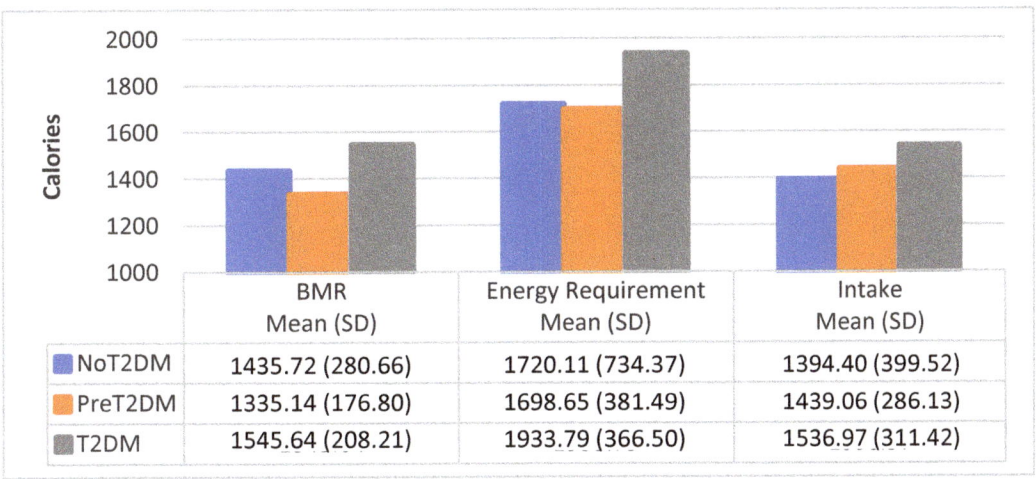

Figure 3. BMR, energy requirement, and caloric intake for all participants by diabetes status.

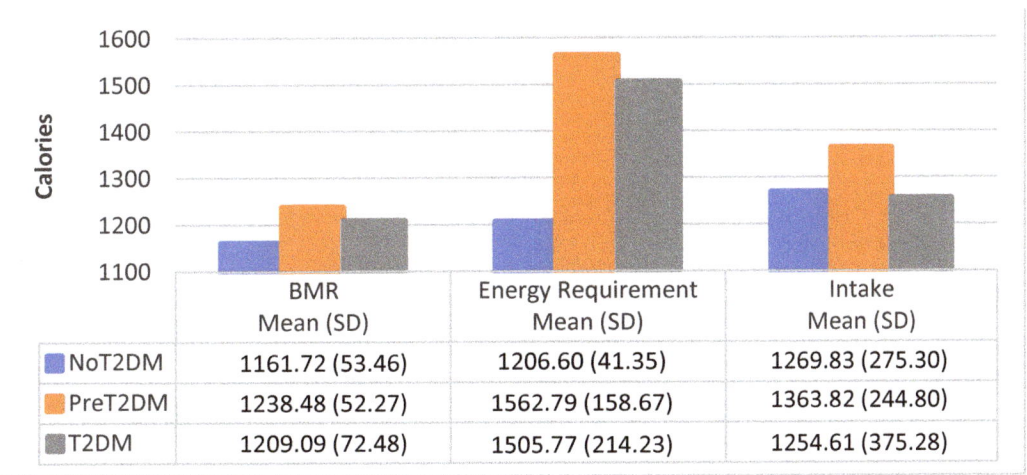

Figure 4. BMR, energy requirement, and caloric intake for female participants by diabetes status.

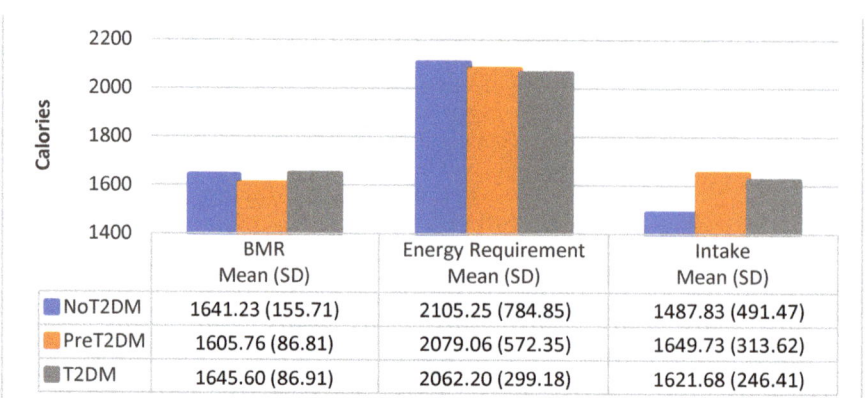

**Figure 5.** BMR, energy requirement, and caloric intake for male participants by diabetes status.

*3.5. Diet Quantity—Macronutrient Distributions—Actual to Needed Calorie Ratios*

Kilocalories required to meet energy needs exceeded caloric intake for all groups, except non-diabetic females; caloric intakes for diabetic females were slightly higher than what is needed to meet energy needs.

The association between macronutrient distribution and diabetes status was examined by looking at the ratio of actual to needed total kilocalories, protein, carbohydrates and fats based on energy needs by gender and diabetes status (Figures 6–9).

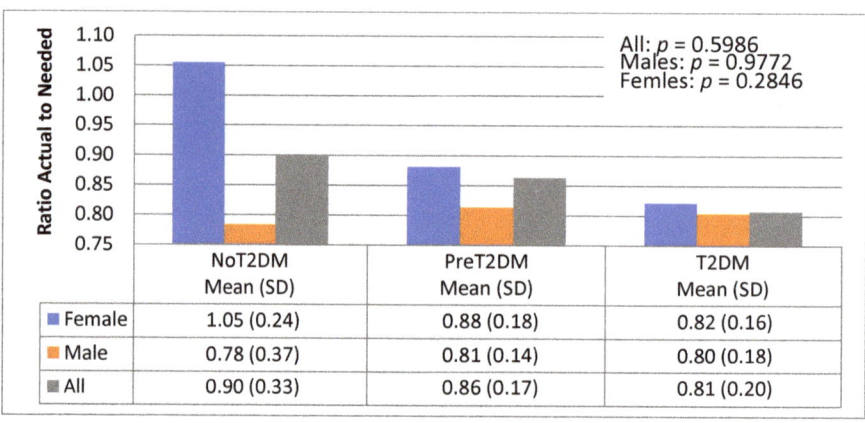

**Figure 6.** Actual to needed total kilocalories by diabetes status and gender.

There were no significant differences noted by diabetes status for total actual to needed kilocalories (Figure 6). However, non-diabetic females did exceed their total needed caloric intake (105%), whereas pre-diabetic and diabetic females consume 81% and 80%, respectively, of their needed kilocalories. Actual to needed ratios of total kilocalories were lower for non-diabetic men (78%) than pre-diabetic (81%) and diabetic men (80%).

Figure 7 shows non-diabetics consuming higher ratios of actual to needed protein than pre-diabetics and diabetics (64%, 59% and 60%, respectively); this difference was not statistically significant ($p = 0.8450$). Non-diabetic females consumed higher ratios of actual to needed protein than pre-diabetic and diabetic females (83%, 61%, and 57%, respectively); this difference was not statistically significant ($p = 0.0699$). Male diabetics consumed the highest ratios of actual to needed protein (61%), followed by pre-diabetics (55%) and then non-diabetics (50%); this difference was not statistically significant ($p = 0.6786$).

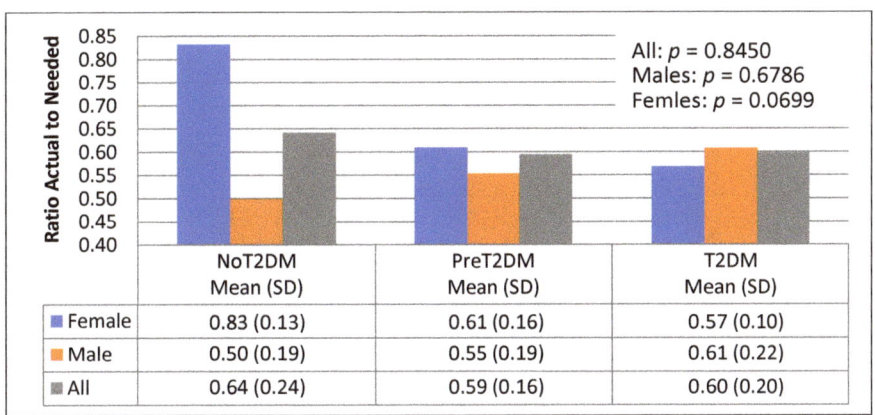

**Figure 7.** Actual to needed kilocalories from protein by diabetes status and gender.

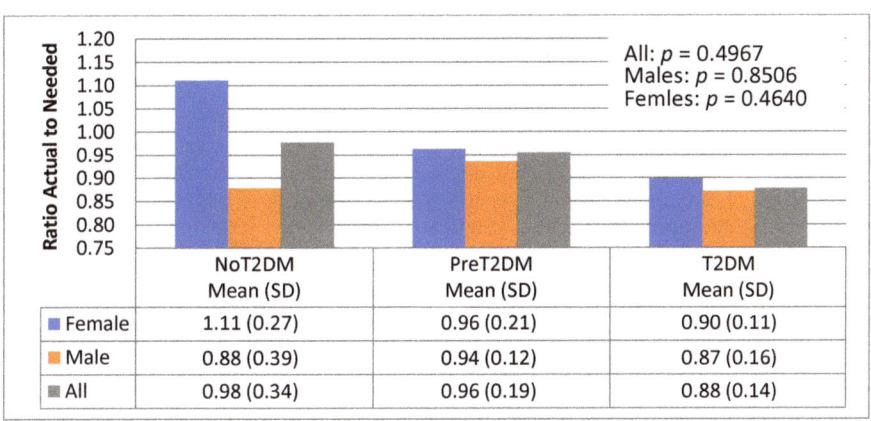

**Figure 8.** Actual to needed kilocalories from carbohydrates by diabetes status and gender.

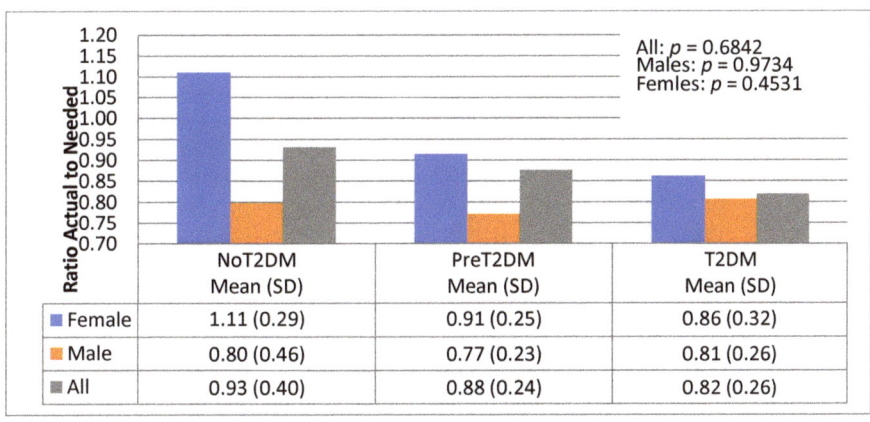

**Figure 9.** Actual to needed kilocalories from fat by diabetes status and gender.

Correlational analysis also showed a significant relationship between diabetes status and actual to needed kilocalories from protein for females ($-0.45$, $p = 0.0458$). This relationship was not seen in males; however, correlational analysis did show a significant relationship for males only between HbA1c level and actual to needed kilocalories from protein (0.51, $p$ = 0.0243); this relationship is in the reverse direction than seen in females.

Figure 8 shows a similar pattern for actual to needed kilocalories from carbohydrates as shown for actual to needed consumption of protein. Non-diabetic females were consuming higher ratios of carbohydrates than pre-diabetics (111% and 96%, respectively); diabetic females consumed the lowest ratios of carbohydrates (90%). The pattern for men is slightly different. Pre-diabetic males consumed the highest ratio of actual to needed carbohydrates (94%), followed by non-diabetic (88%) and finally diabetic males (87%).

Figure 9 shows actual to needed consumption of fat was highest for non-diabetic females, exceeding the daily caloric needed for fat (111%). Pre-diabetics consumed the second highest percent (91%), followed by diabetics (86%). For males, however, diabetics consumed the highest percent of actual to needed fat (81%), followed by non-diabetics (80%) and then pre-diabetics (77%).

*3.6. Diet Quality*

Additional findings from the correlational analysis showed a significant relationship between diabetes status and proportion of trans fats (−0.34034, $p$ = 0.034) and a weak correlation between diabetes status and proportion of insoluble fiber (0.30208, $p$ = 0.0616) for all participants, and a significant correlation between diabetes status and proportion of insoluble fiber (0.45653, $p$ = 0.043) for females only. However, when correlations between HbA1c, macronutrients and other dietary components were examined, percent protein (0.33328, $p$ = 0.0381), proportion of soluble fiber (0.31638, 0.0497), and total kilocalories consumed were significantly correlated with HbA1c levels for all participants. Males did not show any specific significant correlations between diabetes status and any macronutrient, however, when looking at the correlations between HbA1c, macronutrients and other dietary components, percent protein (0.50846, $p$ = 0.0262), and proportion of insoluble fiber (0.50401, $p$ = 0.0278), were significantly correlated, while proportion of soluble fiber was weakly correlated with diabetes status for males (0.45357, $p$ = 0.0511).

*3.7. Predicting Diabetes Status*

A multiple linear regression model was performed to test how well macronutrient independent variables, that were correlated with diabetes status, could predict diabetes status. With diabetes status as the dependent variable the initial model included actual to needed kilocalories from protein, actual to needed kilocalories from carbohydrates, actual to needed kilocalories from fat, proportion of trans fat, proportion of cholesterol, proportion of soluble and insoluble fiber, percent protein as independent variables. The resulting model was significant (F = 2.58, $p$ = 0.0282). All independent variables were significant predictors of diabetes status, except proportion of trans fat and proportion of soluble fiber. However, when these variables were removed from the model, the model was no longer significant, so these variables were retained in the overall model. Table 3 provides the test statics for this multiple regression model. Table 4 shows the results when the same independent variables were tested to predict HbA1c level, the overall model was also significant (F = 4.39, $p$ = 0.0013). The model's performance was improved by removing proportion of cholesterol from the model. The result was a significant regression for the remaining variables (F = 2.66, $p$ = 0.0012), with an $R^2$ of 0.4165.

Table 3. Parameter Estimates for Predicting Diabetes Status.

| Variable | DF | Parameter Estimate | Standard Error | t Value | Pr > \|t\| | Standardized Estimate |
|---|---|---|---|---|---|---|
| Intercept | 1 | 8.24 | 2.74 | 3.01 | 0.01 * | 0.00 |
| Ratio of Actual to Needed Kilocalories from Protein | 1 | 9.68 | 3.75 | 2.58 | 0.02 * | 2.51 |
| Ratio of Actual to Needed Kilocalories from Carbohydrates | 1 | −4.60 | 1.68 | −2.73 | 0.01 * | −1.35 |
| Ratio of Actual to Needed Kilocalories from Fat | 1 | −2.18 | 1.02 | −2.14 | 0.04 * | −0.86 |
| Proportion of Trans Fat (of Total Fat) | 1 | −39.61 | 19.41 | −2.04 | 0.05 | −0.32 |
| Proportion of Cholesterol (of Total Fat) | 1 | −0.19 | 0.10 | −1.91 | 0.07 | −0.33 |
| Proportion of Soluble Fiber (of Total Carbohydrates) | 1 | −61.04 | 29.21 | −2.09 | 0.04 * | −0.75 |
| Proportion of Insoluble Fiber (of Total Carbohydrates) | 1 | 60.82 | 22.42 | 2.71 | 0.01 * | 0.91 |
| Percent Protein (of Total Kilocalories) | 1 | −0.45 | 0.18 | −2.5 | 0.02 * | −1.43 |

* Indicates a significant $p$-value ($p < 0.05$).

Table 4. Parameter Estimates for Predicting A1c Level.

| Variable | DF | Parameter Estimate | Standard Error | t Value | Pr > \|t\| | Standardized Estimate |
|---|---|---|---|---|---|---|
| Intercept | 1 | 14.41 | 3.39 | 4.25 | <<0.01 * | 0 |
| Ratio of Actual to Needed Kilocalories from Protein | 1 | 15.50 | 4.73 | 3.28 | <0.01 * | 2.74 |
| Ratio of Actual to Needed Kilocalories from Carbohydrates | 1 | −6.54 | 2.10 | −3.12 | <0.01 * | −1.31 |
| Ratio of Actual to Needed Kilocalories from Fat | 1 | −3.37 | 1.31 | −2.57 | 0.01 * | −0.90 |
| Proportion of Trans Fat (of Total Fat) | 1 | −61.91 | 25.17 | −2.46 | 0.02 * | −0.34 |
| Proportion of Soluble Fiber (of Total Carbohydrates) | 1 | −57.59 | 34.42 | −1.67 | 0.10 | −0.49 |
| Proportion of Insoluble Fiber (of Total Carbohydrates) | 1 | 75.27 | 27.56 | 2.73 | 0.01 * | 0.77 |
| Percent Protein (of Total Kilocalories) | 1 | −0.64 | 0.23 | −2.75 | 0.01 * | −1.37 |

* Indicates a significant $p$-value ($p < 0.05$); < indicate $p < 0.005$; << indicates $p < 0.0005$.

## 4. Discussion

This study established an association between diet as measured by actual to needed macronutrients and diabetes status. Pre-diabetics and diabetics consumed lower ratios of actual to needed protein, carbohydrates and fats relative their energy requirements than non-diabetics. This is consistent with recommendations normally given to patients with IR, pre-diabetes or diabetes; eat less to lose weight [33]. In addition, participants with pre-diabetes and diabetes ate smaller proportions of insoluble and higher proportions of soluble fiber. Consistent with typical AI diets, refined carbohydrates are preferred over whole grains, however, non-diabetics consumption of higher amounts of insoluble fiber may suggest that carbohydrate quality may be beneficial in this population.

This study also shows that Asian Indian pre-diabetics and diabetics recognize the benefit of physical activity and caloric restriction, as they relate to their diabetes status and as recommended for diabetes management by health care providers; and establishes a pattern of decreased overall caloric intake, and decreased intake for each macronutrient (protein, carbohydrate and fat), below required levels based on energy requirements for pre-diabetics and diabetics in the United States. Additionally, it is not known if the combination of increased physical activity and decreased caloric intake discovered in this population can be viewed as contributing to health or negatively impacting diabetes status.

Understanding associations between diabetes status and dietary intake related to diabetes may provide evidenced based strategies to reduce risk of T2DM in this population. As would be the norm in traditional Indian families, females in this population were responsible for cooking and had control over dietary consumption for themselves as well as their families. Additionally, as 72% of participants were married couples, it was noted that of those participants, 70% of the females did not have diabetes or had pre-diabetes while their spouses had diabetes. Along with females being responsible for the household cooking, this suggests a level of control over dietary options that may have an impact on their spouses' diabetes status.

Contrary to the normal pattern of low physical activity among AIs, levels of physical activity by diabetes status in this study population suggest participants may be recognizing the need for physical activity as a strategy to manage diabetes.

These findings suggest that although AIs may be implementing strategies typically recommended to patients with IR, pre-diabetes and diabetes, those strategies may not be improving disease status in this population. Perhaps a focus on macronutrient balance with sufficient caloric intake to meet energy needs, with increased protein intake, and reduced intake of highly refined carbohydrates in this population would be more effective. A recent comparison of various diets, such as the Mediterranean, Dietary Approaches to Stop Hypertension (DASH), plant-based, low and very low carbohydrate, low-fat, and high protein, aimed at improving metabolic syndrome, T2DM, Cardiovascular Disease (CVD), and hypertension, illustrates that a balance of both macronutrient proportions and quality are needed. In particular, it can be inferred that the macronutrient proportions studied here (50:30:20) provide a starting point from which minor adjustments can be made for individuals' management of T2DM. In addition, the quality of those macronutrients play an important role (e.g., whole grains as compared to processed carbohydrates, fresh fruits and vegetables, plant-based proteins, and unsaturated fats) [31,34]. Additionally, because carbohydrates and fats are primarily implicated in metabolic disorders, studies vary fat and carbohydrate intake (high fat: low carbohydrate vs. low fat: high carbohydrate) and hold protein intake constant. These studies generally show little difference between these two intake conditions [35]. As suggested in this study, in terms of macronutrient proportions, the key may be in moderating carbohydrates and fats, while adjusting protein intake, as well as ensuring quality of macronutrients consumed. Similarly, one additional study looking at regional differences in dietary patterns in Asian Indians in India, suggests that this strategy may be the most beneficial in the management of T2DM [36].

Notable limitations of this study include that generalization of findings to all AIs, or Gujaratis, was not possible because this study used a convenience sample, and most participants were from a specific cohort of AIs; first generation older Gujarati adults with high levels of education, income and acculturation. Additionally, the cross-sectional design of the current study only allowed for examination of associations between diet and diabetes status, and do not imply causality.

Notable strengths of this study include that this is the first study to examine and identify a relationship between diabetes status and macronutrient composition; suggesting a greater adherence to an optimal macronutrient composition (50:30:20; for percent of total kilocalories from carbohydrates, fat and protein) in non-diabetics than in pre-diabetics or diabetics.

The prevalence of type 2 diabetes and its associated co-morbidities within AI populations, especially Gujaratis, in the US and elsewhere is at extremely high levels and is continuing to rise. As such, further research in this population is needed to more thoroughly study the relationship between diet quality and diabetes status to develop evidence-based strategies helpful in the prevention and management of diabetes in this high-risk population. Specifically, further examination is needed on whether the 50:30:20 macronutrient distribution with caloric intakes consistent with energy needs and improved macronutrient quality has an impact on diabetes status and whether adjustments to diet in these ways could impact diabetes related outcomes.

## 5. Conclusions

AIs are at high risk for insulin resistance (IR) leading to impaired glucose tolerance (IGT) and T2DM and their sequelae. Future research is needed to establish the association between diet quality and diabetes status; however, the findings of this study suggest that those at risk for T2DM may benefit from adhering to a macronutrient distribution of approximately 50:30:20 percent of total kilocalories from carbohydrates, fat and protein, or from a higher intake of dietary protein, while ensuring the quality of those macronutrients. Finally, the implications of near universal female responsibility for cooking, in households where a spouse or other family members are diagnosed with either pre-diabetes or diabetes, are intriguing. Targeted education to AI females about preparing meals that adhere to optimal dietary choices, may have a potential benefit to the entire family including those with diabetes and prediabetes.

The current study is the first to investigate a relationship between the consumption of macronutrients in general and in specific relative proportion (50:30:20) and diabetes status in an AI population. These relationships can be further explored to develop a recommended diet for AIs that is quantitatively and qualitatively supportive metabolically for those with IR, pre-diabetes or diabetes.

## 6. Study Limitations

This study lacked sufficient funding to enable laboratory testing to establish hemoglobin A1c levels for group assignment. Therefore, the study leveraged an annual health fair event at the data collection site which provided for this laboratory testing at no cost to the participants. In cases where study participants did not participate in the health fair or their diabetes status did not indicate laboratory testing by a physician, Hemoglobin A1c levels were supplemented by use of the Bayer A1cNow+ POC monitor for group assignment by diabetes status.

**Author Contributions:** This research was conducted by A.P. as part of a graduate thesis project. M.M. advised and assisted in all aspects of the project. K.S. provided support on various aspects of the project as well. Conceptualization, A.P., M.M., and K.S.; methodology, A.P and M.M.; software, A.P.; validation, A.P.; formal analysis, A.P.; investigation, A.P.; resources, A.P.; data curation, A.P.; writing—original draft preparation, A.P.; writing—review and editing, M.M., A.P., K.S.; visualization, A.P.; supervision, M.M.; project administration, A.P.; funding acquisition, M.M. All authors have read and agreed to the published version of the manuscript.

**Funding:** This research received no external funding. The University of Maryland provided internal funds for publication.

**Institutional Review Board Statement:** The study was conducted according to the guidelines of the Declaration of Helsinki, and approved by the Institutional Review Board (or Ethics Committee) of The University of Maryland (771334-3, 3 June 2016).

**Informed Consent Statement:** Informed consent was obtained from all subjects involved in the study.

**Data Availability Statement:** The data presented in this study are available upon request from the corresponding author.

**Acknowledgments:** This research project would not have been possible without the interest, support and participation of the leaders and community of the Mangal Mandir in Spencerville, Maryland, the consultation, support, and nutrient analysis services provided by the Population Health Research Institute (PHRI) located in Canada, the support and understanding of my loving family, and support from my advisor and committee. I wish to thank the religious leadership of the temple as well as all of the volunteer physicians providing free health screens and laboratory analysis for members of the AI community for all their time, encouragement, support and facilitation in recruiting participants for my study as well as providing a venue to administer my study. I wish to thank the Population Health Research Institute (PHRI) for providing both permission for me to use the Food Frequency

Questionnaire (FFQ) for South Asians (SA), which PHRI adapted from the Study of Health Assessment and Risk in Ethnic groups (SHARE) FFQ instrument, and provision of the nutrient analysis for all participants who completed the FFQ-SA in my study. I wish to thank Dipika Desai for her consult and guidance through the process of instituting the student research data use agreement, which provided me the use of the instrument and the nutrient analysis at no charge, and Karleen Schulze, who provide both consult and guidance in the delivery and interpretation of the nutrient data files as well as consult on use of the FFQ to calculate Healthy Eating Index scores. I wish to thank Roche Diagnostics for donating glucometers and test strips for my study.

**Conflicts of Interest:** The authors declare no conflict of interest.

## References

1. Weber, M.B.; Oza-Frank, R.; Staimez, L.R.; Ali, M.K.; Venkat Narayan, K.M. Type 2 Diabetes in Asians: Prevalence, Risk Factors, and Effectiveness of Behavioral Intervention at Individual and Population Levels. *Annu. Rev. Nutr.* **2012**, *32*, 417–439. [CrossRef]
2. International Diabetes Federation, I.D.F. IDF Diabetes Atlas. 2015. Cited 2016; Sseventh. Available online: www.diabetesatlas.org (accessed on 17 April 2017).
3. Venkataraman, R.; Nanda, N.C.; Baweja, G.; Parikh, N.; Bhatia, V. Prevalence of diabetes mellitus and related conditions in Asian Indians living in the United States. *Am. J. Cardiol.* **2004**, *94*, 977–980. [CrossRef] [PubMed]
4. Bhardwaj, S.; Misra, A.; Misra, R.; Goel, K.; Bhatt, S.P.; Rastogi, K.; Vikram, N.K.; Gulati, S. High Prevalence of Abdominal, Intra-Abdominal and Subcutaneous Adiposity and Clustering of Risk Factors among Urban Asian Indians in North India. *PLoS ONE* **2011**, *6*, e24362. [CrossRef]
5. Joshi, S.R. Diabetes Care in India. *Ann. Glob. Health* **2016**, *81*, 830–838. [CrossRef]
6. Bhopal, R.S. A four-stage model explaining the higher risk of Type 2 diabetes mellitus in South Asians compared with European populations. *Diabet. Med.* **2013**, *30*, 35–42. [CrossRef]
7. Staimez, L.R.W.; Mary, B.; Ranjani, H.; Ali, M.K.; Echouffo-Tcheugui, J.B.; Phillips, L.S.; Mohan, V.; Narayan, K.M.V. Evidence of Reduced B-Cell Function in Asian Indians With Mild Dysglycemia. *Diabetes Care* **2013**, *36*, 2772–2778. [CrossRef] [PubMed]
8. Lovegrove, J.A. CVD risk in South Asians: The importance of defining adiposity and influence of dietary polyunsaturated fat. *Proc. Nutr. Soc.* **2007**, *66*, 286–298. [CrossRef] [PubMed]
9. Wulan, S.N.; Westerterp, K.R.; Plasqui, G. Ethnic differences in body composition and the associated metabolic profile: A comparative study between Asians and Caucasians. *Maturitas* **2010**, *65*, 315–319. [CrossRef]
10. Misra, A.; Vikram, N.K. Insulin Resistance Syndrome (Metabolic Syndrome) and Obesity in Asian Indians: Evidence and Implications. *Nutrition* **2004**, *20*, 482–491. [CrossRef] [PubMed]
11. Vikram, N.K.; Pandey, R.M.; Misra, A.; Sharma, R.; Devi, J.R.; Khanna, N. Non-obese (body mass index < 25 kg/m$^2$) Asian Indians with normal waist circumference have high cardiovascular risk. *Nutrition* **2003**, *19*, 503–509. [CrossRef]
12. Misra, A.; Singhal, N.; Sivakumar, B.; Bhagat, N.; Jaiswal, A.; Khurana, L. Nutrition transition in India: Secular trends in dietary intake and their relationship to diet-related non-communicable diseases. *J. Diabetes* **2011**, *3*, 278–292. [CrossRef]
13. Holmboe-Ottesen, G.; Wandel, M. Changes in dietary habits after migration and consequences for health: A focus on South Asians in Europe. *Food Nutr. Res.* **2012**, *56*, 1–13. [CrossRef]
14. Jiang, F.; Hou, X.; Lu, J.; Zhou, J.; Lu, F.; Kan, K.; Tang, J.; Bao, Y.; Jia, W. Assessment of the Performance of A1CNow1 and Development of an Error Grid Analysis Graph for Comparative Hemoglobin A1c Measurements. *Diabetes Technol. Ther.* **2014**, *16*, 363–369. [CrossRef]
15. Hirst, J.A.; McLellan, J.; Price, C.P.; English, E.; Feakins, B.; Stevens, R.J.; Farmer, A.J. Performance of point-of-care HbA1c test devices: Implications for use in clinical practice—A systematic review and meta-analysis. *Clin. Chem. Lab. Med.* **2017**, *55*, 167–180. [CrossRef] [PubMed]
16. Walicka, M.; Jozwiak, J.; Rzeszotarski, J.; Zonenberg, A.; Masierek, M.; Bijos, P.; Franek, E. Diagnostic Accuracy of Glycated Haemoglobin and Average Glucose Values in Type 2 Diabetes Mellitus Treated wtih Premixed Insulin. *Diabetes Ther.* **2019**, *10*, 587–596. [CrossRef] [PubMed]
17. Gülçin Şahingöz Erdal, N.I.; Murat, K.; Nursel, K. Hemoglobin A1c Measurement Using Point of Care Testing. *Istanb. Med. J.* **2020**, *21*, 37–41. [CrossRef]
18. Mattewal, A.; Aldasouqi, S.; Solomon, D.; Gossain, V.; Koller, A. A1cNow® InView™: A New Simple Method for Office-Based Glycohemoglobin Measurement. *J. Diabetes Sci. Technol.* **2007**, *1*, 879–884. [CrossRef]
19. Wang, E.T.; Koning Ld Kanaya, A.M. Higher Protein Intake Is Associated with Diabetes Risk in South Asian Indians: The Metabolic Syndrome and Atherosclerosis in South Asians Living in America (MASALA) Study. *J. Am. Coll. Nutr.* **2010**, *29*, 130–135. [CrossRef] [PubMed]
20. Kelemen, L.E.; Anand, S.S.; Vuksan, V.; Yi, Q.; Teo, K.K.; Devanesen, S.; Yusuf, S. Development and evaluation of cultural food frequency questionnaires for South Asians, Chinese, and Europeans in North America. *J. Am. Diet. Assoc.* **2003**, *103*, 1178–1184. [CrossRef]
21. Joseph, M.; Gupta, R.D.; Prema, L.; Inbakumari, M.; Thomas, N. Are Predictive Equations for Estimating Resting Energy Expenditure Accurate in Asian Indian Male Weightlifters? *Indian J. Endocrinol. Metab.* **2017**, *21*, 515–519.

22. Song, L.; Venkataraman, K.; Gluckman, P.; Chong, Y.S.; Chee, M.-W.L.; Khoo, C.M.; Leow, M.-K.S.; Lee, Y.S.; Tai, E.S.; Khoo, E.Y.H. Smaller size of high metabolic rate organs explains lower resting energy expenditure in Asian-Indian than Chinese men. *Int. J. Obes.* **2016**, *40*, 633–638. [CrossRef] [PubMed]
23. Varte, L.R.; Pal, M. Predictive equation for basal metabolic rate of young Indian soldiers. *Asian J. Med Sci.* **2016**, *7*, 26–31. [CrossRef]
24. Hasson, R.E.; Howe Cheryl, A.; Jones Bryce, L.; Jones Freedson Patty, S. Accuracy of four resting metabolic rate prediction equations: Effects of sex, body mass index, age, and race/ethnicity. *J. Sci. Med. Sport* **2011**, *14*, 344–351. [CrossRef]
25. Miller, S.; Milliron, B.-J.; Woolf, K. Common Prediction Equations Overestimate Measured Resting Metabolic Rate in Young Hispanic Women. *Top. Clin. Nutr.* **2013**, *28*, 120–135. [CrossRef] [PubMed]
26. Frankenfield, D.; Roth-Yousey, L.; Compher, C. Comparison of Predictive Equations for Resting Metabolic Rate in Healthy Nonobese and Obese Adults: A Systematic Review. *J. Am. Diet. Assoc.* **2005**, *105*, 775–788. [CrossRef] [PubMed]
27. Song, T.; Venkataraman, K.; Gluckman, P.; Seng, C.Y.; Meng, K.C.; Khoo, E.Y.; Leow, M.K.; Seng, L.Y.; Shyong, T.E. Validation of prediction equations for resting energy expenditure in Singaporean Chinese men. *Obes. Res. Clin. Pract.* **2015**, *8*, 283–290. [CrossRef]
28. Noakes, M.; Foster Paul, R.; Keogh Jennifer, B.; James Anthony, P.; Mamo John, C.; Clifton Peter, M. Comparison of isocaloric very low carbohydrate/high saturated fat and high carbohydrate/low saturated fat diets on body composition and cardiovascular risk. *Nutr. Metab.* **2006**, *3*, 1–13. [CrossRef]
29. Schwingshackl, L.; Georg, H. Comparison of the long-term effects of high-fat v. low-fat diet consumption on cardiometabolic risk factors in subjects with abnormal glucose metabolism: A systematic review and meta-analysis. *Br. J. Nutr.* **2014**, *111*, 2047–2058. [CrossRef]
30. Pesta, D.H.; Samuel, V.T. A high-protein diet for reducing body fat: Mechanisms and possible caveats. *Nutr. Metab.* **2014**, *11*, 1–8. [CrossRef]
31. Sara Castro-Barquero, A.M.R.-L.; Maria Sierra-Pérez, R.E.; Rosa, C. Dietary Strategies for Metabolic Syndrome: A Comprehensive Review. *Nutrients* **2020**, *12*, 2983. [CrossRef]
32. National Institutes of Medicine, F.a.N.B. *Dietary Reference Intakes (DRI) for Energy, Carbohydrate, Fiber, Fat, Fatty Acids, Cholesterol, Protein, and Amino Acids (Macronutrients)*; The National Academies Press: Washington, DC, USA, 2005.
33. Lawton, J.; Ahmad, N.; Hanna, L.; Douglas, M.; Bains, H.; Hallowell, N. 'We should change ourselves, but we can't': Accounts of food and eating practices amongst British Pakistanis and Indians with type 2 diabetes. *Ethn. Health* **2008**, *13*, 305–319. [CrossRef]
34. Venn, B.J. Macronutrients and Human Health for the 21st Century. *Nutrients* **2020**, *12*, 2363. [CrossRef] [PubMed]
35. Ma, Y.; Fu, Y.; Tian, Y.; Gou, W.; Miao, Z.; Yang, M.; Ordovás, J.M.; Zheng, J.S. Individual Postprandial Glycemic Responses to Diet in n-of-1 Trials: Westlake N-of-1 Trials for Macronutrient Intake (WE-MACNUTR). *J. Nutr.* **2021**, *151*, 3158–3167. [CrossRef] [PubMed]
36. Edward JMJoy, R.G.; Sutapa, A.; Lukasz, A.; Liza, B.; Sanjay, K.; Jennie IMacdiarmid, A.H.; Alan, D.D. Dietary patterns and non-communicable disease risk in Indian adults: Secondary analysis of Indian Migration Study data. *Public Health Nutr.* **2017**, *20*, 1963–1972.

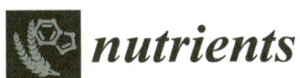 

Article

# Effects of Different Types of Carbohydrates on Arterial Stiffness: A Comparison of Isomaltulose and Sucrose

Ryota Kobayashi [1,*], Miki Sakazaki [2], Yukie Nagai [2], Kenji Asaki [3], Takeo Hashiguchi [4] and Hideyuki Negoro [5,6]

1. Center for Fundamental Education, Teikyo University of Science, Tokyo 120-0045, Japan
2. Research & Development Division, Mitsui Sugar Co., Ltd., Tokyo 103-8423, Japan; Miki.Sakazaki@mitsui-sugar.co.jp (M.S.); Yukie.Nagai@mitsui-sugar.co.jp (Y.N.)
3. Department of Tokyo Judo Therapy, Teikyo University of Science, Tokyo 120-0045, Japan; k-asaki@ntu.ac.jp
4. Department of School Education, Teikyo University of Science, Tokyo 120-0045, Japan; hasiguti@ntu.ac.jp
5. Harvard PKD Center for Polycystic Kidney Disease Research, Boston, MA 02115, USA; oystercope@gmail.com
6. Faculty of Medicine, Nara Medical University, Nara 634-8521, Japan
* Correspondence: rkobayashi.teika@gmail.com; Tel.: +81-80-9193-3605

**Abstract:** Increased arterial stiffness during acute hyperglycemia is a risk factor for cardiovascular disease, but the type of carbohydrate that inhibits it is unknown. The purpose of this study was to determine the efficacy of low-glycemic-index isomaltulose on arterial stiffness during hyperglycemia in middle-aged and older adults. Ten healthy middle-aged and older adult subjects orally ingested a solution containing 25 g of isomaltulose (ISI trial) and sucrose (SSI trial) in a crossover study. In the SSI trial, the brachial–ankle (ba) pulse wave velocity (PWV) increased 30, 60, and 90 min after ingestion compared with that before ingestion ($p < 0.01$); however, in the ISI trial, the baPWV did not change after ingestion compared with that before ingestion. Blood glucose levels 30 min after intake were lower in the ISI trial than in the SSI trial ($p < 0.01$). The baPWV and systolic blood pressure were positively correlated 90 min after isomaltulose and sucrose ingestion ($r = 0.640$, $p < 0.05$). These results indicate that isomaltulose intake inhibits an acute increase in arterial stiffness. The results of the present study may have significant clinical implications on the implementation of dietary programs for middle-aged and elderly patients.

**Keywords:** arterial stiffness; glucose ingestion; middle-aged and older patients; isomaltulose; sucrose

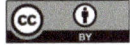

## 1. Introduction

Previous studies have reported acute hyperglycemia as an independent risk factor for cardiovascular disease [1]. An increased postprandial blood glucose level is also a risk factor for cardiovascular disease and exerts a greater effect than the fasting blood glucose level [2]. Moreover, increased arterial stiffness owing to impaired vascular endothelial function underlies the increased risk of cardiovascular disease in acute hyperglycemia [3]. Gordin et al. [4] suggested that arterial stiffness increased with increasing postprandial blood glucose levels in healthy middle-aged and older individuals. Furthermore, we previously demonstrated that systemic arterial stiffness increased in middle-aged and older people after the ingestion of a 25 g glucose solution [5]. Since postprandial blood glucose increases with age [6] and arterial stiffness progresses, there is a significant relationship between arterial stiffness and postprandial blood glucose levels [7]. Japan has a super-aging society [8]; it is important to control the progression of arterial stiffness during acute hyperglycemia in older Japanese individuals.

The increase in arterial stiffness occurs immediately after food intake [7] and may be influenced by the glycemic index (GI) value of the cardiovascular disease indices [9]. In fact, vascular endothelial function, the underlying mechanism of arterial stiffness, varies with GI [10]. A previous study reported that arterial stiffness increased in middle-aged and older people consuming a glucose solution, but the changes differed between different carbohydrate intakes [5]. A high-GI diet has been shown to increase arterial stiffness compared with a low-GI diet. In other words, a low-GI diet may reduce the acute adverse effects on arterial stiffness [11]. For example, isomaltulose is a natural carbohydrate found in honey that has a low GI and is certified as a novel food (European Food Safety Authority) because of its nutritional quality [12]. Isomaltulose has similar amounts of sweetness and energy to sucrose; however, the rate at which it is broken down in the small intestine is slower than that of sucrose, which moderates the rise in blood glucose levels after ingestion [13]. In a previous study, a comparison of acute changes in blood glucose levels after the ingestion of isomaltulose or sucrose in 10 healthy subjects showed that the highest blood glucose levels were lower in patients who ingested isomaltulose than in those who ingested sucrose [14]. In addition, when 10 patients with type 2 diabetes were asked to consume either isomaltulose or sucrose and the changes in blood glucose levels after ingestion were examined, it was found that the blood glucose levels rose rapidly after sucrose ingestion and increased gradually after isomaltulose ingestion, with the peak values being lower for isomaltulose than for sucrose [13]. In other words, isomaltulose, which has a lower GI than sucrose, is expected to reduce the increase in arterial stiffness. However, the changes in arterial stiffness after ingestion of isomaltulose compared with that after the ingestion of sucrose are not sufficiently clear. Therefore, it is necessary to investigate whether arterial stiffness is altered after isomaltulose intake in healthy middle-aged and older people.

In this study, we hypothesized that sucrose intake will increase arterial stiffness with increasing blood glucose levels, but isomaltulose intake will not influence arterial stiffness. To test this hypothesis, we investigated the acute effects of isomaltulose and sucrose intake on arterial stiffness.

## 2. Materials and Methods

### 2.1. Participants

The participants were 10 healthy middle-aged and older adults (five men and five women). Participants were recruited by distributing flyers for research cooperation with residents of the Teikyo University of Science. Finally, we received 20 applications, from which we selected 10 participants who met the following conditions. All participants were normotensive (Japanese standard: <140/90 mmHg), non-smokers, no obvious disease on electrocardiogram or other diagnostic tests, and no exercise habit before the study according to the physical activity questionnaire. Patients with abnormalities in blood tests, urine tests, chest radiographs, or electrocardiograms in the year prior to the study; with diabetes mellitus (American Diabetes Association/ European Association for the Study of Diabetes diagnostic criteria); and who had problems with exercise (e.g., those with musculoskeletal injuries) were excluded from the study. This study was conducted in compliance with the Declaration of Helsinki in terms of ethics, human rights, and protection of participants' personal information. Ethical approval for this study was obtained from the Ethics Committee of Teikyo University of Science (approval no. 20A013). In addition, this study was registered with the University Hospital Medical Information Network Center (UMIN Center; Study No. UMIN000041622). All hardcopy (paper) study data were stored in a locked filing cabinet, and electronic data were stored on a secured network drive, accessible only to those working in the laboratory. The study was conducted in accordance with the guidelines for human experimentation published by the Institutional Review Board.

### 2.2. Study Design

The participants were 10 healthy middle-aged and older adults. They were instructed to maintain a normal diet and activities of daily living for the duration of the study. Intense exercise (training and activities of daily living), caffeine, and alcohol consumption were prohibited for 24 h prior to the experiment. Fasting (10–12 h) was started at 9:00 p.m. the day before the start of the experiment. Arterial stiffness, blood pressure (BP) at the level of the brachial artery and at the ankle, heart rate (HR), and blood glucose (BG) levels were measured before (baseline) and 30, 60, and 90 min after 25-g isomaltulose or sucrose loading. Before each measurement, the subjects were asked to rest in a supine position (Figure 1).

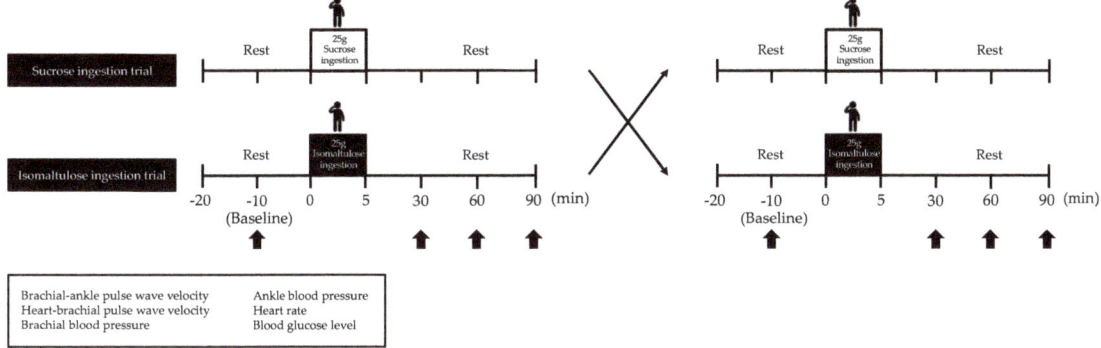

**Figure 1.** Study design. Arterial stiffness, BP, HR, and BG levels were measured at baseline and at 30, 60, and 90 min after isomaltulose or sucrose ingestion. The participants rested in a supine position for 10 min before the test. BP, blood pressure; HR, heart rate; BG, blood glucose.

### 2.3. Body Composition

Height was measured using a height meter in increments of 0.1 cm. Body weight, body fat percentage, and body mass index (BMI) were measured in 0.1 kg increments using a precision instrument body-composition analyzer (WB-150 PMA, Tanita, Tokyo, Japan).

### 2.4. Arterial Stiffness

Pulse wave velocity (PWV) at the brachial and ankle (ba) and at the brachial and heart (hb) of all participants was measured using an automated oscillometric device (PWV/Ankle Brachial Index (ABI), Colin Medical Technology, Komaki, Japan) as previously described [15]. All measurements were performed in a supine position in a quiet room at baseline and 30, 60, and 90 min after isomaltulose solution and sucrose solution ingestion. The daily coefficients of variation in our laboratory were $3 \pm 1\%$ and $3 \pm 2\%$ for baPWV and hbPWV, respectively.

### 2.5. Upper Arm and Ankle Blood Pressure

Systolic blood pressure (SBP), mean blood pressure (MBP), diastolic blood pressure (DBP), and pulse pressure (PP) of the upper arm and ankle were measured in the supine position using an automated oscillometric PWV/ABI device (Omron Colin, Tokyo, Japan) over the brachial and posterior tibial arteries [15]. All measurements were performed in the supine position in a quiet room at baseline and 30, 60, and 90 min after isomaltulose solution and sucrose solution ingestion. The coefficients of variation per day in our laboratory were $2 \pm 1\%$ and $2 \pm 2\%$ for brachial blood pressure and ankle blood pressure, respectively.

### 2.6. Heart Rate

HR was measured in the supine position using an automated oscillometric PWV/ABI device (Omron Colin, Tokyo, Japan) [15]. All measurements were performed in the supine position in a quiet room at baseline and 30, 60, and 90 min after the ingestion of isomaltulose and sucrose solutions. The coefficient of variation per day in our laboratory was $2 \pm 1\%$.

## 2.7. Blood Glucose

Venous blood was collected from the participants' left fingertips. Blood glucose levels were measured by the flavin-adenine dinucleotide glucose dehydrogenase method using a Glutest Neo Alpha glucometer (Sanwa Kagaku Kenkyusho, Tokyo, Japan) [16]. Measurements were taken before and 30, 60, and 90 min after ingestion of isomaltulose and sucrose solutions. The interday coefficient of variation of blood glucose levels was 3 ± 1%.

## 2.8. Isomaltulose Solution and Sucrose Solution Ingestion

Each participant orally ingested 25 g of isomaltulose (ISI trial) or 25 g of sucrose (SSI trial) in 200 mL of water within 5 min, since the new World Health Organization guidelines recommend that adults consume less than 25 g of free sugars per day [17]. Each subject waited approximately 3 days after the completion of one test before taking the next test.

## 2.9. Statistical Analysis

Data are presented as means ± standard deviation. Normality of the data and homogeneity of variance were examined using the Shapiro–Wilk and Levene tests, respectively. Changes in each measurement before and after the intervention are presented as mean values and 95% confidence intervals for each group. Parametric analysis was performed using two-way analysis of variance with repeated measures (time*group) for the measurements taken. When the assumption of sphericity was violated (Mauchly's test), the analysis was adjusted using the Greenhouse–Geisser correction. The Bonferroni method was used with post hoc tests for changes in each intervention. The total area under the curve at 90 min (AUC) was calculated using the trapezoidal formula and analyzed using the corresponding $t$-test. The correlation between baPWV and brachial SBP levels 90 min after consumption was examined using the Pearson product-moment correlation coefficient. SPSS (version 25, IBM Corp., Armonk, NY, USA) was used for the statistical analysis. Statistical significance was set at $\alpha = 0.05$, and all $\alpha$ values were two-sided. To examine the magnitude of the differences, the effect size was calculated based on Cohen's d.

## 3. Results

### 3.1. Physical Characteristics

The mean age of the participants was 62.8 ± 4.4 years; the mean height was 162.5 ± 2.9 cm; the mean weight was 60.9 ± 3.0 kg; the mean BMI was 23.1 ± 1.1 kg/m$^2$; and the mean body fat percentage was 27.7 ± 2.7% (Table 1).

Table 1. Baseline characteristics of the participants.

|  | Value |
| --- | --- |
| Age, years | 62.8 ± 4.4 |
| Height, cm | 162.5 ± 2.9 |
| Weight, kg | 60.9 ± 3.0 |
| BMI, kg/m$^2$ | 23.1 ± 1.1 |
| Body fat, % | 27.7 ± 2.7 |
| Brachial SBP, mmHg | 123.5 ± 6.2 |
| Ankle SBP, mmHg | 153.8 ± 8.6 |
| Heart rate, bpm | 62.0 ± 3.7 |
| Fasting blood glucose, mg/dL | 98.8 ± 4.2 |

Values are mean ± SD. BMI, body mass index; SBP, systolic blood pressure; SD, standard deviation.

### 3.2. Arterial Stiffness

In the SSI trial, the baPWV increased 30, 60, and 90 min after ingestion compared with that before ingestion ($p < 0.01$); however, in the ISI trial, the baPWV did not change after ingestion compared with that before ingestion. The baPWV was not significantly different between the trials before ingestion (Figure 2A). The baPWV AUC was lower ($p < 0.01$) in the ISI trial than in the SSI trial (Figure 2B).

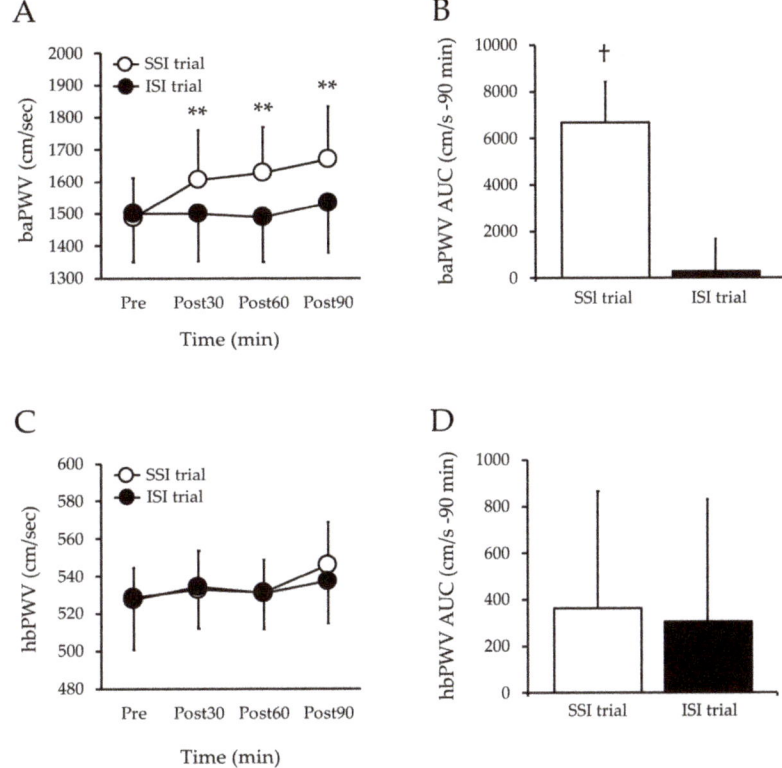

**Figure 2.** Changes in arterial stiffness at baseline and post-ingestion in both trials. Values are mean ± SD. ** $p < 0.01$ vs. baseline. † $p < 0.01$ vs. ISI trial. baPWV, brachial–ankle pulse wave velocity; hbPWV, heart–brachial pulse wave velocity; SSI, sucrose solution intake; ISI, isomaltulose solution intake; AUC, area under the curve; SD, standard deviation; Figure A, baPWV; Figure B, baPWV AUC; Figure C, hbPWV; Figure D, hbPWV AUC.

The hbPWV did not change after ingestion compared with that before ingestion in both the SSI and ISI trials, and the hbPWV was not different between the two trials (Figure 2C). The hbPWV AUC did not differ between the trials (Figure 2D).

### 3.3. Heart Rate

The HR did not change after sucrose ingestion compared with that before sucrose ingestion. Moreover, the HR did not change after isomaltulose ingestion compared with that before isomaltulose ingestion. Furthermore, there was no difference between the trials (Table 2).

### 3.4. Brachial Blood Pressure

The SBP and PP of the upper arm in the SSI trial increased 90 min after ingestion compared with those before ingestion ($p < 0.05$), whereas the SBP and PP of the upper arm in the ISI trial did not change after ingestion compared with those before ingestion. There was no difference between the trials. The MBP and DBP of the upper arm in the SSI trial did not change after ingestion compared with those before ingestion. The MBP and DBP of the upper arm in the ISI trial did not change after ingestion compared with those before ingestion. There was no difference between trials (Table 2).

Table 2. Changes in brachial SBP, MBP, DBP, and HR before and after the ingestion of isomaltulose and sucrose.

| Variable | Trial | Baseline | Post 30 min | Post 60 min | Post 90 min | p-Value (Group) |
|---|---|---|---|---|---|---|
| Brachial SBP, mmHg | SSI trial | 123.5 ± 6.2 | 128.6 ± 6.3 | 131.0 ± 6.1 | 134.4 ± 5.9 * | 0.93 |
|  | ISI trial | 124.2 ± 4.6 | 127.1 ± 4.1 | 129.4 ± 6.1 | 126.1 ± 5.3 |  |
| Brachial MBP, mmHg | SSI trial | 88.2 ± 2.9 | 90.5 ± 3.2 | 91.5 ± 2.9 | 93.4 ± 3.1 | 0.85 |
|  | ISI trial | 88.6 ± 2.9 | 89.8 ± 2.7 | 91.8 ± 3.8 | 90.4 ± 3.4 |  |
| Brachial DBP, mmHg | SSI trial | 70.6 ± 2.5 | 71.5 ± 2.3 | 71.7 ± 2.2 | 72.8 ± 3.0 | 0.80 |
|  | ISI trial | 70.8 ± 2.6 | 71.1 ± 2.6 | 73.0 ± 3.3 | 72.6 ± 3.0 |  |
| Brachial PP, mmHg | SSI trial | 52.9 ± 6.0 | 57.0 ± 5.3 | 59.3 ± 5.7 | 61.6 ± 6.2 * | 0.80 |
|  | ISI trial | 53.4 ± 3.8 | 56.0 ± 3.7 | 56.4 ± 4.9 | 53.6 ± 4.2 |  |
| HR, beats/min | SSI trial | 62.0 ± 3.7 | 60.8 ± 2.7 | 58.1 ± 3.1 | 58.7 ± 2.5 | 0.50 |
|  | ISI trial | 58.1 ± 4.1 | 54.7 ± 3.2 | 55.4 ± 2.7 | 57.4 ± 3.0 |  |

Values are mean ± SD. * $p < 0.05$, vs. baseline. SSI, sucrose solution intake; ISI, isomaltulose solution intake; SBP, systolic blood pressure; MBP, mean blood pressure; DBP, diastolic blood pressure; PP, pulse pressure; HR, heart rate; SD, standard deviation.

### 3.5. Ankle Blood Pressure

The SBP, MBP, and PP of the ankle in the SSI trial increased 90 min after ingestion compared with those before ingestion ($p < 0.05$), and the SBP, MBP, and PP of the ankle in the ISI trial did not change after ingestion compared with those before ingestion. There were no differences between the trials.

The DBP of the ankle in the SSI trial did not change after ingestion compared with that before ingestion, and the DBP and HR of the ankle in the ISI trial did not change after ingestion compared with those before ingestion. There were no differences between the trials (Table 3).

Table 3. Changes in ankle SBP, MBP, and DBP before and after the ingestion of isomaltulose and sucrose.

| Variable | Trial | Baseline | Post 30 min | Post 60 min | Post 90 min | p-Value (Group) |
|---|---|---|---|---|---|---|
| Ankle SBP, mmHg | SSI trial | 153.8 ± 8.6 | 160.6 ± 8.8 | 165.3 ± 10.2 | 167.4 ± 8.0 * | 0.93 |
|  | ISI trial | 147.9 ± 9.9 | 155.1 ± 8.2 | 154.0 ± 8.1 | 155.7 ± 9.6 |  |
| Ankle MBP, mmHg | SSI trial | 99.0 ± 3.1 | 102.4 ± 3.5 | 104.1 ± 3.4 | 106.3 ± 3.2 * | 0.85 |
|  | ISI trial | 95.4 ± 4.7 | 99.9 ± 3.3 | 99.8 ± 3.8 | 100.0 ± 4.4 |  |
| Ankle DBP, mmHg | SSI trial | 71.6 ± 1.7 | 73.2 ± 1.7 | 73.6 ± 2.0 | 75.8 ± 2.8 | 0.80 |
|  | ISI trial | 69.2 ± 3.2 | 72.2 ± 2.6 | 72.7 ± 2.9 | 72.2 ± 3.1 |  |
| Ankle PP, mmHg | SSI trial | 82.2 ± 8.8 | 87.4 ± 8.4 | 91.7 ± 10.7 | 91.6 ± 8.5 * | 0.80 |
|  | ISI trial | 78.7 ± 8.9 | 82.9 ± 8.5 | 81.3 ± 7.6 | 83.4 ± 9.1 |  |

Values are mean ± SD. * $p < 0.05$, vs. baseline. SSI, sucrose solution intake; ISI, isomaltulose solution intake; SBP, systolic blood pressure; MBP, mean blood pressure; DBP, diastolic blood pressure; PP, pulse pressure; SD, standard deviation.

### 3.6. Blood Glucose

The blood glucose levels in the SSI trial increased 30 and 60 min after ingestion compared with those before ingestion ($p < 0.01$). The blood glucose levels in the ISI trial increased 30 min after ingestion compared with those before ingestion ($p < 0.05$). The blood glucose levels 30 min after intake were lower in the ISI trial than in the SSI trial ($p < 0.01$, (Figure 3A). The AUC of blood glucose level was lower in the ISI trial than in the SSI trial (Figure 3B).

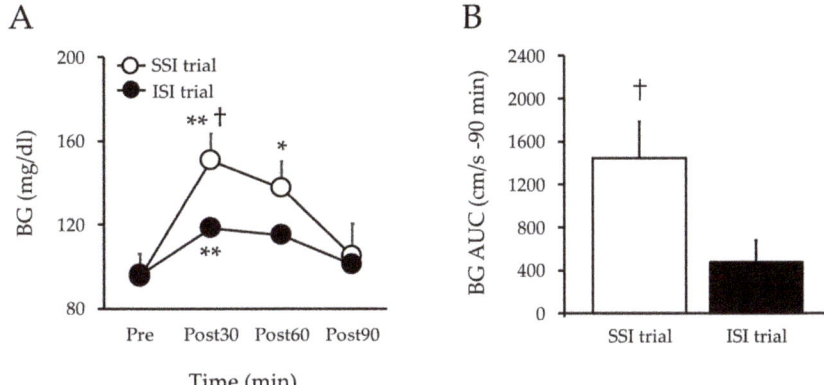

**Figure 3.** Changes in blood glucose at baseline and post-ingestion in both trials. Values are mean ± SD. ** $p < 0.01$ and * $p < 0.05$, vs. baseline. † $p < 0.05$, vs. ISI. BG, blood glucose; SSI, sucrose solution intake; ISI, isomaltulose solution intake; SD, standard deviation; Figure 3A, blood glucose; Figure 3B, blood glucose AUC.

*3.7. Arterial Stiffness and Brachial SBP at 90 Min after Sucrose and Isomaltulose Solution Ingestion*

The baPWV and brachial SBP were positively correlated 90 min after isomaltulose and sucrose ingestion ($r = 0.640$, $p < 0.05$) (Figure 4).

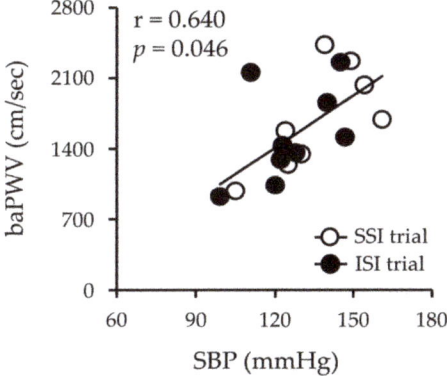

**Figure 4.** Correlation between arterial stiffness and brachial SBP at 90 min after sucrose and isomaltulose intake. Values are mean ± SD. $r = 0.640$ and $p = 0.046$. SBP, systolic blood pressure; SSI, sucrose solution intake; ISI, isomaltulose solution intake; SD, standard deviation.

## 4. Discussion

The main finding of this study was that the baPWV and SBP did not change after isomaltulose intake compared to before. This confirms our hypothesis. These results suggest that isomaltulose could be used as an alternative to sucrose, given the neutral effect on the PWV and SBP.

A rapid increase in blood glucose levels after a meal is an independent risk factor for cardiovascular disease and a greater risk factor than fasting glucose [18]. Therefore, it is necessary to control the rapid increase in blood glucose levels after meals to prevent cardiovascular diseases. There is a consensus that eating high-GI foods results in rapid carbohydrate absorption, whereas low-GI foods result in milder carbohydrate absorption and consequently milder insulin secretion [19]. For example, a previous study of 10 healthy individuals showed a slower increase in blood glucose and insulin levels after consuming isomaltulose compared with that after sucrose consumption [14]. Our results are in agreement with these findings. Blood glucose levels after ingestion were lower in the ISI trial than in the SSI trial. Therefore, isomaltulose may slow down the rise in blood glucose levels after a meal compared with sucrose, the main component of sugar.

A number of studies have shown that arterial stiffness increases during hyperglycemia [4,19,20]. Moreover, previous studies have shown that the baPWV increases during acute hyperglycemia [5]. Our previous study also found an increase in the baPWV after glucose ingestion. The present results are in agreement with these findings, in which the baPWV increased 30, 60, and 90 min after sucrose ingestion compared with before sucrose ingestion, but no increase was observed in the ISI trial. In addition, the AUC of the baPWV was lower in the ISI trial than in the SSI trial. Therefore, isomaltulose can be expected to inhibit the increase in arterial stiffness compared with the consumption of other carbohydrates, such as sucrose and glucose, making it possible to create food products that are both tasty and healthy.

Diabetes mellitus induces peripheral arterial disease in the limbs [21] and it has been found that peripheral arterial stiffness increases after the 75-g glucose-tolerance test compared with before the test [22]. Previous studies have reported that the peripheral arterial PWV, especially in the lower limb arteries, increases during acute hyperglycemia [23]. In the current SSI study, the baPWV increased after ingestion compared to before sucrose ingestion, while the hbPWV did not change. Previous studies have reported that the baPWV reflects arterial stiffness in the distal (mainly abdominal) aorta and lower limbs [24], while the hbPWV reflects arterial stiffness in the proximal aorta and upper limbs [25]. In addition, the MBP and PP, which reflect aortic and peripheral arterial stiffness, are elevated after sucrose ingestion. Therefore, in middle-aged and older people, an increase in arterial stiffness during acute hyperglycemia is likely to affect the abdominal aorta and lower-limb arteries. However, in the current study, we were unable to measure arterial stiffness in detail by site. In future studies, we plan to further investigate the increase in arterial stiffness during acute hyperglycemia by site.

This study did not examine the mechanism by which arterial stiffness was not altered after isomaltulose ingestion, but there are several possible explanations. In the present study, in the SSI test, the SBP increased 90 min after compared to before sucrose intake. In previous studies, the SBP and baPWV were found to be correlated [26]. In the present study, there was a correlation between the SBP and baPWV in the upper arm after 90 min of ingestion ($r = 0.640$, $p < 0.05$). This suggests that increased systemic arterial stiffness may be responsible for the increase in the SBP. In this study, there was no correlation between the baPWV and the blood glucose level at 90 min, when the increase in the baPWV was highest. In other words, the blood glucose level may not be directly involved in the increase in the baPWV during acute hyperglycemia. Furthermore, sympathetic hyperactivity, increased oxidative stress, and decreased vascular endothelial function associated with increased blood glucose levels may be related in parallel. Increased sympathetic nerve activity has been implicated in the increase in the baPWV [27]. Sympathetic nerve activity has been found to increase after eating [28]. The sympathetic ratio after a meal shows a sustained elevation lasting at least one hour, which has been suggested to be primarily due to a decrease in vagal activity [28]. Thus, the increase in the baPWV after sucrose consumption in the present study may be due to increased sympathetic nerve activity. However, since sympathetic nerve activity was not measured in this study, it should be assessed in the future. Decreased vascular function (PWV and FMD) after a meal has been proven to be dependent on oxidative stress [3]. For example, 2-thiobarbituric-acid-reactive substances (TBARS), an indicator of oxidative stress, have been shown to increase after acute hyperglycemia [29]. Oxidative stress is thought to reduce vascular function by increasing asymmetric dimethylarginine (ADMA) [30]. Hyperglycemia-induced vascular dysfunction after an oral glucose challenge was found to be associated with increased plasma ADMA/Arg [30]. Therefore, it is likely that acute hyperglycemia increased TBARS and induced vascular endothelial dysfunction via increased ADMA, which caused the increase in the PWV. However, oxidative stress was not measured in this study and should be measured in future studies.

Regarding the application of the study results, the use of isomaltulose as a sweetener in everyday cooking may reduce arterial stiffness and blood pressure increases during acute hyperglycemia compared with the use of other carbohydrates. We believe that the need for isomaltulose to prevent arteriosclerosis and elevated blood pressure will increase, especially as people are increasingly cooking for themselves as a way of preventing new coronavirus infections and as they become more conscious of nutritional balance.

Nevertheless, this study has certain limitations. One limitation was the relatively small number of participants. However, the sample size was statistically significant. Furthermore, we believe that the findings are not generalizable to different populations (e.g., young people and people with diabetes) because the study was conducted in older people, and we will therefore examine different groups of people in the future. In addition, although insulin and endothelial dysfunction may alter the PWV, insulin levels and endothelial function biomarkers were not measured in the present study.

## 5. Conclusions

The main finding of this study was that the baPWV and SBP did not change after isomaltulose intake compared to before. This confirms our hypothesis. These results suggest that isomaltulose could be used as an alternative to sucrose, given the neutral effect on the PWV and SBP.

**Author Contributions:** R.K. designed the study; R.K. and K.A. collected the data and conducted the study; R.K. performed the statistical analysis; R.K. drafted the manuscript; M.S., Y.N., K.A., T.H., and H.N. provided a critical review of the manuscript; R.K. had primary responsibility for the final content. All authors have read and agreed to the published version of the manuscript.

**Funding:** This study was supported by a joint research grant from Mitsui Sugar Co., Ltd.

**Institutional Review Board Statement:** This study was conducted in compliance with the Declaration of Helsinki on the basis of ethics, human rights, and the protection of the personal information of participants. Ethical approval for this study was obtained from the Ethics Committee of Teikyo University of Science (approval number 20A024, September 30, 2020). This study was also registered at the University Hospital Medical Information Network Center (UMIN Center; Study No. UMIN000041622).

**Informed Consent Statement:** Informed consent was obtained from all subjects involved in the study.

**Data Availability Statement:** The data presented in this study are available from the corresponding author upon request.

**Conflicts of Interest:** The authors declare no conflict of interest.

## References

1. Tominaga, M.; Eguchi, H.; Manaka, H.; Igarashi, K.; Kato, T.; Sekikawa, A. Impaired Glucose Tolerance Is a Risk Factor for Cardiovascular Disease, but Not Impaired Fasting Glucose. The Funagata Diabetes Study. *Diabetes Care* **1999**, *22*, 920–924. [CrossRef] [PubMed]
2. DECODE Study Group, the European Diabetes Epidemiology Group. Glucose Tolerance and Cardiovascular Mortality: Comparison of Fasting and 2-Hour Diagnostic Criteria. *Arch. Intern. Med.* **2001**, *161*, 397–405. [CrossRef] [PubMed]
3. Jacome-Sosa, M.; Parks, E.J.; Bruno, R.S.; Tasali, E.; Lewis, G.F.; Schneeman, B.O.; Rains, T.M. Postprandial Metabolism of Macronutrients and Cardiometabolic Risk: Recent Developments, Emerging Concepts, and Future Directions. *Adv. Nutr.* **2016**, *7*, 364–374. [CrossRef] [PubMed]
4. Gordin, D.; Saraheimo, M.; Tuomikangas, J.; Soro-Paavonen, A.; Forsblom, C.; Paavonen, K.; Steckel-Hamann, B.; Vandenhende, F.; Nicolaou, L.; Pavo, I.; et al. Influence of Postprandial Hyperglycemic Conditions on Arterial Stiffness in Patients With Type 2 Diabetes. *J. Clin. Endocrinol. Metab.* **2016**, *101*, 1134–1143. [CrossRef] [PubMed]
5. Kobayashi, R.; Sato, K.; Sakazaki, M.; Nagai, Y.; Iwanuma, S.; Ohashi, N.; Hashiguchi, T. Acute Effects of Difference in Glucose Intake on Arterial Stiffness in Healthy Subjects. *Cardiol. J.* **2021**, *28*, 446–452. [CrossRef]

6. Ko, G.T.C.; Wai, H.P.S.; Tang, J.S.F. Effects of Age on Plasma Glucose Levels in Non-Diabetic Hong Kong Chinese. *Croat. Med. J.* **2006**, *47*, 709–713.
7. Tsuboi, A.; Ito, C.; Fujikawa, R.; Yamamoto, H.; Kihara, Y. Association between the Postprandial Glucose Levels and Arterial Stiffness Measured According to the Cardio-Ankle Vascular Index in Non-Diabetic Subjects. *Intern. Med.* **2015**, *54*, 1961–1969. [CrossRef] [PubMed]
8. Arai, H.; Ouchi, Y.; Toba, K.; Endo, T.; Shimokado, K.; Tsubota, K.; Matsuo, S.; Mori, H.; Yumura, W.; Yokode, M.; et al. Japan as the Front-Runner of Super-Aged Societies: Perspectives from Medicine and Medical Care in Japan. *Geriatr. Gerontol. Int.* **2015**, *15*, 673–687. [CrossRef]
9. Kelsch, E.; Diana, J.C.; Burnet, K.; Hanson, E.D.; Fryer, S.F.; Credeur, D.P.; Stone, K.J.; Stoner, L. Arterial Stiffness Responses to Prolonged Sitting Combined with a High-Glycemic-Index Meal: A Double-Blind, Randomized Crossover Trial. *J. Appl. Physiol. (1985)* **2021**, *131*, 229–237. [CrossRef]
10. Gaesser, G.A.; Rodriguez, J.; Patrie, J.T.; Whisner, C.M.; Angadi, S.S. Effects of Glycemic Index and Cereal Fiber on Postprandial Endothelial Function, Glycemia, and Insulinemia in Healthy Adults. *Nutrients* **2019**, *11*, 2387. [CrossRef]
11. Sanchez-Aguadero, N.; Patino-Alonso, M.C.; Mora-Simon, S.; Gomez-Marcos, M.A.; Alonso-Dominguez, R.; Sanchez-Salgado, B.; Recio-Rodriguez, J.I.; Garcia-Ortiz, L. Postprandial Effects of Breakfast Glycemic Index on Vascular Function among Young Healthy Adults: A Crossover Clinical Trial. *Nutrients* **2017**, *9*, 712. [CrossRef]
12. Low, N.H.; Nelson, D.L.; Sporns, P. Carbohydrate Analysis of Western Canadian Honeys and Their Nectar Sources to Determine the Origin of Honey Oligosaccharides. *J. Apic. Res.* **1988**, *27*, 245–251. [CrossRef]
13. Kawai, K.; Yoshikawa, H.; Murayama, Y.; Okuda, Y.; Yamashita, K. Usefulness of Palatinose as a Caloric Sweetener for Diabetic Patients. *Horm. Metab. Res.* **1989**, *21*, 338–340. [CrossRef]
14. Kawai, K.; Okuda, Y.; Yamashita, K. Changes in Blood Glucose and Insulin after an Oral Palatinose Administration in Normal Subjects. *Endocrinol. Jpn* **1985**, *32*, 933–936. [CrossRef] [PubMed]
15. Kobayashi, R.; Sato, K.; Takahashi, T.; Asaki, K.; Iwanuma, S.; Ohashi, N.; Hashiguchi, T. Arterial Stiffness during Hyperglycemia in Older Adults with High Physical Activity vs Low Physical Activity. *J. Clin. Biochem. Nutr.* **2019**, *65*, 146–152. [CrossRef] [PubMed]
16. Kobayashi, R.; Sato, K.; Takahashi, T.; Asaki, K.; Iwanuma, S.; Ohashi, N.; Hashiguchi, T. Effects of a Short-Term Increase in Physical Activity on Arterial Stiffness during Hyperglycemia. *J. Clin. Biochem. Nutr.* **2020**, *66*, 238–244. [CrossRef]
17. *Guideline: Sugars Intake for Adults and Children*; WHO Guidelines Approved by the Guidelines Review Committee; World Health Organization: Geneva, Switzerland, 2015; ISBN 978-92-4-154902-8.
18. Bonora, E. Postprandial Peaks as a Risk Factor for Cardiovascular Disease: Epidemiological Perspectives. *Int. J. Clin. Pract. Suppl.* **2002**, 5–11.
19. Wolever, T.M.; Jenkins, D.J.; Ocana, A.M.; Rao, V.A.; Collier, G.R. Second-Meal Effect: Low-Glycemic-Index Foods Eaten at Dinner Improve Subsequent Breakfast Glycemic Response. *Am. J. Clin. Nutr.* **1988**, *48*, 1041–1047. [CrossRef]
20. Fang, F.-S.; Liu, M.-Y.; Cheng, X.-L.; Zhong, W.-W.; Miao, X.-Y.; Li, J.; Li, C.-L.; Tian, H. Insulin Resistance Correlates with the Arterial Stiffness before Glucose Intolerance. *Intern. Med.* **2014**, *53*, 189–194. [CrossRef]
21. Yokoyama, H.; Shoji, T.; Kimoto, E.; Shinohara, K.; Tanaka, S.; Koyama, H.; Emoto, M.; Nishizawa, Y. Pulse Wave Velocity in Lower-Limb Arteries among Diabetic Patients with Peripheral Arterial Disease. *J. Atheroscler. Thromb.* **2003**, *10*, 253–258. [CrossRef] [PubMed]
22. Kobayashi, R.; Yoshida, S.; Okamoto, T. Arterial Stiffness after Glucose Ingestion in Exercise-Trained versus Untrained Men. *Appl. Physiol. Nutr. Metab.* **2015**, *40*, 1151–1156. [CrossRef]
23. Tucker, W.J.; Sawyer, B.J.; Jarrett, C.L.; Bhammar, D.M.; Ryder, J.R.; Angadi, S.S.; Gaesser, G.A. High-Intensity Interval Exercise Attenuates but Does Not Eliminate Endothelial Dysfunction after a Fast Food Meal. *Am. J. Physiol. Heart. Circ. Physiol.* **2018**, *314*, H188–H194. [CrossRef]
24. Sugawara, J.; Tanaka, H. Brachial-Ankle Pulse Wave Velocity: Myths, Misconceptions, and Realities. *Pulse* **2015**, *3*, 106–113. [CrossRef] [PubMed]
25. Sugawara, J.; Tomoto, T.; Tanaka, H. Heart-to-Brachium Pulse Wave Velocity as a Measure of Proximal Aortic Stiffness: MRI and Longitudinal Studies. *Am. J. Hypertens* **2019**, *32*, 146–154. [CrossRef] [PubMed]
26. Li, B.; Gao, H.; Li, X.; Liu, Y.; Wang, M. Correlation between Brachial-Ankle Pulse Wave Velocity and Arterial Compliance and Cardiovascular Risk Factors in Elderly Patients with Arteriosclerosis. *Hypertens Res.* **2006**, *29*, 309–314. [CrossRef]
27. Nakao, M.; Nomura, K.; Karita, K.; Nishikitani, M.; Yano, E. Relationship between Brachial-Ankle Pulse Wave Velocity and Heart Rate Variability in Young Japanese Men. *Hypertens Res.* **2004**, *27*, 925–931. [CrossRef] [PubMed]
28. Lu, C.L.; Zou, X.; Orr, W.C.; Chen, J.D. Postprandial Changes of Sympathovagal Balance Measured by Heart Rate Variability. *Dig. Dis. Sci.* **1999**, *44*, 857–861. [CrossRef]
29. Takei, Y.; Tomiyama, H.; Tanaka, N.; Yamashina, A. Close Relationship between Sympathetic Activation and Coronary Microvascular Dysfunction during Acute Hyperglycemia in Subjects with Atherosclerotic Risk Factors. *Circ. J.* **2007**, *71*, 202–206. [CrossRef]
30. Mah, E.; Noh, S.K.; Ballard, K.D.; Matos, M.E.; Volek, J.S.; Bruno, R.S. Postprandial Hyperglycemia Impairs Vascular Endothelial Function in Healthy Men by Inducing Lipid Peroxidation and Increasing Asymmetric Dimethylarginine:Arginine. *J. Nutr.* **2011**, *141*, 1961–1968. [CrossRef]

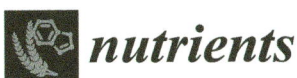

*Article*

# Macronutrient Intake and Insulin Resistance in 5665 Randomly Selected, Non-Diabetic U.S. Adults

Larry A. Tucker

College of Life Sciences, Brigham Young University, Provo, UT 84602, USA; tucker@byu.edu; Tel.: +1-801-422-4927

**Abstract:** The main goal of this investigation was to evaluate the relationships between several macronutrients and insulin resistance in 5665 non-diabetic U.S. adults. A secondary objective was to determine the extent to which the associations were influenced by multiple potential confounding variables. A cross-sectional design and 8 years of data from the 2011–2018 National Health and Nutrition Examination Survey (NHANES) were used to answer the research questions. Ten macronutrients were evaluated: total carbohydrate, starch, simple carbohydrate, dietary fiber, total protein, total fat, saturated, polyunsaturated, monounsaturated, and total unsaturated fat. The homeostatic model assessment (HOMA), based on fasting glucose and fasting insulin levels, was used to index insulin resistance. Age, sex, race, year of assessment, physical activity, cigarette smoking, alcohol use, and waist circumference were used as covariates. The relationships between total carbohydrate intake (F = 6.7, $p$ = 0.0121), simple carbohydrate (F = 4.7, $p$ = 0.0344) and HOMA-IR were linear and direct. The associations between fiber intake (F = 9.1, $p$ = 0.0037), total protein (F = 4.4, $p$ = 0.0393), total fat (F = 5.5, $p$ = 0.0225), monounsaturated fat (F = 5.5, $p$ = 0.0224), and total unsaturated fat (F = 6.5, $p$ = 0.0132) were linear and inversely related to HOMA-IR, with 62 degrees of freedom. Starch, polyunsaturated fat, and saturated fat intakes were not related to HOMA-IR. In conclusion, in this nationally representative sample, several macronutrients were significant predictors of insulin resistance in U.S. adults.

**Keywords:** carbohydrate; protein; fat; unsaturated fat; saturated fat; sugar; starch; fiber; diabetes

**Citation:** Tucker, L.A. Macronutrient Intake and Insulin Resistance in 5665 Randomly Selected, Non-Diabetic U.S. Adults. *Nutrients* **2022**, *14*, 918. https://doi.org/10.3390/nu14050918

Academic Editors: Silvia V. Conde and Fatima O. Martins

Received: 14 January 2022
Accepted: 19 February 2022
Published: 22 February 2022

**Publisher's Note:** MDPI stays neutral with regard to jurisdictional claims in published maps and institutional affiliations.

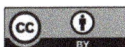

**Copyright:** © 2022 by the author. Licensee MDPI, Basel, Switzerland. This article is an open access article distributed under the terms and conditions of the Creative Commons Attribution (CC BY) license (https:// creativecommons.org/licenses/by/ 4.0/).

## 1. Introduction

Insulin resistance is a pathological condition in which body cells manifest reduced sensitivity to insulin. Insulin promotes the distribution of glucose across muscle and fat tissues and decreases the liver's release of glucose by decreasing the breakdown of glycogen, and gluconeogenesis. Additionally, insulin represses the release of non-esterified fatty acids from fat tissue by decreasing lipolysis [1]. Because of insulin resistance, glucose is not transported into cells at the correct rate, resulting in elevated blood glucose levels. As blood glucose levels increase, the body responds by increasing circulating insulin levels. Consequently, individuals who are insulin resistant often have elevated insulin levels.

Some of the most common chronic diseases in developed societies are linked to insulin resistance. For example, the relationship between insulin resistance and the risk of developing cardiovascular disease is strong [2–4]. Endothelial dysfunction and the development of atherosclerosis is also closely tied to insulin resistance [5,6], along with stroke [7], hypertension [8], dyslipidemia [9], neurodegenerative diseases [10,11], metabolic syndrome [12], and type 2 diabetes [13], to name a few.

Although there are many factors that contribute to insulin resistance, obesity is one of the strongest driving factors [14], even in children [15]. Abdominal obesity seems to pose a greater risk of metabolic disease than an elevated body mass index [16]. Although challenging, weight loss increases insulin sensitivity and reduces the risk of developing insulin resistance and diabetes.

Regular physical activity also plays a significant role in reducing the likelihood of insulin resistance [17], even in those with abdominal obesity [18]. Furthermore, exercise and physical activity also reduce the risk of developing type 2 diabetes [19].

Although obesity and physical inactivity often lead to metabolic impairment, several other lifestyle factors also contribute to metabolic health. For example, research indicates that diet is a key modifiable variable that can be targeted to counter the rising rates of insulin resistance and diabetes. Research indicates that diet composition can be manipulated to improve insulin sensitivity and reduce the risk of diabetes.

To date, dozens of investigations have been conducted to evaluate the relationship between diet composition and metabolic disease, particularly insulin resistance. Study designs and methods have varied substantially, and findings have been mixed. Due to the inconsistent findings in the literature, additional investigations are needed to assess the relationship between diet composition and insulin resistance. Moreover, most investigations in this area have been conducted using small samples and have resulted in few generalizable findings. Hence, the chief goal of the present study was to determine the extent to which differences in diet composition, particularly macronutrient intake, account for differences in insulin resistance in a large sample of adults representing the U.S. population. Another objective was to ascertain the role of several potential confounding factors, including age, sex, race, year of assessment, smoking, alcohol, physical activity, and waist circumference, on the relationship between macronutrient intake and insulin resistance. Effect modification was also evaluated across tertiles of the primary macronutrients and levels of physical activity.

## 2. Materials and Methods

### 2.1. Study Design and Sample

The U.S. National Health and Nutrition Examination Survey (NHANES) database was used to answer the research questions. NHANES is an ongoing government-run survey, administered by the National Center for Health Statistics (NCHS) and the Centers for Disease Control and Prevention (CDC). NHANES data were gathered through the use of extensive interviews, questionnaires, blood samples, and physical examinations performed by trained professionals on individuals selected randomly from the U.S. population.

Before data were collected, each individual in the sample provided written informed consent. The Ethics Review Board for the NCHS approved the data collection protocol and the data files, containing no confidential information, that were published on the NHANES website for public use [20].

This investigation used NHANES data gathered during an 8-year period, from 2011–2018. Data from 2019–2020 were not available due to the COVID pandemic limiting the NHANES data collection process. The codes signifying ethical approval for NHANES data collected from 2011–2018 are: Protocol #2011–17 and Protocol #2018-01.

A total of 5665 adults were included in this study, ages 18–75 years. A 4-stage strategy was employed to randomly select non-institutionalized, civilian U.S. adults. Census information was utilized so that counties, then blocks, then dwelling units, and finally individuals were randomly selected, so that the final data are nationally representative [21].

Individuals who reported that they were diabetic, or took oral medication or insulin to control their blood sugar levels, or were found to have a fasting blood glucose concentration of 126 mg/dL or higher, were excluded from the sample. Those with hypoglycemia (fasting glucose < 70 mg/dL) were also excluded. Additionally, subjects who did not consume any kilocalories (kcal) during either of the two 24-h dietary recall assessments (i.e., they fasted) were excluded. Participants with extreme HOMA-IR levels ($\geq 4$ standard deviations above the mean) were excluded, and individuals who were underweight (BMI < 18.5) were excluded because of the likelihood of an eating disorder, severe frailty, or a serious disease.

## 2.2. Instrumentation and Measurement Methods

Macronutrient intake was the exposure variable for this study. A total of 10 macronutrients were studied. The outcome variable was insulin resistance, indexed using the homeostatic model assessment for insulin resistance (HOMA-IR). Age, sex, race, year of assessment, physical activity, cigarette smoking, alcohol use, and waist circumference were included as covariates, so their influence on the association between the exposure and outcome variables could be minimized.

### 2.2.1. Insulin Resistance

HOMA-IR is the most frequently used method of assessing insulin resistance. Over 18,600 published journal articles available in PUBMED include the term "HOMA" or "HOMA-IR." The HOMA-IR calculation was based on fasting plasma glucose and fasting insulin levels., specifically: fasting insulin ($\mu$U/mL) $\times$ fasting glucose (mg/dL) $\div$ 405. Subjects who were randomly assigned to attend a morning data collection session were asked to fast for 9 h for the fasting blood draw. Comprehensive information is provided by NHANES on their website about the glucose and insulin measurement protocols [22,23].

### 2.2.2. Macronutrient Intake

Two 24-h dietary recall assessments were used to gather the macronutrient data. The first diet interview occurred in-person. Data for the second recall interview was collected by telephone 3 to 10 days later. The average of the two assessments was used. Both dietary assessments gathered detailed information about all foods and beverages eaten during the 24-h period prior to the interview (midnight to midnight). Individuals reporting that they did not eat during one or both of the 24-h dietary assessment periods were not included in the analyses.

According to Willett, one 24-h dietary recall may be adequate if sample sizes are sufficiently large. He also states that, to estimate within-person variability, "it is statistically most efficient to increase the number of individuals in the sample, rather than to increase the number of days beyond 2 days per individual" (page 55) [24]. Given that the present study included over 5000 randomly selected adults, with each completing two 24-h dietary recalls 3–10 days apart, the assessment methods employed were more than satisfactory to secure quality estimates of dietary intake.

The diet recall interviewers were thoroughly trained in preparation for administering the diet assessments. They each had at least 10 college credits in nutrition courses, and each was a graduate in Food and Nutrition or Home Economics. Each of the individuals administering the diet recalls was bilingual and the dietary data collection occurred in a private setting in the NHANES mobile examination center (MEC). Interviewers were guided by scripts, and the computer-based program afforded a standard interview protocol. The diet assessments followed a multi-pass format called the Automated Multiple Pass Method (AMPM), available online [25]. The diet recall included food probes that have been used in previous United States Department of Agriculture (USDA) and NHANES surveys.

To help the participant, the in-person interviews included a number of real-life examples, such as different sized glasses, bowls, mugs, bottles, spoons, cups, plates, etc. After completing the first (in-person) diet interview, subjects were given sample cups, spoons, etc. and a food model booklet to take home to assist them during the telephone diet interview.

The present investigation included 10 macronutrients in order to study their relationship with insulin resistance: total carbohydrate, starch, simple carbohydrate, and fiber; total protein; total fat, polyunsaturated fat, monounsaturated fat, saturated fat, and total unsaturated fat. Except for dietary fiber intake, each of the macronutrients was reported as a percentage of the total energy consumed by the participant. Hence, total energy intake was taken into account for each macronutrient and for each participant. For fiber intake, the value was expressed as grams per 1000 kcal.

*2.3. Covariates*

NHANES classifies race into six categories: Mexican American, Non-Hispanic Black, Non-Hispanic White, Non-Hispanic Asian, Other Hispanic, or Other Race/Multi-racial. The NHANES racial categories were used as a covariate in the present study.

Waist circumference was utilized to index abdominal or central adiposity. Abdominal adiposity tends to be a better predictor of insulin resistance and diabetes than general obesity [16]. The measurement was taken by trained specialists. The procedures used by those performing the assessment were evaluated regularly to ensure high-quality performance. Measurement of the waist was taken in a customized room in the mobile examination center (MEC). Those taking the measurements were assisted by a trained recorder. The person taking the measurement and the assistant worked together to position, assess, and record the values precisely. The measuring tape was put around the body in a horizontal plane immediately above the top border of the ilium. To safeguard horizontal alignment of the tape, a wall mirror was utilized. The tape was placed snugly around the person, but the skin was not to be compressed. The measurement was finalized at the conclusion of a normal expiration [26].

Differences in physical activity levels were also used as a covariate. Physical activity was measured via interview. Participants were queried about the amount of time they spent in moderate and vigorous activities. Moderate activity was described as physical activity that results in small increases in breathing or heart rate, such as walking, carrying light loads or casual bike riding. Vigorous physical activity was explained as activity resulting in large increases in breathing or heart rate, such as jogging or running, walking up a moderate or steep incline, or lifting heavy loads.

Physical activity (PA) was assessed using specific questions asked by the NHANES interviewer: "In a typical week, on how many days do you do moderate-intensity sports, fitness, or recreational activities?" Also, "How much time do you spend doing moderate-intensity sports, fitness, or recreational activities on a typical day?" These questions, with slight alterations, were also used to assess vigorous PA. For the two intensities, days and minutes were multiplied together to produce the total minutes of moderate and total minutes of vigorous physical activity. These minutes were summed together to give total time (minutes) spent doing moderate and vigorous physical activity (MVPA).

The relationship between each of the primary macronutrients and insulin resistance was evaluated within three different sex-specific categories of physical activity. Participants who reported 0–30 min of activity per week were placed into the Low physical activity category. This category comprised approximately 45% of the sample. The remaining participants were divided equally between the Moderate and High physical activity categories. Specifically, females who reported 40 or more minutes and less than 180 min of activity per week were placed in the Moderate physical activity category. Males who reported 40 or more minutes and less than 240 min of activity per week were also placed in the Moderate physical activity category. Women reporting 180 min or more and men reporting 240 min or more of activity were placed in the High physical activity category.

Statistical adjustments were also made for differences in alcohol use in the current study. As part of the two 24-h dietary recall interviews, participants were asked to report their alcoholic beverage consumption. Those who reported that they did not drink any beverages containing alcohol were given a zero and alcohol consumers were assigned values based on the percentage of their total energy intake derived from alcohol.

Differences in cigarette smoking were also controlled statistically in this study. Smoking was measured by assessing the typical number of cigarettes smoked per day during the past month. An NHANES interviewer specifically asked, "During the past 30 days, on the days that you smoked, about how many cigarettes did you smoke?" Non-smokers were given the value of 0, whereas smokers had values up to 95 [27].

*2.4. Data Analysis*

A multi-level sampling technique was employed in this study so that the findings can be generalized to the U.S. adult population. To accomplish this, strata, clusters and individual sample weights were included in each statistical model.

With a sample size of 5665 individuals, a high level of statistical power would be expected in each statistical model. However, given the sampling strategy employed, degrees of freedom (df) were based on the number of clusters (121) minus the number of strata (58), resulting in 62 df, instead of 5665 df in the denominator.

There was one outcome variable (HOMA-IR) and 10 exposure variables (macronutrient intake) evaluated separately using multiple regression. A number of covariates were controlled statistically to reduce their influence on the relationship between the macronutrients and insulin resistance, specifically age, sex, race, year of assessment, physical activity, smoking, alcohol use, and waist circumference. Macronutrients could not be employed as covariates to determine their influence on the key relationships because of multicollinearity, tested by using the SAS variance inflation factor option (VIF). The VIF was 3.8 for total carbohydrate intake and 3.5 for total fat intake when in the same model. A VIF $\geq 2.5$ is considered problematic [28].

Two statistical analysis strategies were employed to measure the associations between the macronutrients and HOMA-IR. First, linear relationships were tested by treating both the exposure and outcome measures as continuous variables and using multiple regression and the SAS SurveyReg procedure. Second, one-way analysis of variance (ANOVA) was employed using the SAS SurveyReg procedure to measure mean differences in HOMA-IR across each macronutrient divided into tertiles. Tertile cut-points were: Total Carbohydrate: <44.10, 44.11–51.85, >51.85; Simple carbohydrate: <16.52, 16.53–23.59, >23.59%; Starch: <24.23, 24.24–29.51, >29.51; Fiber: <6.43, 6.44–9.31, >9.31; Total protein: <13.94, 13.95–17.24, >17.24; Total fat: 31.47, 31.48–37.44, >37.44; Saturated fat: <9.70, 9.71–12.36, >12.36; Unsaturated fat: <20.93, 20.94–25.20, >25.20; Monounsaturated fat: <10.60, 10.61–13.07, >13.07; Polyunsaturated fat: <6.70, 6.71–8.82, >8.82. The macronutrient categories were based on tertiles calculated using percentage of total kilocalories, so energy intake was taken into account for each macronutrient and each participant. Tertiles of total fiber consumption were categorized based on grams consumed per 1000 kilocalories (kcal).

Covariates were controlled using multiple regression and partial correlation, and the Least Squares Means (LSMeans) procedure was used to produce adjusted means. Effect modification was tested by dividing the macronutrients into tertiles and then analyzing the relationships between each primary macronutrient and HOMA-IR within the individual tertiles. Effect modification was also evaluated with physical activity divided into three categories and then analyzing the associations between each primary macronutrient and HOMA-IR within the three categories separately. Physical activity could not be divided into tertiles because over 40% of the subjects reported participating in no regular physical activity each week.

SAS version 9.4 (SAS Institute, Inc., Cary, NC, USA) was used to organized and examine the data. All the statistical tests were two-sided, and alpha was fixed at <0.05 to define statistical significance.

## 3. Results

The sampling strategy used by NHANES included 59 strata and 121 clusters selected randomly. There were 5665 subjects in the sample spread evenly from 2011–2018. Mean age ($\pm$ SE) was 43.7 $\pm$ 0.4 years. Mean ($\pm$ SE) energy intake for the two independent 24-h recall assessments was 2130 $\pm$ 14.0 kilocalories (kcals) per 24 h. Average ($\pm$ SE) HOMA-IR was 2.76 $\pm$ 0.05. Moreover, mean ($\pm$ SE) intake of the primary macronutrients, expressed as a percentage of total energy intake, was: total carbohydrate (48.0 $\pm$ 0.2), total protein (16.1 $\pm$ 0.1), and total fat (34.4 $\pm$ 0.1). Fiber intake averaged ($\pm$ SE) 8.5 $\pm$ 0.1 g per 1000 kcals. Mean ($\pm$ SE) waist circumference was 98.4 ($\pm$0.4) cm. Table 1 shows the distribution of values across percentiles for each of the key continuous variables.

Table 1. Percentile values of the key variables for 5665 adults representing the U.S. population.

| Variable | Percentile | | | | |
|---|---|---|---|---|---|
| | 10th | 25th | 50th | 75th | 90th |
| HOMA-IR | 0.86 | 1.30 | 2.06 | 3.43 | 5.37 |
| Energy Intake (kilocalories) | 1224 | 1570 | 2032 | 2585 | 3168 |
| Carbohydrate intake (% of kcal) | 36.10 | 41.94 | 48.06 | 54.05 | 59.93 |
| Starch intake (% of kcal) | 19.16 | 22.81 | 26.88 | 31.06 | 35.57 |
| Sugar intake (% of kcal) | 10.29 | 14.49 | 19.97 | 25.89 | 32.28 |
| Fiber intake (grams per 1000 kcal) | 4.37 | 5.86 | 7.73 | 10.34 | 13.49 |
| Protein intake (% of kcal) | 11.21 | 13.16 | 15.53 | 18.38 | 21.66 |
| Fat intake (% of kcal) | 25.32 | 29.64 | 34.48 | 39.11 | 43.41 |
| Saturated fat intake (% of kcal) | 7.18 | 9.04 | 10.99 | 13.19 | 15.25 |
| Polyunsaturated fat intake (% of kcal) | 4.94 | 6.16 | 7.76 | 9.49 | 11.57 |
| Monounsaturated fat intake (% of kcal) | 8.29 | 9.91 | 11.79 | 13.81 | 15.98 |
| Alcohol intake (% of kcal) | 0 | 0 | 0 | 3.26 | 9.78 |
| Smoking (cigarettes per day) | 0 | 0 | 0 | 0 | 9.37 |
| Physical activity (minutes of MVPA per wk) | 0 | 0 | 59 | 238 | 478 |
| Waist circumference (cm) | 78.74 | 86.65 | 96.57 | 107.73 | 119.00 |
| Age (years) | 22.26 | 30.04 | 42.73 | 55.85 | 65.02 |

HOMA-IR is the homeostatic model of assessment. % of kcal is the percentage of total kilocalories derived from the listed macronutrient. MVPA is moderate to vigorous physical activity.

Race and sex were treated as categorical variables in this investigation. Results indicated that 66.2% were Non-Hispanic White, 11.0% were Non-Hispanic Black, 8.4% were Mexican American, 6.2% were Other Hispanic, 4.7% were Non-Hispanic Asian, and 3.4% were Other-race or Multi-racial. The sample was comprised of 52.4% women and 47.6% men.

### 3.1. Dietary Carbohydrate and Insulin Resistance

The linear relationship between carbohydrate intake and HOMA-IR was studied with carbohydrate intake and insulin resistance both treated as continuous variables. After adjusting for the covariates (i.e., age, sex, race, year of assessment, smoking, alcohol, physical activity, and waist circumference) total carbohydrate intake was a significant predictor of HOMA-IR with 62 degrees of freedom. Specifically, as percent of kilocalories (kcal) from total carbohydrate increased, HOMA-IR increased linearly ($F = 6.7$, $p = 0.0121$), as shown in Table 2. Level of simple carbohydrate consumption was also positively and linearly related to HOMA-IR ($F = 4.7$, $p = 0.0344$). However, percentage of kcals from starch was not predictive of insulin resistance ($F = 1.8$, $p = 0.1886$). Grams of total fiber intake per 1000 kcals were inversely associated with HOMA-IR ($F = 9.1$, $p = 0.0037$). As fiber consumption increased, insulin resistance tended to decrease in a linear fashion (Table 2), after adjusting for the covariates.

The association between total carbohydrate consumption and HOMA-IR was also evaluated by comparing mean differences in HOMA-IR across tertile levels of carbohydrate intake (Table 3). As displayed in Table 3, results showed that adults in the lowest tertile of total carbohydrate intake had significantly less insulin resistance compared to the other two tertiles ($F = 10.4$, $p = 0.0001$). Similarly, those in the lowest tertile of simple carbohydrate consumption had lower HOMA-IR levels than the other two tertiles ($F = 4.8$, $p = 0.0117$). However, mean HOMA-IR levels did not differ across tertiles of starch intake. Finally, those in the highest one-third of fiber intake had significantly less insulin resistance than the other two tertiles ($F = 3.3$, $p = 0.0436$), as displayed in Table 3.

**Table 2.** Linear relationship between macronutrient consumption and HOMA-IR in a randomly selected sample of 5665 adults representing the U.S. population.

| Dietary Intake Variable | HOMA-IR | | | |
|---|---|---|---|---|
| | Regression Coefficient (Slope) | SE | F | p |
| Total Carbohydrate | 0.011 | 0.004 | 6.7 | 0.0121 |
| Simple Carbohydrate | 0.008 | 0.004 | 4.7 | 0.0344 |
| Starch | 0.008 | 0.006 | 1.8 | 0.1886 |
| Fiber | −0.023 | 0.008 | 9.1 | 0.0037 |
| Total Protein | −0.016 | 0.008 | 4.4 | 0.0393 |
| Total Fat | −0.013 | 0.005 | 5.5 | 0.0225 |
| Polyunsaturated Fat | −0.017 | 0.011 | 2.6 | 0.1102 |
| Monounsaturated Fat | −0.030 | 0.013 | 5.5 | 0.0224 |
| Unsaturated Fat | −0.016 | 0.006 | 6.5 | 0.0132 |
| Saturated Fat | −0.018 | 0.013 | 2.1 | 0.1513 |

Note: Each of the dietary intake variables was reported as the percentage of total kilocalories consumed by the participant. For example, if an individual consumed an average of 2000 kilocalories per day for the two 24-h dietary recall assessments, and the person averaged 250 g of carbohydrate intake per day, then the individual's total carbohydrate intake would be 50% of total kcals (250 g × 4 kcal = 1000 kcal; 1000/2000 = 0.50). The covariates for each model were age, sex, race, year of assessment, smoking, alcohol, physical activity, and waist circumference. There were 62 degrees of freedom (df) in the denominator for each model.

**Table 3.** Differences in mean HOMA-IR levels across tertiles of macronutrient intake in 5665 U.S. adults, after adjusting for covariates.

| Macronutrient | Macronutrient Category (Tertiles) | | | | |
|---|---|---|---|---|---|
| | Low | Moderate | High | | |
| | HOMA Mean ± SE | HOMA Mean ± SE | HOMA Mean ± SE | F | p |
| Total Carbohydrate | 2.7 [a] ± 0.06 | 3.1 [b] ± 0.06 | 3.0 [b] ± 0.07 | 10.4 | 0.0001 |
| Simple Carbohydrate | 2.8 [a] ± 0.06 | 3.0 [b] ± 0.07 | 3.0 [b] ± 0.07 | 4.8 | 0.0117 |
| Starch | 2.8 [a] ± 0.08 | 2.9 [a] ± 0.06 | 3.0 [a] ± 0.06 | 1.0 | 0.3759 |
| Fiber | 3.0 [a] ± 0.08 | 3.0 [a] ± 0.07 | 2.8 [b] ± 0.06 | 3.3 | 0.0436 |
| Total Protein | 3.0 [a] ± 0.08 | 3.0 [a] ± 0.06 | 2.8 [a] ± 0.05 | 1.5 | 0.2336 |
| Total Fat | 3.0 [a] ± 0.07 | 3.0 [a] ± 0.06 | 2.7 [b] ± 0.06 | 6.4 | 0.0030 |
| Saturated Fat | 3.0 [a] ± 0.07 | 2.9 [a] ± 0.06 | 2.8 [a] ± 0.06 | 1.6 | 0.2180 |
| Unsaturated Fat | 3.0 [a] ± 0.06 | 3.0 [a] ± 0.06 | 2.8 [b] ± 0.06 | 4.1 | 0.0218 |
| Monounsaturated Fat | 3.0 [a] ± 0.08 | 3.0 [a] ± 0.07 | 2.8 [a] ± 0.06 | 2.2 | 0.1194 |
| Polyunsaturated Fat | 3.0 [a] ± 0.06 | 3.0 [a] ± 0.06 | 2.8 [a] ± 0.06 | 1.8 | 0.1752 |

[a,b] Means on the same row with the same superscript letter do not differ significantly. The difference in HOMA-IR between the moderate and high fiber groups was borderline significant ($p = 0.0915$). All means were adjusted for differences in the covariates: age, sex, race, year of assessment, physical activity, smoking, alcohol, and waist circumference. Tertile cut-points were: Total Carbohydrate: <44.10%, 44.10–51.85%, >51.85; Sugar: <16.52%, 16.53–23.59%, >23.59%; Starch: <24.23, 24.24–29.51, >29.51; Fiber: <6.43, 6.44–9.31, >9.31; Total protein: <13.94, 13.95–17.24, >17.24; Total fat: 31.47, 31.48–37.44, >37.44; Saturated fat: <9.70, 9.71–12.36, >12.36; Unsaturated fat: <20.93, 20.94–25.20, >25.20; Monounsaturated fat: <10.60, 10.61–13.07, >13.07; Polyunsaturated fat: <6.70, 6.71–8.82, >8.82. The macronutrient categories were based on tertiles calculated using percentage of total kilocalories. Tertiles of fiber intake were categorized based on grams consumed per 1000 kilocalories.

### 3.2. Dietary Protein and Insulin Resistance

Percent of kcals derived from dietary protein was also a significant predictor of insulin resistance ($F = 4.4$, $p = 0.0393$). The association was linear and inverse. As total protein consumption increased, insulin resistance tended to decrease (Table 2). However, when mean HOMA-IR levels were compared across tertiles of total protein intake, mean differences were not significant (Table 3).

### 3.3. Dietary Fat and Insulin Resistance

As displayed in Table 2, total dietary fat intake, recorded as a percentage of total kcals, was a significant predictor of HOMA-IR ($F = 5.5$, $p = 0.0225$), with 62 df and both measures treated as continuous variables. The relationship was linear and inverse. Specifically, as total fat intake increased, insulin resistance decreased, after controlling for the potential confounding variables. Conversely, the association between polyunsaturated fat consumption and HOMA-IR was not statistically significant (F = 2.6, $p$ = 0.1102). However, the relationship between monounsaturated fat and insulin resistance was significant and inverse (F = 5.5, $p$ = 0.0224). Additionally, with polyunsaturated and monounsaturated fat intake combined, the association between unsaturated fat intake and HOMA-IR was significant and inverse (F = 6.5, $p$ = 0.0132). Level of saturated fat consumption was not predictive of HOMA-IR (F = 2.1, $p$ = 0.1513), with the covariates controlled.

With total fat consumption divided into equal categories, mean HOMA-IR levels differed significantly across the tertiles (F = 6.4, $p$ = 0.0030), as shown in Table 3. Specifically, subjects in the highest tertile of total fat intake had significantly less insulin resistance compared to those in the middle or lowest tertile of fat consumption. However, mean levels of insulin resistance did not differ significantly across tertiles of saturated, polyunsaturated, or monounsaturated fat intakes (Table 3). However, with poly- and monounsaturated fat intakes combined, mean HOMA-IR levels differed significantly across tertiles of unsaturated fat (F = 4.1, $p$ = 0.0218). Specifically, adults in the highest tertile of unsaturated fat intake had significantly lower levels of HOMA-IR compared to the other two tertiles.

### 3.4. Effect Modification

Isolating the association between macronutrient consumption and insulin resistance is challenging. Consuming more of some foods typically results in consuming less of others. Macronutrients are intercorrelated. Using multiple regression and partial correlation to control statistically for differences in a macronutrient, such as dietary fat intake, when studying the relationship between carbohydrate consumption and insulin resistance, typically results in problems associated with multicollinearity, making the findings invalid or uncertain. Although different from partial correlation, testing for effect modification can help clarify the interaction between each macronutrient and insulin resistance.

As displayed in Table 4, when delimited to individual tertiles of total dietary fat intake, carbohydrate consumption was not related to HOMA-IR. Similarly, total protein intake and dietary fat consumption were not associated with insulin resistance within any of the fat intake tertiles (Table 4).

**Table 4.** Linear relationships between the primary macronutrients and HOMA-IR within tertiles of dietary fat intake, after controlling for the covariates.

| | Total Dietary Fat Intake | | | | | | | | |
|---|---|---|---|---|---|---|---|---|---|
| | Lowest Tertile Only | | | Middle Tertile Only | | | Highest Tertile Only | | |
| Predictor | Regression Coefficient ± SE | F | $p$ | Regression Coefficient ± SE | F | $p$ | Regression Coefficient ± SE | F | $p$ |
| Carbohydrate | 0.001 ± 0.007 | 0.0 | 0.9274 | 0.010 ± 0.012 | 0.7 | 0.4056 | 0.009 ± 0.008 | 1.5 | 0.2203 |
| Protein | −0.011 ± 0.010 | 1.1 | 0.2901 | −0.019 ± 0.014 | 2.3 | 0.1390 | −0.019 ± 0.014 | 1.9 | 0.1725 |
| Fat | −0.010 ± 0.014 | 0.5 | 0.4795 | −0.012 ± 0.033 | 0.1 | 0.7213 | −0.006 ± 0.012 | 0.2 | 0.6415 |

SE = standard error of the regression coefficient. Total dietary fat intake was divided into tertiles. The relationships between insulin resistance (HOMA-IR) and consumption of total carbohydrate, total protein, and total fat were evaluated separately within each of the three dietary fat tertiles. Age, sex, race, year of assessment, physical activity, smoking, alcohol, and waist circumference were the covariates. Each of the analyses had 62 degrees of freedom (df) in the denominator.

According to Table 5, none of the primary macronutrients were significantly related to insulin resistance within the lowest tertile of protein intake. Similarly, none were associated with insulin resistance when the sample was delimited to the middle tertile of protein consumption. On the other hand, total carbohydrate, protein, and fat intakes were each related to HOMA-IR in adults reporting a high protein diet. The carbohydrate and HOMA-IR association was positive (direct), and the protein and fat intake correlations were negative (inverse).

**Table 5.** Linear relationships between the primary macronutrients and HOMA-IR within tertiles of dietary protein intake, after controlling for the covariates.

|  | Total Protein Intake | | | | | | | | |
|---|---|---|---|---|---|---|---|---|---|
|  | Lowest Tertile Only | | | Middle Tertile Only | | | Highest Tertile Only | | |
| Predictor | Regression Coefficient ± SE | F | p | Regression Coefficient ± SE | F | p | Regression Coefficient ± SE | F | p |
| Carbohydrate | 0.005 ± 0.008 | 0.4 | 0.5384 | 0.006 ± 0.008 | 0.5 | 0.4800 | 0.021 ± 0.007 | 10.0 | 0.0025 |
| Protein | 0.025 ± 0.035 | 0.5 | 0.4821 | −0.077 ± 0.060 | 1.7 | 0.1969 | −0.028 ± 0.011 | 6.4 | 0.0137 |
| Fat | −0.009 ± 0.008 | 1.5 | 0.2262 | −0.005 ± 0.008 | 0.5 | 0.5054 | −0.022 ± 0.007 | 8.7 | 0.0045 |

SE = standard error of the regression coefficient. Total dietary protein intake was divided into tertiles. The relationships between insulin resistance (HOMA-IR) and consumption of total carbohydrate, total protein, and total fat were evaluated separately within each of the three dietary protein tertiles. Age, sex, race, year of assessment, physical activity, smoking, alcohol, and waist circumference were the covariates. Each of the analyses had 62 degrees of freedom (df) in the denominator.

As revealed in Table 6, among adults reporting a high carbohydrate diet (highest tertile), none of the primary macronutrients were related to HOMA-IR. With the sample delimited to adults in the middle tertile of carbohydrate intake, fat intake was inversely related to HOMA-IR. Among those eating a low carbohydrate diet, protein intake was inversely related and carbohydrate intake was directly associated with insulin resistance. The carbohydrate correlation was borderline significant.

**Table 6.** Linear relationships between the primary macronutrients and HOMA-IR within tertiles of dietary carbohydrate intake, after controlling for the covariates.

|  | Total Carbohydrate Intake | | | | | | | | |
|---|---|---|---|---|---|---|---|---|---|
|  | Lowest Tertile Only | | | Middle Tertile Only | | | Highest Tertile Only | | |
| Predictor | Regression Coefficient ± SE | F | p | Regression Coefficient ± SE | F | p | Regression Coefficient ± SE | F | p |
| Carbohydrate | 0.018 ± 0.009 | 3.7 | 0.0585 | −0.006 ± 0.030 | 0.1 | 0.8310 | 0.006 ± 0.010 | 0.4 | 0.5459 |
| Protein | −0.023 ± 0.011 | 5.1 | 0.0281 | 0.031 ± 0.017 | 3.2 | 0.0775 | −0.014 ± 0.016 | 0.8 | 0.3861 |
| Fat | −0.001 ± 0.009 | 0.0 | 0.8874 | −0.034 ± 0.017 | 4.1 | 0.0476 | −0.005 ± 0.010 | 0.2 | 0.6419 |

SE = standard error of the regression coefficient. Total carbohydrate intake was divided into tertiles. The relationships between insulin resistance (HOMA-IR) and consumption of total carbohydrate, total protein, and total fat were evaluated separately within each of the three dietary carbohydrate tertiles. Age, sex, race, year of assessment, physical activity, smoking, alcohol, and waist circumference were the covariates. Each of the analyses had 62 degrees of freedom (df) in the denominator.

As shown in Table 7, there were no significant relationships between macronutrient consumption and insulin resistance in the Moderate or High physical activity categories. However, among participants who reported Low physical activity, dietary fat intake was inversely related to HOMA-IR and total carbohydrate consumption was associated with HOMA-IR in a direct and significant relationship. Protein intake was not related to insulin resistance within any of the physical activity categories, Low, Moderate, or High.

Table 7. Linear relationships between the primary macronutrients and HOMA-IR within 3 categories of physical activity, after controlling for the covariates.

| | Physical Activity Category | | | | | | | | |
|---|---|---|---|---|---|---|---|---|---|
| | Low Physical Activity | | | Moderate Physical Activity | | | High Physical Activity | | |
| Predictor | Regression Coefficient ± SE | F | p | Regression Coefficient ± SE | F | p | Regression Coefficient ± SE | F | p |
| Carbohydrate | 0.013 ± 0.006 | 4.0 | 0.0497 | 0.009 ± 0.006 | 2.6 | 0.1156 | 0.009 ± 0.007 | 1.4 | 0.2466 |
| Protein | −0.009 ± 0.013 | 0.5 | 0.5033 | −0.018 ± 0.011 | 2.3 | 0.1309 | −0.015 ± 0.009 | 2.1 | 0.1487 |
| Fat | −0.017 ± 0.007 | 5.7 | 0.0203 | −0.010 ± 0.008 | 1.3 | 0.2551 | −0.009 ± 0.008 | 1.2 | 0.2801 |

SE = standard error of the regression coefficient. Total physical activity was divided into 3 categories. Adults with Low weekly physical activity (30 min or less per week) comprised 45% of the sample. The remaining 55% was divided into sex-specific equal categories with approximately 27.5% of the sample in each. For females, the cut-point dividing between Moderate and High physical activity was 180 min per week. For males, the cut-point was 240 min per week. The relationships between the primary macronutrients and insulin resistance (HOMA-IR) were evaluated separately within each of the three physical activity categories. Age, sex, race, year of assessment, smoking, alcohol, and waist circumference were the covariates. Each of the analyses had 62 degrees of freedom (df) in the denominator.

## 4. Discussion

The chief objective of the present study was to evaluate the relationships between multiple dietary macronutrient intakes and insulin resistance, measured using HOMA-IR, in 5665 randomly selected U.S. adults. Several potential confounding variables were controlled statistically to help isolate the association between the macronutrient intakes and HOMA-IR. Effect modification across tertiles of the primary macronutrients and physical activity were also evaluated.

There were seven major outcomes in this study: (1) Macronutrient intake was predictive of insulin resistance measured by HOMA-IR in U.S. adults. (2) Both total carbohydrate and simple carbohydrate intakes were positively and linearly related to HOMA-IR, but starch consumption was not associated with HOMA-IR. (3) Fiber intake was inversely related to HOMA-IR. (4) Protein intake was inversely associated with HOMA-IR when both variables were treated as continuous, but protein consumption was not associated with HOMA-IR when protein intake was divided into tertiles. (5) Total fat consumption was linearly and inversely related to HOMA-IR, along with monounsaturated fat intake, when both were treated as continuous measures. However, polyunsaturated and saturated fats were not related to HOMA-IR. Unsaturated fat intake (poly- and monounsaturated fats combined) was linearly and inversely related to HOMA-IR, whether or not the association was analyzed with both variables treated as continuous or with unsaturated fat intake divided into tertiles. (6) With dietary fat intake divided into tertiles, none of the primary macronutrients were predictive of HOMA-IR when confined within the tertiles. (7) None of the primary macronutrients were predictive of HOMA-IR within the Moderate or High physical activity categories, but only within the Low physical activity group.

### 4.1. Dietary Carbohydrate

In the present investigation, as carbohydrate consumption increased, insulin resistance increased in a linear fashion. Simple carbohydrate intake followed a similar pattern, but starch intake was not related to insulin resistance. Numerous scientists have studied the relationship between carbohydrate intake and insulin resistance. However, findings focusing on this relationship vary widely [29].

In a cross-sectional analysis of the Framingham Offspring Study by McKeown et al. with 2834 participants, total carbohydrate intake was not associated with HOMA-IR [30], conflicting with the present findings. On the other hand, whole grain intake and fiber consumption were significantly related to lower levels of insulin resistance. When high glycemic index foods were consumed in larger amounts (i.e., typically indicating more simple carbohydrate intake), HOMA-IR was also significantly higher. On the other hand, in a cross-sectional study of 173 south Asian and European men, elevated insulin levels were directly related to carbohydrate intake ($p = 0.001$) [31], similar to this investigation.

Findings from the Inter99 study revealed that grams of sucrose, glucose, and fructose were each inversely related to HOMA-IR, whereas the association was positively associated with daily lactose intake [32]. Each of these relationships was significant or borderline significant. Note that in the Inter99 investigation, simple sugar intakes were expressed as grams per day, not as a percent of total energy intake.

Randomized controlled trials afford a different perspective. For example, Borkman et al. compared the effect of a high carbohydrate diet or a high fat diet (mostly saturated fat) on insulin sensitivity over three weeks [33]. The diets were administered in random order. Whole body glucose uptake using euglycemic glucose clamps revealed no change or difference in the effects of the diets on insulin sensitivity. Similarly, Garg et al. studied eight men with mild diabetes using a randomized cross-over investigation [34]. Diets were isocaloric and either high carbohydrate (60% of kcal) or low carbohydrate (35% of kcal). The low carbohydrate diet was high in monounsaturated fat. Plasma glucose and insulin responses were equal and insulin sensitivity via clamp at the end of each period were not different.

There is evidence that postprandial glycemic and insulinemic responses to foods differ based on the amount and characteristics of the carbohydrate ingested [35–37]. As shown in the McKeown investigation above, the glycemic index (GI) can be used to study the degree to which glucose levels are affected by carbohydrate type [36]

According to a randomized cross-over study in diabetic men by Rizkalla et al., four-weeks on a low glycemic diet produced lower postprandial glucose and insulin levels and areas under the curve than 4-weeks on a high GI diet [38]. Overall, whole-body glucose use, assessed using the euglycemic clamp, favored the low glycemic diet [38]. Similarly, Juanola-Falgarona et al. directed a six-month study of 122 overweight or obese adults to evaluate the effect of two moderate-carbohydrate diets or a low-fat diet, each with energy restriction, and different glycemic index scores, on a variety of cardio-metabolic outcomes, including HOMA-IR [39]. Results showed that insulin resistance was decreased more in the low-GI group than the low-fat group.

Several prospective investigations have studied the relationship between the dietary glycemic index and the development of type II diabetes, a common consequence of insulin resistance [40]. Specifically, Villegas et al. studied a cohort of over 64,000 Chinese women with no history of diabetes or other chronic disease for almost five years [41]. Divided into quintiles, the highest GI group had 21% greater risk of developing diabetes than the lowest quintile, and 34% greater risk based on glycemic load. When the focus was simply on carbohydrate intake rather than glycemic index, the highest quintile had 28% higher risk of developing diabetes than the lowest quintile [41]. On the other hand, in a smaller cohort study of Japanese men, Sakurai showed that men in the upper quintile of the glycemic index had 80% higher risk of developing diabetes compared to the lowest quintile, although the fourth and fifth quintiles based on glycemic load did not differ from the lowest quintile [42].

In a five-year prospective study of older Australians by Barclay et al., consumption of total carbohydrate, sugar, starch, and fiber, evaluated separately, were not predictive of the development of type 2 diabetes. However, in adults younger than 70 years old, higher intake levels on the glycemic index were predictive of higher incidence of diabetes over time [43].

Three large prospective cohort investigations, the Nurses' Health Study [44], the Health Professionals Follow-up Study [45], and the Iowa Women's Health Study [46] investigated the extent to which total carbohydrate intake influences risk of developing diabetes over time. None of these investigations found an association between total carbohydrate consumption and diabetes incidence. On the other hand, Swishburn et al. designed a five-year prospective cohort investigation which showed that a low fat, moderately high carbohydrate diet was correlated with reduced insulin resistance and decreased risk of developing diabetes in adults with diminished glucose tolerance [47].

*4.2. Dietary Fiber*

Fiber intake and insulin resistance were strongly and inversely related. Similar to the current study, many investigations indicate that diets with high fiber content have beneficial effects on insulin sensitivity. Specifically, Fukagawa et al. studied 12 healthy individuals before and after 3–4 weeks of a high carbohydrate and high fiber diet [48]. Glucose disposal using the euglycemic clamp was measured. The high carbohydrate and high fiber diet reduced fasting glucose and insulin levels substantially and glucose disposal rates were also improved significantly. Similarly, Pereira et al. looked at the effect of a whole grain compared to a refined grain diet on insulin sensitivity using a randomized crossover design in 11 overweight, hyper-insulinemic adults [49]. Energy needs were balanced to prevent weight gain. Insulin sensitivity was significantly better when on the whole grain compared to the refined grain diet.

Using a cross-sectional design and baseline values from the Inter99 study, Lau et al. employed Danish adults to study the association between fiber consumption and HOMA-IR [32]. A food frequency questionnaire (FFQ) was utilized to assess fiber intake. Fiber was reported in total grams, not grams per 1000 kcal. Even after controlling for a variety of covariates, the relationship between fiber intake per day and HOMA-IR remained significant and inverse.

Lutsey et al. studied the association between whole grain intake and HOMA-IR in the MESA (Multi-Ethnic Study of Atherosclerosis) investigation [50]. Findings indicated that as whole grain intake increased, HOMA-IR decreased, even after adjusting for potential mediating factors.

Cross-sectional outcomes were also the focus of the Insulin Resistance Atherosclerosis Study by Liese et al. [51]. Fiber intake was measured by a food frequency questionnaire. Fiber consumption was not reported as grams per 1000 kcal. Findings revealed that fiber intake was associated directly with insulin sensitivity.

In general, it appears that the link between fiber intake and insulin resistance is strong and consistent. Current dietary recommendations in the United States encourage significant amounts of whole-grains and high-fiber foods, consistent with the literature [52].

*4.3. Dietary Protein*

Fewer studies have investigated the relationship between protein intake compared to carbohydrate consumption and insulin resistance. Overall, findings have been mixed. In a large, cross-sectional study that included 5675 non-diabetic subjects, a food frequency questionnaire (FFQ) was employed to measure total protein intake [32]. Across quartiles of insulin resistance, mean protein intake levels, reported as a percentage of total energy, increased as HOMA-IR increased ($p = 0.001$), after adjusting for potential confounders.

Protein consumption has an insulinotropic effect. In short, protein intake results in insulin release, which leads to increased glucose clearance from the blood. Despite these predictable outcomes, insulin resistance findings of short-term intervention trials vary, depending on the characteristics of the sample and the source of the protein. For example, according to Kahleova et al., in a 16-week randomized controlled trial, plant-based protein intake was predictive of reduced insulin resistance, whereas animal protein had the opposite effects [53]. However, most of the protein and insulin resistance associations of Kahleova's study were no longer significant after controlling for changes in BMI and energy intake, suggesting that nearly all the relationships were driven by weight loss. On the other hand, according to Adevia-Andany et al., the association between animal protein intake and insulin resistance is independent of body mass index [54].

Several other short-term trials show that protein intake has no effect on insulin resistance when the sample is healthy [55,56]. However, not all studies agree. Some indicate that protein consumption reduces plasma insulin levels [57].

In obese subjects, the influence of protein on insulin resistance is unpredictable. As shown in a review by Rietman et al., some investigations indicate that protein intake improves insulin resistance, whereas other studies indicate there is no effect [55]. Still others suggest that the outcome is dependent on whether or not weight is lost [55].

Prospective cohort investigations have also produced varied results. In a cohort study with 1205 subjects, Asghari et al. determined that intake of several individual branch-chain amino acids was related to increased risk of developing insulin resistance over 2.3 years [58]. However, total branch-chain amino acid consumption was not related to incident insulin resistance.

In another prospective cohort investigation, Chen et al. followed 6822 participants for over 20 years [59]. Baseline protein intake, particularly animal protein consumption, was positively related to HOMA-IR, increased risk of pre-diabetes, and diabetes. Total plant protein was not associated with any of the metabolic problems, including insulin resistance or diabetes [59].

According to Rietman et al., increasing amino acid levels in the blood by consuming protein can lead to insulin resistance by preventing muscle glucose transport and phosphorylation of glucose with ensuing decreased glycogen synthesis [55]. Hence, protein intake can contribute to alterations in insulin sensitivity and promote insulin resistance [60]. Long-term investigations are likely to capture this process better than studies of short duration or cross-sectional studies.

### 4.4. Dietary Fat

Research findings also vary concerning the relationship between dietary fat intake and insulin resistance. In a high-quality intervention by Samaha et al., after six months on a high fat diet, insulin sensitivity improved among obese subjects [61]. In another investigation, Bisschop et al. designed a cross-over study using six healthy men [62]. Subjects ate each of three isocaloric diets for 11 days. The diets were low-fat with high carbohydrate, intermediate fat and intermediate carbohydrate, and high fat with low carbohydrate. Insulin sensitivity was measured using the clamp method. The ratio of fat to carbohydrate in the diets had no effect on glucose uptake. However, glucose disposal tended to increase as the fat to carbohydrate ratios in the diets increased.

Bradley et al. used a RCT to test the effect of a low-fat versus a low-carbohydrate weight reduction diet ($-500$ kcals) on insulin resistance in 24 overweight/obese adults over an 8-week period [63]. Insulin action was measured using the clamp method. Significant weight loss occurred in both groups but there was no difference between the two groups in insulin resistance at the conclusion of the study.

Using a cross-sectional design and 7-day weighed food records, no relationship was found between saturated fat intake and serum insulin concentrations in nearly 200 middle-aged men [31]. However, in a sample of 389 older men, ages 70–89, intake of polyunsaturated fats was inversely associated with insulin levels and saturated fat intake was directly related to insulin concentrations [64]. Additionally, using cross-sectional data from the Inter99 study, total fat intake, expressed as a percentage of total kcal, was not related to quartiles of HOMA-IR [32].

According to Rivellese et al., animal studies indicate that insulin action is not only affected by the amount of fat consumed, but the type of fat also has a significant influence [65]. Specifically, saturated fatty acids tend to increase insulin resistance, whereas long- and short-chain omega-3 fatty acids tend to enhance insulin sensitivity.

As part of the multicenter KANWU study, 162 healthy subjects were fed an isoenergetic diet for 3-months with either a high level of saturated or monounsaturated fatty acids [66]. Insulin sensitivity was 12.5% lower on the saturated fat diet and 8.8% higher when the focus was on monounsaturated fat intake. The difference in insulin sensitivity was not present when total fat intake was high.

In a 16-week RCT by Kahleova and Fleeman et al., overweight subjects were randomized to follow a randomized low-fat vegan ($n = 38$) or control diet ($n = 37$) [67]. HOMA-IR was used to index insulin resistance. The authors concluded that even after adjusting for differences in energy intake and body mass, decreased intakes of saturated and trans fats and increased consumption of polyunsaturated fats decreased fat mass and insulin resistance.

High quality clinical studies designed to assess the effect of dietary fat on insulin resistance typically use isocaloric substitution methods to prevent changes in body weight. This safeguard is crucial for accurately determining the influence of dietary fat on insulin sensitivity. However, one of the most important contributors to insulin resistance is weight gain and obesity. Hence, inhibiting weigh gain by using an isoenergetic diet may result in false judgments about the effect of dietary fat on insulin resistance because weight gain is prevented. In the general public, ad libitum, high fat diets often lead to weight gain [68–70]. In short, it is likely that many dietary fat and insulin resistance intervention studies have questionable external validity because of the use of this common substitution strategy.

### 4.5. Effect Modification

Rarely have researchers studied the relationship between diet composition and insulin resistance across tertiles of carbohydrate, protein, and fat intake considered separately. Nor have researchers evaluated the association between diet composition and insulin resistance across categories of physical activity. In the present study, there were several unique effect modification findings. For example, none of the primary macronutrients were related to insulin resistance when evaluated within fat intake tertiles. Specifically, total carbohydrate consumption was not related to insulin resistance in adults when the focus was only on those reporting a low-fat, a moderate-fat, or a high-fat diet. Yet, total carbohydrate consumption was directly associated with insulin resistance when participants were not restricted to fat intake tertiles. These results suggest that the relationship between carbohydrate intake and insulin resistance is partly due to the wide-ranging variation in fat intake across the U.S. diet. In short, when delimited to individual tertiles of fat intake, the shared variation necessary for the carbohydrate and insulin resistance association to manifest itself is not sufficient, but when differences in fat intake are not restricted, carbohydrate intake is a significant predictor of insulin resistance.

The same pattern appears to be true for both protein and fat intakes. Specifically, there was no relationship between either of these primary macronutrients and insulin resistance when the associations were confined to fat intake tertiles. However, like carbohydrate consumption, protein and fat intakes were each significant predictors of insulin resistance when the wide-spread variation in fat intake was not restricted to tertiles. Apparently, differences in total fat intake play an important role in the relationships between macronutrient consumption and insulin resistance in U.S. adults.

Effect modification across tertiles of carbohydrate and protein also seems to affect the macronutrient and insulin resistance associations. This is logical because of the intercorrelations among the macronutrients. However, confining subjects to tertiles of carbohydrate or tertiles of protein appears to have less influence on the macronutrient and HOMA-IR relationships than restricting subjects to tertiles of dietary fat.

Also of interest, each of the three primary macronutrients were related to HOMA-IR, but only within the highest protein intake tertile. Macronutrient consumption was not predictive of insulin resistance in adults reporting low or moderate protein intake.

Effect modification was also tested within three categories of physical activity. Only two of the nine associations were significant and both relationships, carbohydrate and fat, were within the low physical activity category. These findings suggest that macronutrient intake may not play as significant a role in insulin resistance when physical activity levels are moderate or high. It could be that if physical activity levels are sufficient, macronutrient consumption may be less important to the development of insulin resistance.

### 4.6. Application of the Results

As shown in Tables 2 and 3, total carbohydrate and simple carbohydrate consumption were related directly to insulin resistance in U.S. adults. However, fiber, protein, and dietary fat consumption, particularly unsaturated fat, were inversely related to HOMA-IR. Consequently, the temptation would be to conclude that a diet with less carbohydrate, particularly fewer simple carbohydrates, and with more fiber, protein, and unsaturated fat, should be recommended. Of course, such advice would be overreaching the cross-sectional design of this study. Instead, the present results should be considered as additional evidence supporting other investigations that have found similar dietary patterns associated with insulin resistance.

*4.7. Intricacies of the Diet and Insulin Resistance Relationship*

Dietary relationships are complex. An inherent issue associated with the study of diet composition is that higher consumption of one macronutrient usually translates into lower intake of another. For example, when dietary fat is decreased in the diet, carbohydrate intake is usually increased. Foods are not eaten in isolation. The obvious question is whether the outcome is caused by the increased intake of carbohydrates or the decreased consumption of dietary fat, or some other combination? Randomized controlled trials (RCT) are especially vulnerable to this issue because diets are assigned and manipulated. Compliance is also a concern and can have a significant influence on findings.

Insulin resistance is not a simple phenotype. It appears that different tissues have different levels of sensitivity to insulin. Without question, the complexity surrounding the biology of insulin action has led to multiple interpretations of the relationships between diet composition and insulin resistance [1].

There are a number of investigations in the literature about diet composition and insulin resistance. Comparing these investigations is challenging for a variety of reasons. For example, was the study design cross-sectional, prospective, or based on an intervention? Was it short-term or long-term? Was there a control group? What was the composition of the control diet? Did participants gain weight or lose weight? What was the protein source, animal or plant? What was the composition of the dietary fat, saturated or unsaturated? What was the composition of the carbohydrate, simple or complex? How much fiber was in the diet? Was the fiber soluble or insoluble? Were participants younger or older, normal weight, overweight, or obese? Were subjects diabetic or non-diabetic? Clearly, studies focusing on the relationship between diet composition and insulin resistance have produced mixed results partly because investigations that look similar on the surface often have important differences in their samples, designs, and measurement methods.

*4.8. Weaknesses and Strengths of the Study*

The present investigation had multiple weaknesses. Because the study was based on a cross-sectional design, cause-and-effect conclusions cannot be applied. Additionally, there was only a single measure of protein consumption, i.e., total protein intake. It was not divided by NHANES into animal-derived or plant-based protein. Similarly, fiber intake was not categorized by NHANES as soluble or insoluble, but only as total grams of fiber. Moreover, although two 24-h dietary recalls were obtained from each subject, and the sample was very large (>5000 individuals), in general, the more dietary assessments, the more representative the dietary data will tend to be.

This investigation also had several strengths. First, participants were randomly selected using a four-stage sampling model, making the results generalizable to the U.S. civilian, non-institutionalized adult population. Second, a large ($n$ = 5665), multi-racial sample was utilized, including subjects who were Mexican American, Non-Hispanic Black, Non-Hispanic White, Non-Hispanic Asian, Other Hispanic, or Other Race/Multi-racial. Third, carbohydrate intake was divided into total carbohydrate, starch, simple carbohydrate, and fiber. Fat was broken into total fat, polyunsaturated, monounsaturated, unsaturated, and saturated fat. Fourth, a number of potential confounding factors, demographic and lifestyle, were controlled statistically to minimize their influence on the results. Fifth, although the cross-sectional design employed in this study has weaknesses, in correlational research, dietary intake can be studied using an ad libitum perspective because usual macronutrient intake is the focus. The present investigation took advantage of this strength. Participants were required to report what they had eaten during the previous 24 h, on two different days. As a result, degree of insulin resistance was evaluated based on usual macronutrient consumption, without concern for artificial manipulation of intake, or lack of compliance among participants.

## 5. Conclusions

In conclusion, evidence from the present investigation, conducted using participants representing the U.S. adult population, clearly shows that diet composition accounts for differences in insulin resistance. Higher intakes of carbohydrate predicted higher levels of insulin resistance. However, a closer look indicated that starch consumption was not related to insulin resistance, and fiber intake fits hand-in-hand with increased insulin sensitivity. Furthermore, elevated consumption of simple carbohydrates was predictive of higher levels of insulin resistance. Additionally, higher intakes of protein predicted lower levels of insulin resistance, but not with protein intake divided into tertiles. Also, higher amounts of fat consumption, particularly unsaturated fat, predicted lower levels of insulin resistance. Adjusting for differences in many demographic and lifestyle variables seemed to have little influence on the relationships. However, testing for effect modification indicated that the wide-range of dietary fat intake in the U.S. may play an important role in the macronutrient and insulin resistance associations. Moreover, evaluation of effect modification also showed that moderate to high levels of physical activity may reduce the role of macronutrient intake on insulin resistance. Overall, because numerous studies focusing on diet composition and insulin resistance have been conducted to date with broadly differing results, more investigations are needed to untangle the complex associations between diet composition and insulin resistance.

**Funding:** This research received no external funding.

**Institutional Review Board Statement:** The study was conducted according to the guidelines of the Declaration of Helsinki and approved by the Institutional Review Board of the National Center for Health Statistics, now referred to as the Ethics Review Board (ERB). The ethical approval codes for NHANES data collection for 2011–2018 are: Protocols #2011-17, #2018-01.

**Informed Consent Statement:** Written informed consent was obtained from all subjects involved in the study.

**Data Availability Statement:** All data supporting reported results can be found online as part of the National Health and Nutrition Examination Survey (NHANES). The data are free and can be found at the following website: https://wwwn.cdc.gov/nchs/nhanes/Default.aspx. (accessed on 21 February 2022).

**Acknowledgments:** Much appreciation is extended to the NHANES technicians who performed the measurements and gathered the data. Also, to those who participated as subjects in the survey.

**Conflicts of Interest:** The author declares no conflict of interest.

## References

1. Bessesen, D.H. The role of carbohydrates in insulin resistance. *J. Nutr.* **2001**, *131*, 2782S–2786S. [CrossRef] [PubMed]
2. Gast, K.B.; Tjeerdema, N.; Stijnen, T.; Smit, J.W.; Dekkers, O.M. Insulin resistance and risk of incident cardiovascular events in adults without diabetes: Meta-analysis. *PLoS ONE* **2012**, *7*, e52036. [CrossRef] [PubMed]
3. Pyorala, K. Relationship of glucose tolerance and plasma insulin to the incidence of coronary heart disease: Results from two population studies in Finland. *Diabetes Care* **1979**, *2*, 131–141. [CrossRef] [PubMed]
4. Despres, J.P.; Lamarche, B.; Mauriege, P.; Cantin, B.; Dagenais, G.R.; Moorjani, S.; Lupien, P.J. Hyperinsulinemia as an independent risk factor for ischemic heart disease. *N. Engl. J. Med.* **1996**, *334*, 952–957. [CrossRef] [PubMed]
5. Janus, A.; Szahidewicz-Krupska, E.; Mazur, G.; Doroszko, A. Insulin Resistance and Endothelial Dysfunction Constitute a Common Therapeutic Target in Cardiometabolic Disorders. *Mediat. Inflamm.* **2016**, *2016*, 3634948. [CrossRef]
6. Bornfeldt, K.E.; Tabas, I. Insulin resistance, hyperglycemia, and atherosclerosis. *Cell Metab.* **2011**, *14*, 575–585. [CrossRef]
7. Deng, X.L.; Liu, Z.; Wang, C.; Li, Y.; Cai, Z. Insulin resistance in ischemic stroke. *Metab. Brain Dis.* **2017**, *32*, 1323–1334. [CrossRef]

8. Falkner, B.; Hulman, S.; Tannenbaum, J.; Kushner, H. Insulin resistance and blood pressure in young black men. *Hypertension* **1990**, *16*, 706–711. [CrossRef]
9. Ormazabal, V.; Nair, S.; Elfeky, O.; Aguayo, C.; Salomon, C.; Zuniga, F.A. Association between insulin resistance and the development of cardiovascular disease. *Cardiovasc. Diabetol.* **2018**, *17*, 122. [CrossRef]
10. Morris, J.K.; Vidoni, E.D.; Perea, R.D.; Rada, R.; Johnson, D.K.; Lyons, K.; Pahwa, R.; Burns, J.M.; Honea, R.A. Insulin resistance and gray matter volume in neurodegenerative disease. *Neuroscience* **2014**, *270*, 139–147. [CrossRef]
11. Luchsinger, J.A. Insulin resistance, type 2 diabetes, and AD: Cerebrovascular disease or neurodegeneration? *Neurology* **2010**, *75*, 758–759. [CrossRef] [PubMed]
12. Ebron, K.; Andersen, C.J.; Aguilar, D.; Blesso, C.N.; Barona, J.; Dugan, C.E.; Jones, J.L.; Al-Sarraj, T.; Fernandez, M.L. A Larger Body Mass Index is Associated with Increased Atherogenic Dyslipidemia, Insulin Resistance, and Low-Grade Inflammation in Individuals with Metabolic Syndrome. *Metab. Syndr. Relat. Disord.* **2015**, *13*, 458–464. [CrossRef] [PubMed]
13. Lorenzo, C.; Hazuda, H.P.; Haffner, S.M. Insulin resistance and excess risk of diabetes in Mexican-Americans: The San Antonio Heart Study. *J. Clin. Endocrinol. Metab.* **2012**, *97*, 793–799. [CrossRef]
14. Barazzoni, R.; Gortan Cappellari, G.; Ragni, M.; Nisoli, E. Insulin resistance in obesity: An overview of fundamental alterations. *Eat. Weight Disord.* **2018**, *23*, 149–157. [CrossRef] [PubMed]
15. Tagi, V.M.; Chiarelli, F. Obesity and insulin resistance in children. *Curr. Opin. Pediatr.* **2020**, *32*, 582–588. [CrossRef] [PubMed]
16. Wang, Y.; Rimm, E.B.; Stampfer, M.J.; Willett, W.C.; Hu, F.B. Comparison of abdominal adiposity and overall obesity in predicting risk of type 2 diabetes among men. *Am. J. Clin. Nutr.* **2005**, *81*, 555–563. [CrossRef]
17. Gill, J.M. Physical activity, cardiorespiratory fitness and insulin resistance: A short update. *Curr. Opin. Lipidol.* **2007**, *18*, 47–52. [CrossRef]
18. Fowler, J.R.; Tucker, L.A.; Bailey, B.W.; LeCheminant, J.D. Physical Activity and Insulin Resistance in 6,500 NHANES Adults: The Role of Abdominal Obesity. *J. Obes.* **2020**, *2020*, 3848256. [CrossRef]
19. Colberg, S.R.; Sigal, R.J.; Yardley, J.E.; Riddell, M.C.; Dunstan, D.W.; Dempsey, P.C.; Horton, E.S.; Castorino, K.; Tate, D.F. Physical Activity/Exercise and Diabetes: A Position Statement of the American Diabetes Association. *Diabetes Care* **2016**, *39*, 2065–2079. [CrossRef]
20. NHANES. NCHS Ethics Review Board Approval. Available online: https://www.cdc.gov/nchs/nhanes/irba98.htm (accessed on 17 February 2022).
21. Centers for Disease Control and Prevention. NHANES Questionnaire, Datasets, and Related Documentation. Available online: https://wwwn.cdc.gov/nchs/nhanes/Default.aspx (accessed on 17 February 2022).
22. NHANES. Laboratory Procedure Manual: Insulin. Available online: https://wwwn.cdc.gov/nchs/data/nhanes/2017-2018/labmethods/INS-J-MET-508.pdf (accessed on 17 February 2022).
23. NHANES. Laboratory Procedure Manual: Glucose. Available online: https://wwwn.cdc.gov/nchs/data/nhanes/2017-2018/labmethods/GLU-J-MET-508.pdf (accessed on 17 February 2022).
24. Willett, W. *Nutritional Epidemiology*, 2nd ed.; Oxford University Press: New York, NY, USA, 1998; p. xiv. 514p.
25. U.S. Department of Agriculture. Food Surveys Research Group: AMPM, USDA Automated Multiple-Pass Method. Available online: https://www.ars.usda.gov/northeast-area/beltsville-md-bhnrc/beltsville-human-nutrition-research-center/food-surveys-research-group/docs/ampm-usda-automated-multiple-pass-method/ (accessed on 17 February 2022).
26. NHANES. Anthropometry Procedures Manual. Available online: https://www.cdc.gov/nchs/data/nhanes/nhanes_11_12/Anthropometry_Procedures_Manual.pdf (accessed on 17 February 2022).
27. NHANES. Data Documentation, Codebook, and Frequencies. Available online: https://wwwn.cdc.gov/Nchs/Nhanes/2013-2014/PAQ_H.htm (accessed on 17 February 2022).
28. Johnston, R.; Jones, K.; Manley, D. Confounding and collinearity in regression analysis: A cautionary tale and an alternative procedure, illustrated by studies of British voting behaviour. *Qual. Quant.* **2018**, *52*, 1957–1976. [CrossRef]
29. Wolever, T.M. Dietary carbohydrates and insulin action in humans. *Br. J. Nutr.* **2000**, *83* (Suppl. 1), S97–S102. [CrossRef] [PubMed]
30. McKeown, N.M.; Meigs, J.B.; Liu, S.; Saltzman, E.; Wilson, P.W.; Jacques, P.F. Carbohydrate nutrition, insulin resistance, and the prevalence of the metabolic syndrome in the Framingham Offspring Cohort. *Diabetes Care* **2004**, *27*, 538–546. [CrossRef] [PubMed]
31. Sevak, L.; McKeigue, P.M.; Marmot, M.G. Relationship of hyperinsulinemia to dietary intake in south Asian and European men. *Am. J. Clin. Nutr.* **1994**, *59*, 1069–1074. [CrossRef] [PubMed]
32. Lau, C.; Faerch, K.; Glumer, C.; Tetens, I.; Pedersen, O.; Carstensen, B.; Jorgensen, T.; Borch-Johnsen, K.; Inter, S. Dietary glycemic index, glycemic load, fiber, simple sugars, and insulin resistance: The Inter99 study. *Diabetes Care* **2005**, *28*, 1397–1403. [CrossRef]
33. Borkman, M.; Campbell, L.V.; Chisholm, D.J.; Storlien, L.H. Comparison of the effects on insulin sensitivity of high carbohydrate and high fat diets in normal subjects. *J. Clin. Endocrinol. Metab.* **1991**, *72*, 432–437. [CrossRef]
34. Garg, A.; Grundy, S.M.; Unger, R.H. Comparison of effects of high and low carbohydrate diets on plasma lipoproteins and insulin sensitivity in patients with mild NIDDM. *Diabetes* **1992**, *41*, 1278–1285. [CrossRef]
35. Crapo, P.A.; Insel, J.; Sperling, M.; Kolterman, O.G. Comparison of serum glucose, insulin, and glucagon responses to different types of complex carbohydrate in noninsulin-dependent diabetic patients. *Am. J. Clin. Nutr.* **1981**, *34*, 184–190. [CrossRef]
36. Jenkins, D.J.; Wolever, T.M.; Taylor, R.H.; Barker, H.; Fielden, H.; Baldwin, J.M.; Bowling, A.C.; Newman, H.C.; Jenkins, A.L.; Goff, D.V. Glycemic index of foods: A physiological basis for carbohydrate exchange. *Am. J. Clin. Nutr.* **1981**, *34*, 362–366. [CrossRef]

37. Bornet, F.R.; Costagliola, D.; Rizkalla, S.W.; Blayo, A.; Fontvieille, A.M.; Haardt, M.J.; Letanoux, M.; Tchobroutsky, G.; Slama, G. Insulinemic and glycemic indexes of six starch-rich foods taken alone and in a mixed meal by type 2 diabetics. *Am. J. Clin. Nutr.* **1987**, *45*, 588–595. [CrossRef]
38. Rizkalla, S.W.; Taghrid, L.; Laromiguiere, M.; Huet, D.; Boillot, J.; Rigoir, A.; Elgrably, F.; Slama, G. Improved plasma glucose control, whole-body glucose utilization, and lipid profile on a low-glycemic index diet in type 2 diabetic men: A randomized controlled trial. *Diabetes Care* **2004**, *27*, 1866–1872. [CrossRef]
39. Juanola-Falgarona, M.; Salas-Salvado, J.; Ibarrola-Jurado, N.; Rabassa-Soler, A.; Diaz-Lopez, A.; Guasch-Ferre, M.; Hernandez-Alonso, P.; Balanza, R.; Bullo, M. Effect of the glycemic index of the diet on weight loss, modulation of satiety, inflammation, and other metabolic risk factors: A randomized controlled trial. *Am. J. Clin. Nutr.* **2014**, *100*, 27–35. [CrossRef] [PubMed]
40. Wali, J.A.; Solon-Biet, S.M.; Freire, T.; Brandon, A.E. Macronutrient Determinants of Obesity, Insulin Resistance and Metabolic Health. *Biology* **2021**, *10*, 336. [CrossRef] [PubMed]
41. Villegas, R.; Liu, S.; Gao, Y.T.; Yang, G.; Li, H.; Zheng, W.; Shu, X.O. Prospective study of dietary carbohydrates, glycemic index, glycemic load, and incidence of type 2 diabetes mellitus in middle-aged Chinese women. *Arch. Intern. Med.* **2007**, *167*, 2310–2316. [CrossRef]
42. Sakurai, M.; Nakamura, K.; Miura, K.; Takamura, T.; Yoshita, K.; Morikawa, Y.; Ishizaki, M.; Kido, T.; Naruse, Y.; Suwazono, Y.; et al. Dietary glycemic index and risk of type 2 diabetes mellitus in middle-aged Japanese men. *Metabolism* **2012**, *61*, 47–55. [CrossRef] [PubMed]
43. Barclay, A.W.; Flood, V.M.; Rochtchina, E.; Mitchell, P.; Brand-Miller, J.C. Glycemic index, dietary fiber, and risk of type 2 diabetes in a cohort of older Australians. *Diabetes Care* **2007**, *30*, 2811–2813. [CrossRef]
44. Salmeron, J.; Manson, J.E.; Stampfer, M.J.; Colditz, G.A.; Wing, A.L.; Willett, W.C. Dietary fiber, glycemic load, and risk of non-insulin-dependent diabetes mellitus in women. *JAMA* **1997**, *277*, 472–477. [CrossRef]
45. Salmeron, J.; Ascherio, A.; Rimm, E.B.; Colditz, G.A.; Spiegelman, D.; Jenkins, D.J.; Stampfer, M.J.; Wing, A.L.; Willett, W.C. Dietary fiber, glycemic load, and risk of NIDDM in men. *Diabetes Care* **1997**, *20*, 545–550. [CrossRef]
46. Meyer, K.A.; Kushi, L.H.; Jacobs, D.R., Jr.; Slavin, J.; Sellers, T.A.; Folsom, A.R. Carbohydrates, dietary fiber, and incident type 2 diabetes in older women. *Am. J. Clin. Nutr.* **2000**, *71*, 921–930. [CrossRef]
47. Swinburn, B.A.; Metcalf, P.A.; Ley, S.J. Long-term (5-year) effects of a reduced-fat diet intervention in individuals with glucose intolerance. *Diabetes Care* **2001**, *24*, 619–624. [CrossRef]
48. Fukagawa, N.K.; Anderson, J.W.; Hageman, G.; Young, V.R.; Minaker, K.L. High-carbohydrate, high-fiber diets increase peripheral insulin sensitivity in healthy young and old adults. *Am. J. Clin. Nutr.* **1990**, *52*, 524–528. [CrossRef]
49. Pereira, M.A.; Jacobs, D.R., Jr.; Pins, J.J.; Raatz, S.K.; Gross, M.D.; Slavin, J.L.; Seaquist, E.R. Effect of whole grains on insulin sensitivity in overweight hyperinsulinemic adults. *Am. J. Clin. Nutr.* **2002**, *75*, 848–855. [CrossRef] [PubMed]
50. Lutsey, P.L.; Jacobs, D.R., Jr.; Kori, S.; Mayer-Davis, E.; Shea, S.; Steffen, L.M.; Szklo, M.; Tracy, R. Whole grain intake and its cross-sectional association with obesity, insulin resistance, inflammation, diabetes and subclinical CVD: The MESA Study. *Br. J. Nutr.* **2007**, *98*, 397–405. [CrossRef] [PubMed]
51. Liese, A.D.; Schulz, M.; Fang, F.; Wolever, T.M.; D'Agostino, R.B., Jr.; Sparks, K.C.; Mayer-Davis, E.J. Dietary glycemic index and glycemic load, carbohydrate and fiber intake, and measures of insulin sensitivity, secretion, and adiposity in the Insulin Resistance Atherosclerosis Study. *Diabetes Care* **2005**, *28*, 2832–2838. [CrossRef] [PubMed]
52. U.S. Department of Agriculture; U.S. Department of Health and Human Services. Dietary Guidelines for Americans, 2020–2025. Available online: https://www.dietaryguidelines.gov/ (accessed on 17 February 2022).
53. Kahleova, H.; Fleeman, R.; Hlozkova, A.; Holubkov, R.; Barnard, N.D. A plant-based diet in overweight individuals in a 16-week randomized clinical trial: Metabolic benefits of plant protein. *Nutr. Diabetes* **2018**, *8*, 58. [CrossRef]
54. Adeva-Andany, M.M.; Gonzalez-Lucan, M.; Fernandez-Fernandez, C.; Carneiro-Freire, N.; Seco-Filgueira, M.; Pedre-Pineiro, A.M. Effect of diet composition on insulin sensitivity in humans. *Clin. Nutr. ESPEN* **2019**, *33*, 29–38. [CrossRef] [PubMed]
55. Rietman, A.; Schwarz, J.; Blokker, B.A.; Siebelink, E.; Kok, F.J.; Afman, L.A.; Tome, D.; Mensink, M. Increasing protein intake modulates lipid metabolism in healthy young men and women consuming a high-fat hypercaloric diet. *J. Nutr.* **2014**, *144*, 1174–1180. [CrossRef] [PubMed]
56. Walrand, S.; Short, K.R.; Bigelow, M.L.; Sweatt, A.J.; Hutson, S.M.; Nair, K.S. Functional impact of high protein intake on healthy elderly people. *Am. J. Physiol. Endocrinol. Metab.* **2008**, *295*, E921–E928. [CrossRef]
57. Harber, M.P.; Schenk, S.; Barkan, A.L.; Horowitz, J.F. Effects of dietary carbohydrate restriction with high protein intake on protein metabolism and the somatotropic axis. *J. Clin. Endocrinol. Metab.* **2005**, *90*, 5175–5181. [CrossRef]
58. Asghari, G.; Farhadnejad, H.; Teymoori, F.; Mirmiran, P.; Tohidi, M.; Azizi, F. High dietary intake of branched-chain amino acids is associated with an increased risk of insulin resistance in adults. *J. Diabetes* **2018**, *10*, 357–364. [CrossRef]
59. Chen, Z.; Franco, O.H.; Lamballais, S.; Ikram, M.A.; Schoufour, J.D.; Muka, T.; Voortman, T. Associations of specific dietary protein with longitudinal insulin resistance, prediabetes and type 2 diabetes: The Rotterdam Study. *Clin. Nutr.* **2020**, *39*, 242–249. [CrossRef]
60. Krebs, M.; Krssak, M.; Bernroider, E.; Anderwald, C.; Brehm, A.; Meyerspeer, M.; Nowotny, P.; Roth, E.; Waldhausl, W.; Roden, M. Mechanism of amino acid-induced skeletal muscle insulin resistance in humans. *Diabetes* **2002**, *51*, 599–605. [CrossRef] [PubMed]
61. Samaha, F.F.; Iqbal, N.; Seshadri, P.; Chicano, K.L.; Daily, D.A.; McGrory, J.; Williams, T.; Williams, M.; Gracely, E.J.; Stern, L. A low-carbohydrate as compared with a low-fat diet in severe obesity. *N. Engl. J. Med.* **2003**, *348*, 2074–2081. [CrossRef] [PubMed]

62. Bisschop, P.H.; de Metz, J.; Ackermans, M.T.; Endert, E.; Pijl, H.; Kuipers, F.; Meijer, A.J.; Sauerwein, H.P.; Romijn, J.A. Dietary fat content alters insulin-mediated glucose metabolism in healthy men. *Am. J. Clin. Nutr.* **2001**, *73*, 554–559. [CrossRef] [PubMed]
63. Bradley, U.; Spence, M.; Courtney, C.H.; McKinley, M.C.; Ennis, C.N.; McCance, D.R.; McEneny, J.; Bell, P.M.; Young, I.S.; Hunter, S.J. Low-fat versus low-carbohydrate weight reduction diets: Effects on weight loss, insulin resistance, and cardiovascular risk: A randomized control trial. *Diabetes* **2009**, *58*, 2741–2748. [CrossRef]
64. Feskens, E.J.; Loeber, J.G.; Kromhout, D. Diet and physical activity as determinants of hyperinsulinemia: The Zutphen Elderly Study. *Am. J. Epidemiol.* **1994**, *140*, 350–360. [CrossRef]
65. Rivellese, A.A.; De Natale, C.; Lilli, S. Type of dietary fat and insulin resistance. *Ann. N. Y. Acad. Sci.* **2002**, *967*, 329–335. [CrossRef]
66. Vessby, B.; Uusitupa, M.; Hermansen, K.; Riccardi, G.; Rivellese, A.A.; Tapsell, L.C.; Nalsen, C.; Berglund, L.; Louheranta, A.; Rasmussen, B.M.; et al. Substituting dietary saturated for monounsaturated fat impairs insulin sensitivity in healthy men and women: The KANWU Study. *Diabetologia* **2001**, *44*, 312–319. [CrossRef]
67. Kahleova, H.; Hlozkova, A.; Fleeman, R.; Fletcher, K.; Holubkov, R.; Barnard, N.D. Fat Quantity and Quality, as Part of a Low-Fat, Vegan Diet, Are Associated with Changes in Body Composition, Insulin Resistance, and Insulin Secretion. A 16-Week Randomized Controlled Trial. *Nutrients* **2019**, *11*, 615. [CrossRef]
68. Astrup, A.; Grunwald, G.K.; Melanson, E.L.; Saris, W.H.; Hill, J.O. The role of low-fat diets in body weight control: A meta-analysis of ad libitum dietary intervention studies. *Int. J. Obes. Relat. Metab. Disord.* **2000**, *24*, 1545–1552. [CrossRef]
69. Astrup, A.; Ryan, L.; Grunwald, G.K.; Storgaard, M.; Saris, W.; Melanson, E.; Hill, J.O. The role of dietary fat in body fatness: Evidence from a preliminary meta-analysis of ad libitum low-fat dietary intervention studies. *Br. J. Nutr.* **2000**, *83* (Suppl. 1), S25–S32. [CrossRef]
70. Mueller-Cunningham, W.M.; Quintana, R.; Kasim-Karakas, S.E. An ad libitum, very low-fat diet results in weight loss and changes in nutrient intakes in postmenopausal women. *J. Am. Diet. Assoc.* **2003**, *103*, 1600–1606. [CrossRef] [PubMed]

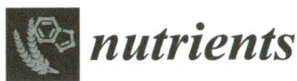

*Review*

# Taurine Supplementation as a Neuroprotective Strategy upon Brain Dysfunction in Metabolic Syndrome and Diabetes

Zeinab Rafiee [1,2], Alba M. García-Serrano [1,2] and João M. N. Duarte [1,2,*]

[1] Department of Experimental Medical Science, Faculty of Medicine, Lund University, 22100 Lund, Sweden; zeinab.rafiee@med.lu.se (Z.R.); albags89@gmail.com (A.M.G.-S.)
[2] Wallenberg Centre for Molecular Medicine, Lund University, 22100 Lund, Sweden
* Correspondence: joao.duarte@med.lu.se

**Abstract:** Obesity, type 2 diabetes, and their associated comorbidities impact brain metabolism and function and constitute risk factors for cognitive impairment. Alterations to taurine homeostasis can impact a number of biological processes, such as osmolarity control, calcium homeostasis, and inhibitory neurotransmission, and have been reported in both metabolic and neurodegenerative disorders. Models of neurodegenerative disorders show reduced brain taurine concentrations. On the other hand, models of insulin-dependent diabetes, insulin resistance, and diet-induced obesity display taurine accumulation in the hippocampus. Given the possible cytoprotective actions of taurine, such cerebral accumulation of taurine might constitute a compensatory mechanism that attempts to prevent neurodegeneration. The present article provides an overview of brain taurine homeostasis and reviews the mechanisms by which taurine can afford neuroprotection in individuals with obesity and diabetes. We conclude that further research is needed for understanding taurine homeostasis in metabolic disorders with an impact on brain function.

**Keywords:** 2-aminoethanesulfonic acid; neurodegeneration; brain metabolism; diabetes; obesity

## 1. Introduction

Taurine, or 2-aminoethanesulfonic acid, was first isolated from ox bile in 1827, by Friedrich Tiedemann and Leopold Gmelin. Taurine is obtained from the diet or results from de novo synthesis through catabolism of the amino acid cysteine (Figure 1). Together with glycine, taurine is well known for bile acid amidation, producing bile salts for excretion. Taurine supplementation has been suggested to have beneficial effects on a number of disorders, for example, hypertension [1,2], congestive heart failure [3], ischemia–reperfusion myocardial injury [4], intracerebral hemorrhage [5], pulmonary fibrosis [6], obesity-induced low-grade inflammation [7]. The neuroprotective effects of taurine have received considerable attention, and there is a plethora of publications showing the ability of exogenously added taurine to prevent toxicity in neurons or astrocytes in vitro, as well as in animal models of neurological disorders (reviewed by Jakaria et al. [8]). Namely, taurine treatments have been shown to protect tissues and cells against oxidative stress (e.g., [9]), mitochondrial stress (e.g., [10]), or inflammation (e.g., [11]). In addition, brain taurine is known as an osmoregulator and neuromodulator [12,13] and is involved in numerous processes, such as the modulation of neuronal excitability, the cerebral control of the cardiorespiratory system, appetite regulation, resistance to hypoxia, osmoregulation, and anti-oxidation [14]. Enzymes that synthetize taurine show low activity in cats, dogs, and foxes, which develop pathologies when fed a taurine-deficient diet, namely, cardiomyopathy and myocardial dysfunction, retinal degeneration, neurological abnormalities, weakened immune response, pregnancy and fetal development complications, as well as gastrointestinal problems (see [15] and references therein). This is clear evidence advocating for the importance of taurine.

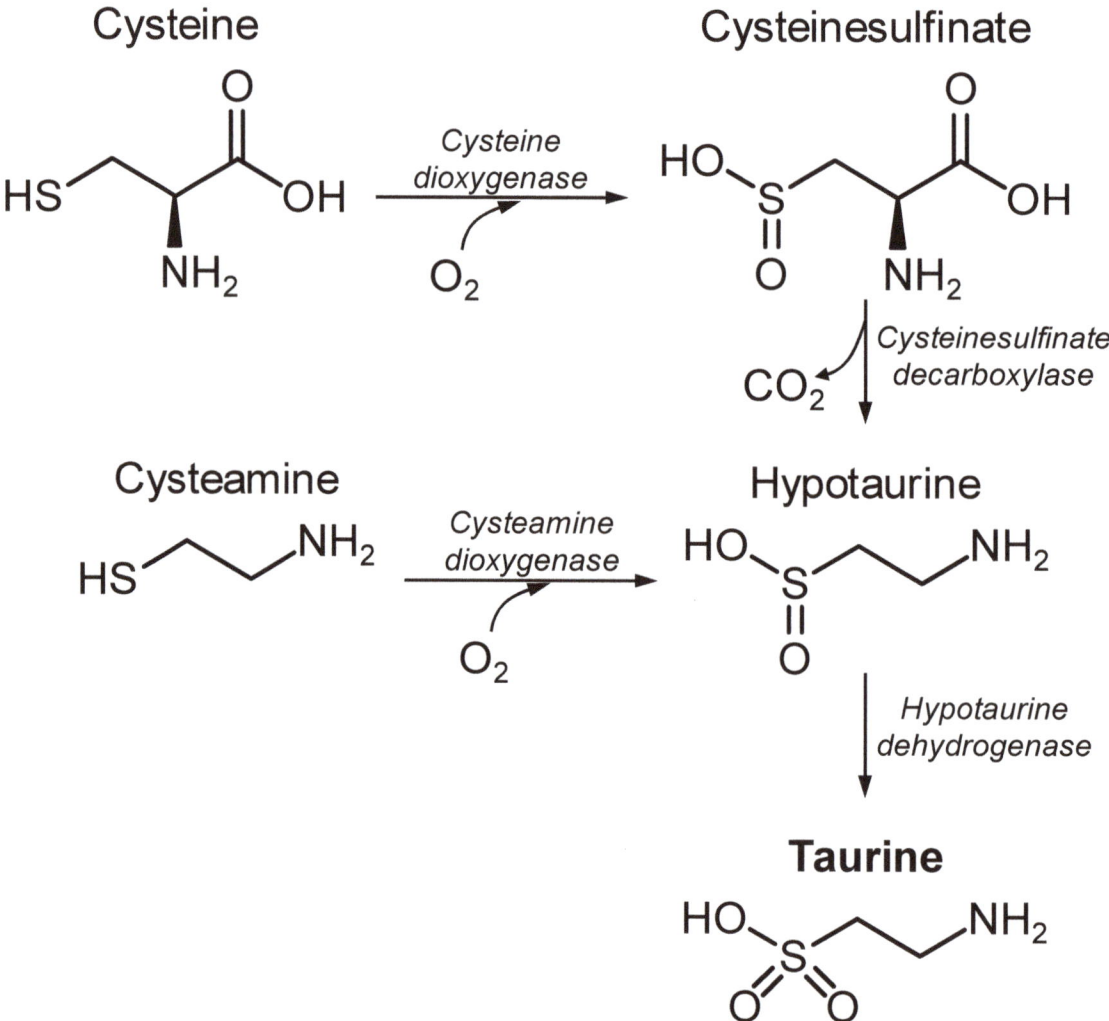

**Figure 1.** Synthesis of taurine in mammals from the sulfur amino acid cysteine.

Taurine is one of the most abundant metabolites in the central nervous system (CNS), whose levels show substantial variations across species, brain areas, and developmental stages (Figure 2). The particularly high concentration of taurine in the developing brain further suggests its developmental importance. Indeed, a relation between plasma taurine and neurodevelopment has been proposed [16]. This role of taurine in CNS development was made clear by experiments on cats fed a taurine-deficient diet [17]. More recent research proposes that taurine has neurotrophic effects, playing an important role in neurite outgrowth, synaptogenesis, and synaptic transmission during the early stages of brain development [18,19].

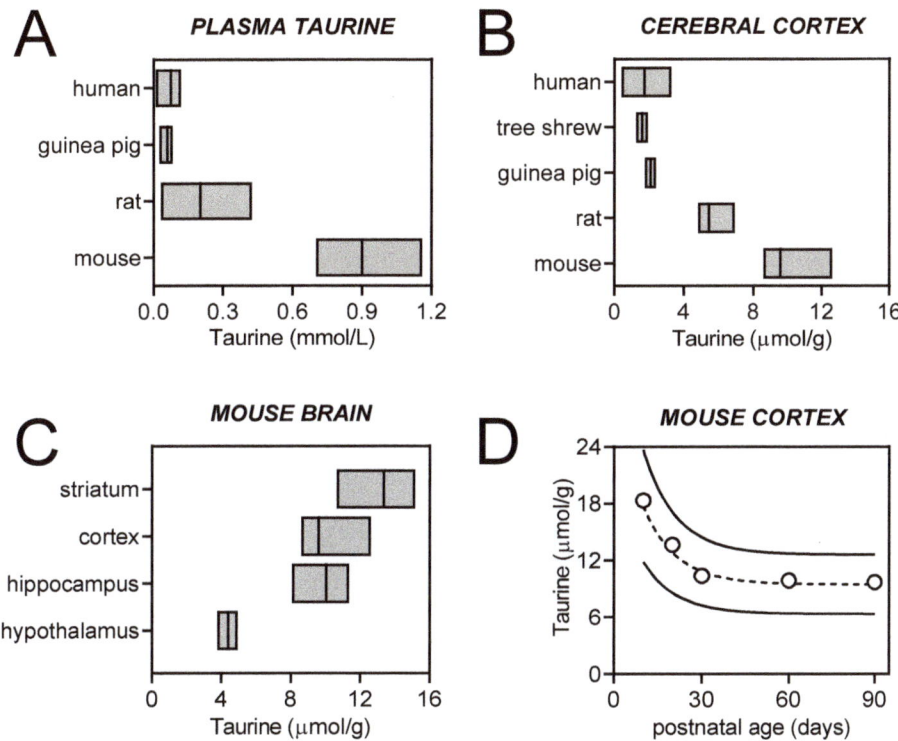

**Figure 2.** Concentrations of taurine in the plasma (**A**) and cerebral cortex of various species (**B**), in different areas of the mouse brain (**C**), and in the mouse cortex during development (**D**). Plasma taurine levels are indicated as mean and range for humans [2,20–27], guinea pigs [28,29], rat [30–36], and mice [37–41]. The plotted brain taurine concentration ranges are based on the concentrations reported in $^1$H MRS studies for humans [42–47], tree shrews [48], guinea pigs [49], Sprague–Dawley rats [50–55], and C57BL/6J mice [38,56–60].

## 2. Taurine Homeostasis

Dietary taurine is absorbed by the gut, released into the blood stream, and excreted by the kidney through urine and by the liver via conjugation to bile acids [14,61]. Submillimolar concentrations of taurine are observed in the plasma (Figure 2A), while much larger concentrations occur in organs with high energy metabolism rates, such as the heart [62–65].

### 2.1. Brain Taurine Transport

Taurine in the brain results from its transport from the periphery (believed to be the main source) and local de novo synthesis. In most mammals, taurine is mainly synthetized in the liver and then actively transported through the blood-brain barrier into the brain parenchyma.

Taurine, as well as hypotaurine, β-alanine, and other β-amino acids, are taken up through the blood–brain barrier into the brain by a high-affinity, low-capacity $Na^+$- and $Cl^-$-dependent transport system [66,67]. The passive diffusion of taurine across the blood-brain barrier is negligible [14]. Taurine uptake or efflux at both luminal and albumen membranes has been proposed to be mediated by SLC6A6 transporter, also called TauT [68]. The blood-brain barrier also expresses the GABA transporter SLC6A13, known as GAT-2, which is capable of carrying taurine across membranes [69,70]. Both TauT and GAT-2 are also able to efficiently carry hypotaurine [71]. Genetic deletion of the taurine transporter (TauT) in mice reduces taurine concentrations in plasma and tissues, including the brain [37]. In contrast, genetic deletion of GAT-2 in mice increases brain taurine levels, suggesting that GAT-2 is mainly functioning as a brain-to-blood efflux system for taurine [69].

TauT is expressed in astrocytes and to a lesser extent in neurons [72,73]. GAT-2 expression appears restricted to leptomeninges and blood vessels [74]. Taurine is also transported by ubiquitously expressed volume-sensitive organic osmolyte–anion channels, commonly called volume-regulated anion channels (VRACs), that are activated by cell swelling (see [75] and references therein). Within the brain parenchyma, it has been proposed that taurine uptake is mediated by TauT, while taurine release is mostly mediated by VRACs. Furukawa et al., have shown that that taurine uptake is blocked by a TauT inhibitor and taurine release is blocked by a VRAC blocker in the developing mouse neocortex [76].

## 2.2. Taurine Metabolism

The synthesis of taurine occurs from the catabolism of cysteine in both neurons and astrocytes (Figure 1) and is limited by the oxidation of hypotaurine [77,78]. Cysteine dioxygenase and cysteine sulfinate decarboxylase are concerted to produce hypotaurine from cysteine. Genetic deletion of cysteine dioxygenase in mice depletes hypotaurine and taurine, while causing the accumulation of cysteine and cysteine-containing metabolites such as glutathione [48]. Genetic deletion of cysteine sulfinate decarboxylase also reduces taurine levels in the brain (four-fold less than in controls), as well as in the plasma and other tissues [79]. Either of these mouse models shows impaired development, including reduced brain volume. Cysteamine can also be converted to hypotaurine via cysteamine dioxygenase. The identity of the enzyme that catalyzes the biosynthesis of taurine from hypotaurine, which is denominated hypotaurine dehydrogenase, has remained elusive. Recently, Veeravalli et al., proposed that the oxygenation of hypotaurine to taurine is mainly catalyzed by flavin-containing monooxygenase 1 [80]. Accordingly, the developmental expression of this enzyme in the mouse brain [81] accompanies the developmental decay of brain taurine levels (Figure 2).

Neurons and astrocytes express taurine transporters (e.g., [82]) and release hypotaurine and/or taurine originating from cysteine oxidation [77,78]. However, it remains to be experimentally determined whether taurine metabolism is interdependently regulated by neurons and astrocytes, as proposed elsewhere (see discussion by Banerjee et al. [83]).

## 2.3. Sulphur-Containing Amino Acids

Taurine is not used for protein synthesis. In contrast, the sulphur-containing amino acids methionine and cysteine are protein components and play important roles in maintaining protein structure. While methionine is a very hydrophobic amino acid that contributes to interactions such as those between proteins and lipid bilayers, cysteine mainly participates in protein folding by the formation of disulfide bonds with other cysteine residues [84]. Methionine can be metabolized to the cofactor S-adenosylmethionine that participates in a number of metabolic pathways by acting as a methyl donor, including epigenetic regulation [85] and catecholamine metabolism (epinephrine synthesis) [86]. Such transmethylation reactions can be funneled to produce homocysteine that generates cysteine through transsulfuration [85,87]. Notably, both methionine and cysteine produced from protein degradation can generate taurine as an end-product [88].

## 3. Taurine in Cellular Physiology

### 3.1. Osmoregulation by Taurine

Cells swell and shrink when challenged with osmotic changes. The regulation of cell volume in response to extracellular or intracellular stimuli or osmotic changes is critical for cellular homeostasis. Neuronal activity is associated with changes in cell membrane polarization as a result of active ion fluxes and involves cell volume regulation (e.g., [89]). Pathological edema resulting from cellular swelling occurs in hypo-osmotic conditions or in the presence of cytotoxic ion imbalance. While water is taken up via aquaporin-

4 mainly expressed in astrocytes, it has been reported that both neurons and astrocytes swell during acute hypo-osmotic stress (e.g., [90]). As a reaction to cell swelling, several low-molecular-weight organic compounds will influence intracellular osmolarity.

Taurine occurs in its zwitterionic form over the physiological pH range, turning into an excellent metabolite for osmolarity regulation [14,91]. Indeed, neurons and astrocytes exposed to exogenous taurine up to 10 mmol/L are able to take up extracellular taurine without changes in cell volume [92]. Consistent with a tight regulation of taurine concentration for its action as an organic osmolyte, exposure of brain cells to cysteine or cysteamine results in elevated hypotaurine, but not taurine, levels [78]. Superfused acute mouse cerebral cortical slices regulate taurine release upon osmotic challenges [93]. Brain taurine levels decline over 2 weeks of hyponatremia in rats in vivo [94], while increasing during hypernatremia [95]. Accordingly, taurine synthesis is stimulated under hypertonic conditions in cultured neurons [78]. Astrocytes in a hyperosmotic medium accumulate taurine [96,97]. This is likely due to the increased expression of TauT for taurine uptake rather than to the stimulation of taurine synthesis [98]. In contrast, astrocytes cultured in a hypo-osmotic medium release taurine [99], a process likely mediated by VRAC [100]. While osmotic pressure is regulated by taurine, there are other effects of this compound on the balance of $K^+$ and $Ca^{2+}$, which might have implications for neurotransmission [92].

### 3.2. Taurine as a Neurotransmitter

Early work reported taurine uptake into synaptosomes and its release upon electrical stimulation [101,102], as well as taurine binding to synaptosomal membranes [103,104]. Such observations suggested a role of taurine as a neurotransmitter in the central nervous system (CNS); in fact, taurine turned out to be a modulator of inhibitory neurotransmission.

γ-Aminobutyric acid (GABA) and glycine are amino acids that mediate inhibitory transmission at chemical synapses. GABAergic synapses employ three types of postsynaptic receptors: the ionotropic $GABA_A$ and $GABA_C$ that are permeable to $Cl^-$ and the metabotropic $GABA_B$. Glycine receptors are also permeable to $Cl^-$ upon ligand binding. Taurine is known to interact with $GABA_A$, $GABA_B$, and glycine receptors (Figure 3; [12,105]). While taurine binding to $GABA_A$ and $GABA_B$ is weaker than to GABA, taurine is a rather potent ligand of the glycine receptor [105].

Intracellular taurine concentration is estimated to be 400-fold higher than the concentration in the extracellular space [30]. Taurine concentration in the brain measured extracellularly using microdialysis is generally below 10 μmol/L, and increases by at least one order of magnitude upon depolarization [106–108]. After release, taurine acts on GABA and glycine receptors and is cleared through sodium-dependent transport (see above). Taurine release does not take place exclusively at synapses but can be of glial origin [109–112] and mediate astrocyte-to-neuron communication [110,113].

Concentrations of taurine below 1 mmol/L are rather selective for glycine receptors, as observed in neurons in the basolateral amygdala [114], supraoptic nucleus [115], hippocampus [116], nucleus accumbens [117], and inferior colliculus [118]. Above 1 mmol/L, taurine also activates GABA receptors. However, taurine was shown to act as an endogenous ligand for extra-synaptic $GABA_A$ receptors at concentrations ranging from 10 to 100 μmol/L [119].

While not modulating glutamatergic neurotransmission, taurine regulates cytoplasmic and intra-mitochondrial $Ca^{2+}$ homeostasis. Therefore, taurine is able to dampen glutamate-induced $Ca^{2+}$ transients in neurons, and thus intracellular $Ca^{2+}$-dependent signaling mediators, and even prevent glutamate excitotoxicity [120–122]. Therefore, inhibitory actions of taurine on neuronal excitability might be attributed to a direct enhancement of GABAergic and glycinergic neurotransmission, as well as to the dampening glutamatergic neurotransmission via intracellular effects (discussed by El Idrissi and Trenkner [123]).

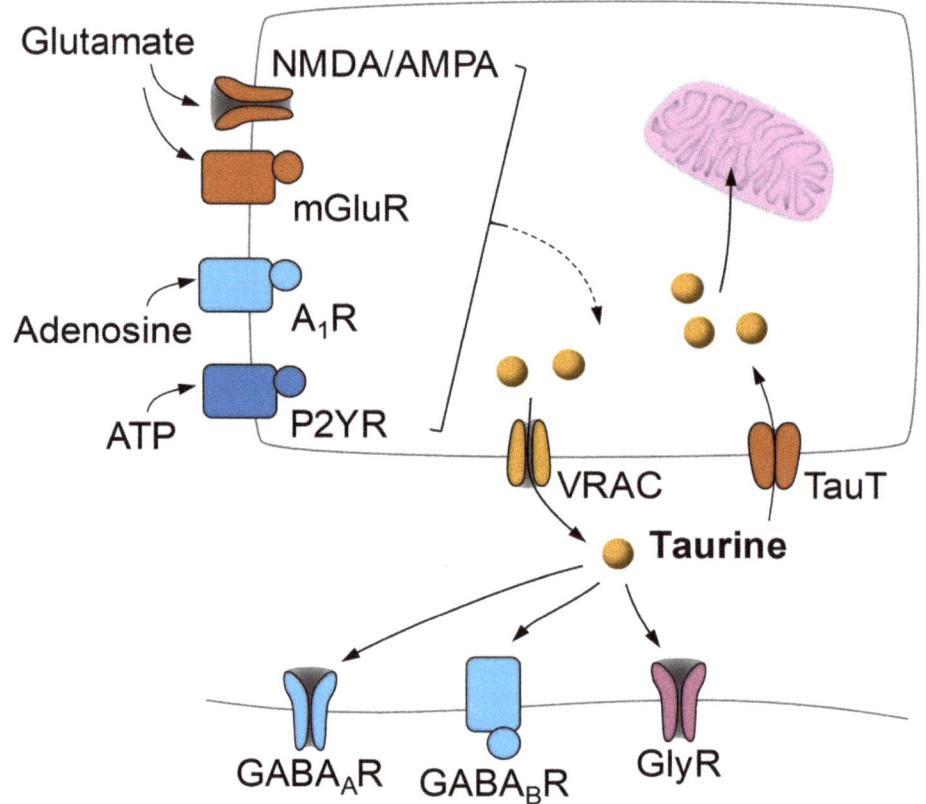

**Figure 3.** Schematic representation of activity-dependent taurine release modulation from neurons or astrocytes by glutamate and purines and action of taurine on inhibitory receptors. Taurine release is mainly mediated by volume-regulated anion channels (VRAC) that are activated by hypo-osmotic conditions and electrical activity and can be stimulated via glutamate metabotropic (mGluR) and ionotropic receptors (mainly NMDA and AMPA), adenosine $A_1$ receptors ($A_1R$), and metabotropic ATP receptors (P2Y). Taurine mediates its neuromodulatory effects by binding to $GABA_A$, $GABA_B$, and glycine receptors. Reuptake of taurine occurs vis the taurine transporter TauT.

### 3.3. Modulation of Taurine Release in the CNS

In the central nervous system, basal taurine release is largely independent of $Ca^{2+}$, and a $Ca^{2+}$-dependent component can be stimulated by glutamate and $K^+$ [124–126]. The facilitation of glutamate-induced taurine release is slow and prolonged, varies across the life span, and is mediated by NMDA and AMPA receptors, as well as by kainate receptors in the developing brain [125]. Metabotropic glutamate receptors have also been proposed to modulate taurine release from acute hippocampal slices [127]. Adenosine has been proposed to modulate both basal and $K^+$-stimulated taurine release from mouse hippocampal slices via $A_1$ receptors [126]. While the activation of adenosine $A_1$ receptors enhanced the basal taurine release and stimulated it in hippocampal slices from the developing mouse, it inhibited the basal but not the stimulated release in adults. Purinergic activation by ATP was also proposed to stimulate taurine efflux in cultured rat hippocampal neurons [128]. ATP caused a dose-dependent loss of taurine mediated by P2Y rather than P2X receptors, which could be blocked by a VRAC inhibitor. In sum, taurine release appears to be physiologically regulated by glutamatergic activity and their modulators (Figure 3), namely, purines.

### 3.4. Taurine in Mitochondria

Taurine concentrations in the brain mitochondria are in the same order of magnitude than those found in other subcellular compartments, such as synaptosomes [129]. Recently, in cultured HeLa cells, taurine concentrations in the mitochondrial matrix were also determined to be similar to those in the whole cell [130]. The authors further found that blocking the complex I with piericidin reduced taurine levels by 40%, but no substantial effects on taurine concentrations in the matrix were found when inhibiting complex II or ATP synthase [130].

Taurine amino group with a pKa of 8.6 at 37 °C is suitable for acting as a mitochondrial matrix pH buffer [131]. The regulation of mitochondrial pH is important for brain function, since mitochondrial metabolism in both neurons and astrocytes responds to brain activity (see [132] and references therein). The proton gradient and mitochondrial membrane potential are the drivers of the proton-motive force that produces ATP. Like other cells, neurons and astrocytes in culture show a mitochondrial matrix pH of 7.5–8 [133–135]. For example, the uptake of glutamate by astrocytes after synaptic release triggers intracellular acidification that spreads over the mitochondrial matrix [134]. The authors further showed that glutamate-induced mitochondrial matrix acidification exceeded cytosolic acidification and dissipated the cytosol-to-mitochondrial matrix pH gradient, which resulted in the modulation of metabolism and oxygen consumption [131,134,136]. On the other hand, the pH in the mitochondrial matrix of neurons increased upon exposure to excitotoxic levels of glutamate [133]. Taurine might counteract extreme mitochondrial pH fluctuations and help preserve mitochondrial physiology. Mohammadi et al., exposed mitochondria isolated from the mouse liver to a wide range of exogenous taurine concentrations and found that taurine participates in regulating mitochondrial potential, $Ca^{2+}$-induced mitochondrial swelling, the activity of mitochondrial dehydrogenases, and ATP concentration [137]. Mitochondria isolated from the mouse brain or liver show inhibited mitochondrial dehydrogenases activity, collapse of mitochondrial membrane potential, induced mitochondrial swelling, and increased levels of reactive oxygen species upon exposure to ammonia, which are all mitigated by taurine [138].

Taurine is not able to act as a radical scavenger [139]. However, beneficial antioxidant effects of taurine in cells have mostly been linked to improved mitochondrial action and reduced generation of mitochondrial superoxide. Taurine administration to isolated mitochondria from liver or brain was shown to mitigate ammonia-induced mitochondrial dysfunction, including preventing or ameliorating the ammonia-induced collapse of mitochondrial membrane potential, mitochondrial swelling, ATP depletion, and increased reactive oxygen species and oxidative stress [138]. Taurine also decreased the activity of glutathione peroxidase and manganese-superoxide dismutase upon tamoxifen toxicity, which contributed to decreasing mitochondrial oxidative stress, measured through lipid peroxidation, protein carbonyl content, and superoxide radical generation [140].

Taurine is a component of mitochondrial tRNAs in taurine-containing modified uridines that are indispensable for protein translation [141,142]. This taurine modification is catalyzed by the enzyme mitochondrial optimization-1, whose deficiency impairs mitochondrial protein translation and ultimately the efficiency of respiration [143]. Several diseases have been directly associated with the lack taurine modification of mitochondrial tRNA [144,145].

In sum, taurine supplementation is proposed to improve the function of the mitochondria, contributing to the preservation of mitochondrial membrane potential, proton gradient, and matrix pH that are critical for energy metabolism and efficient oxidative phosphorylation, as well as intracellular calcium homeostasis.

### 3.5. Taurine as an Inhibitor of Apoptosis

Taurine was found to prevent apoptosis upon many noxious challenges (e.g., [146–148]). The most striking neuroprotective effects of taurine were observed on the reduction of apoptotic rates and the improvement of neurological outcomes upon brain ischemia. The suggested mechanisms include the prevention of mitochondrial and endoplasmic reticulum (ER) stress. Taurine was found to attenuate mitochondria-dependent cell death in the ischemic core and penumbra of stroke models by stimulating the antioxidant machinery, preventing energy charge dampening, inhibiting the reduction of anti-apoptotic Bcl-xL and the increase of the pro-apoptotic Bax, preventing cytochrome C release from the mitochondria, and inhibiting the activation of calpain and caspase-3 [149–151]. Taurine was also found to prevent ischemia/hypoxia-induced endoplasmic reticulum (ER) stress by inhibiting the unfolded protein response via transcription factor 6 (ATF6), protein kinase R-like ER kinase (PERK), and inositol-requiring enzyme 1 (IRE1) pathways [152,153].

## 4. Brain Taurine in Diabetes

Diabetes and many factors of the metabolic syndrome impact the brain, leading to metabolic alterations, synaptic dysfunction, gliosis, and memory impairment [154,155]. MRS studies on rats rendered diabetic by streptozotocin administration showed increased taurine concentrations in the hippocampus (+23%) [156] and cortex (+8%) [157], which is consistent with increased brain taurine uptake in this model [31]. Non-obese, insulin resistant Goto-Kakizaki rats also display increased taurine concentration in the hippocampus (+22%), a brain area involved in learning and memory, relative to Wistar control rats [158]. Brain taurine alterations have also been reported in diet-induced obesity models. Namely, mice fed a lard-based 60%-fat-rich diet for 6 months showed increased taurine in the cortex (+7%), hypothalamus (+9%), and, most prominently, hippocampus (+12%), when compared to low-fat-fed mice [159]. Recently, we further demonstrated that a high-fat and high-sugar diet led to increased hippocampal levels of taurine after 4 weeks, which persisted for several months (ranging from +8% to +14% relative to low-fat-diet-fed controls), which were reversed by diet normalization [38]. Such increase in brain taurine levels in mice with diabetes might have resulted from a compensatory mechanism for cellular protection against metabolic syndrome.

While increased hippocampal taurine concentrations have been reported in the brain of diabetes models, that remains to be demonstrated in individuals with diabetes (reviewed and discussed in [160]). The lack of evidence on alterations of brain taurine levels in diabetes patients is inherent to the relatively low levels of taurine in the human brain (see Figure 2), and to the difficulty in distinguishing taurine peaks at the weak magnetic fields used in clinical MRS studies (discussed in [161]). However, MRS at higher magnetic fields, namely, at 7 T and above, improves the ability to examine taurine in the living human brain. While not many MRS studies on diabetes individuals are available, other neurodegenerative disorders have been more studied, including Alzheimer's disease (AD).

### 4.1. Brain Taurine Levels in Subjects with Alzheimer's Disease

There is a growing body of epidemiological evidence suggesting that obesity and insulin resistance increases the risk of developing age-related cognitive decline, mild cognitive impairment, vascular dementia, and AD, and molecular and metabolic mechanisms linking T2D and AD have been proposed [154,162,163]. While there are limited studies measuring brain taurine in patients with diabetes, research from the AD field might provide additional clues on taurine alterations upon neurodegeneration.

Little attention has been given to taurine concentrations measured by MRS in the brain of AD patients relative to those in healthy individuals ([164,165] and references therein). That is because most MRS studies were conducted at low magnetic fields. In a recent MRS study conducted at 7.0 T, Marjańska et al., found similar concentrations of taurine in AD individuals and age- and gender-matched cognitively healthy controls in the posterior cingulate cortex, a region known to be impacted by AD, and the occipital cortex [166]. Early studies on AD patients also found no substantial changes in cerebrospinal fluid (CSF) taurine levels [167,168] or post-mortem brain taurine levels [169,170]. These studies, however, might be biased by confounding effects from previous medications. Indeed, taurine levels were found reduced (up to −36%) in the CSF of individuals diagnosed with dementia and probable AD who had never been treated with antidepressant or neuroleptic medications [171] and in individuals with advanced symptoms of AD [172]. In another study, CSF taurine levels in AD patients correlated significantly with cognitive scores [168]. Altogether, one might speculate that taurine loss in patients with AD is linked to worsened cognitive deterioration.

### 4.2. Plasma Taurine Levels in Individuals with Dementia and Alzheimer's Disease

Reduced levels of blood taurine ($-23\%$ to $-40\%$) have been observed in subjects with Alzheimer's disease relative to subjects without neurodegenerative symptoms [173]. In another study, low taurine levels were associated with dementia risk but not with AD risk [174]. Therefore, the authors postulated that a low concentration of taurine might be linked to vascular dysfunction (possibly, vascular dementia) rather than to neurodegeneration. Accordingly, low levels of dietary taurine have been linked to hypertension [175], taurine supplementation in a mouse study was implicated in blood flow regulation [176], and a chronic taurine supplementation showed antihypertensive effects in a clinical trial [2]. However, not all studies associate low taurine levels to AD, and higher taurine levels in the plasma have actually been found in patients with mild cognitive impairment (+43%) and Alzheimer's disease (AD) (+49%) compared to control subjects [177].

### 4.3. Brain Taurine Levels in AD Models

The transgenic rat model of AD TgF344-AD rat has been reported to develop age-dependent MRS alterations in brain metabolites, including increased taurine levels in the cortex (+35%) at 18 months of age, but not earlier [178]. Age-dependent increased taurine levels were also observed in the hippocampus (+16% to +21%) and cortex (+25%) of McGill-R-Thy1-APP rats, relative to controls [179]. One study on aged transgenic mice carrying the human Swedish APP mutant Tg2576 showed elevated taurine levels in the cortex (+21%) [180]. However, taurine levels were found unaltered during aging in the brain in many other studies on transgenic mouse models of AD (Refs. [181–183] and references therein). Altogether, we conclude that the current evidence points towards contrasting findings on brain taurine levels in AD patients and animal models of the disease.

## 5. Neuroprotection by Taurine

Neuroprotection by taurine has been reported for many models of brain injury and neurodegeneration. In animal models, taurine treatments have been reported to significantly improve functional recovery after traumatic brain injury [184,185] or ischemic stroke [149,176,186]. Not only taurine has beneficial effects against neurodegeneration, but also it can modulate inflammatory processes. Namely, it has been established that taurine dampens neuroinflammation in animal models of ischemic stroke and traumatic brain injury that develop severe gliosis (e.g., [11,184,186]).

Given its role as an inhibitory transmitter, taurine was shown to reduce seizures in a mouse model of kainite-induced epilepsy and prevent cell death in the hippocampus, as well as microgliosis and astrogliosis [187]. Furthermore, taurine was suggested to protect dopaminergic neurons in a mouse and rat models of Parkinson's disease, namely, by inhibiting neuroinflammation and microgliosis [188,189]. Taurine was found to ameliorate cellular and neurochemical alterations in the hippocampus of rodents exposed to chronic stress induced by repeated immobilization or noise exposure, with substantial improvements on memory performance [190,191]. Taurine supplementation was also suggested to afford neuroprotection and anti-apoptotic activity, as well as to reduce microglia activation, in a rat model of chronic inflammation induced by the repeated administration of lipopolysaccharide that mimics a bacterial infection [192].

In aging mice, taurine administration was reported to stimulate hippocampal neurogenesis by increasing the rate of progenitor cell formation and to induce a shift in microglia from activated to resting states [193].

Taurine has been shown to protect neurons against excitotoxicity induced by amyloid-β or glutamate in vitro [121,194]. Moreover, taurine supplementation was reported to recover spatial memory in the APP/PS1 mouse model [195] and to improve glutamatergic activity in the brain of the 5xFAD mouse model [196]. While in both models taurine failed to reduce the rate of amyloid-β deposition, taurine was reported to have the ability to decrease amyloid-β aggregation, while favoring the formation for tau protein fibrils [197].

## 5.1. Taurine Affords Neuroprotection in Diabetes Models

In streptozotocin-induced diabetic rats (insulin-deficient diabetes), treatment with taurine at a dose of 100 mg/kg i.p. during a month reduced oxidative stress, DNA damage, and inflammatory cytokine levels in the frontal cortex and hippocampus, contributing to improving memory performance [198,199]. A study by Agca et al. [200] demonstrated that a 2% ($w/v$) taurine supplementation in drinking water for 8 weeks administered to streptozotocin-treated rats ameliorated the diabetes-induced increase of the transcription factor NF-κβ, involved in inflammatory processes, and the diabetes-induced reduction of Nrf2 and glucose transporters Glut1 and Glut3 in the brain. Rahmeier et al. [201] further showed anti-apoptotic effects of taurine administration (100 mg/kg daily i.p.) in the brain of streptozotocin-treated rats. Li et al. [202] described taurine as a protector against myelin damage of the sciatic nerve in streptozotocin-treated rats through the inhibition of apoptosis of Schwann cells. In mice fed a fat-rich diet, which develop metabolic syndrome, we recently demonstrated that 3% ($w/v$) taurine supplemented in the drinking water for 2 months prevented memory impairment [203]. Furthermore, magnetic resonance spectroscopy (MRS) for metabolic profiling in vivo showed that taurine treatment prevented the obesity-induced reduction of the neuronal marker N-acetylaspartate in the hippocampus [203]. Energy metabolism impairments were also observed in the hippocampus of high-fat-diet-fed mice in this study but could not be prevented by taurine. However, treatment with N-acetylcysteine, which acts as a cysteine donor for the synthesis of taurine as well as glutathione, fully prevented obesity-induced metabolic alterations in the hippocampus. Interestingly, it has also been proposed that taurine treatment increases brain insulin receptor density, in particular in the hippocampus [204], which could improve brain insulin sensitivity and thus have beneficial effects to counteract cognitive impairment [154,162,163]. Altogether, the available literature supports taurine administration as a way of preventing neuronal dysfunction in patients with obesity and diabetes.

## 5.2. Taurine Effectiveness in Diabetes Management

Taurine supplementation has shown beneficial effects on metabolic syndrome factors in both preclinical and clinical studies. We recently reported a taurine-induced improvement of glucose tolerance in female mice fed a high-fat diet during 2 months, compared to non-taurine-supplemented obese mice [202]. Similar results were described by Ribeiro et al. [205], who used 5% ($w/v$) taurine in drinking water for 6 months.

The plasma levels of taurine were found to be slightly lower in individuals with T2D than in healthy subjects [20,21]. Interestingly, plasma taurine was found to inversely correlate with fasting glycemia but not with glycated hemoglobin $HbA1_c$ levels [206] and to be independent of obesity or body mass index [20,22]. This suggests that taurine is involved in acute metabolic regulation and glucose homeostasis, but not in the etiology of diabetes. Indeed, plasma taurine is reduced during an euglycemic hyperinsulinemic clamp in healthy individuals [23] or during the metabolic response to exercise [207]. According to the roles of taurine in metabolic regulation, we previously observed that taurine concentration in the hippocampus of streptozotocin-treated diabetic rats could be reduced by acute glycemic normalization by means of insulin administration [156].

Given the lower levels of circulating taurine in subjects with diabetes, it has been speculated that dietary taurine supplementation might contribute to diabetes management. Accordingly, several studies on animal models of diabetes have indicated that taurine supplementation lowers glycaemia and improves insulin secretion and sensitivity (e.g., [205,208–212]). Interestingly, it has been proposed that such effects could also be associated with taurine conjugation to bile acids, such as the formation of tauro–ursodeoxycholic acid [213].

Evidence from studies in humans remains controversial, and taurine supplementation has little or no effect on improving metabolic syndrome or T2D and its complications (reviewed in [214]). The source of controversy regarding taurine effects on diabetes might be the poor study design and the low number of subjects tested. For example, a sufficiently powered, double-blinded, randomized, crossover study, based on the administration of a daily taurine supplementation for 8 weeks found no effect on insulin secretion and action and on plasma lipid levels in overweight men with a positive history of T2D [215]. Nevertheless, the beneficial effects of taurine might contribute to protect the various bodily systems from diabetes complications.

## 6. Conclusions

Overfeeding and sedentary lifestyles drive the development of a systemic metabolic imbalance and the emergence of obesity and prediabetes that are strongly associated with all-cause dementia, Alzheimer's disease (AD), and vascular dementia (e.g., [216]). Obesity is associated with comorbidities such as hypertension, cardiovascular disease, metabolic syndrome, and insulin resistance or type 2 diabetes [216,217], which might modulate the genetic susceptibility to neurodegenerative disorders [218] and thus constitute a risk factor for cognitive decline [219,220]. The reported cytoprotective actions of taurine contribute to brain health improvements in subjects with obesity and diabetes through various mechanisms that improve neuronal function, such as the modulation of inhibitory neurotransmission and, therefore, the promotion of an excitatory–inhibitory balance, the stimulation of antioxidant systems, and the stabilization of mitochondria and thus of energy production and $Ca^{2+}$ homeostasis. Taurine supplementation in experimental models of obesity and diabetes provides evidence for its effects in the prevention of metabolic syndrome-associated memory dysfunction, but the exact mechanisms of taurine action remain to be ascertained; this should be addressed in future studies. Based on this literature survey, we conclude that further research is indeed necessary for a clear understanding of taurine homeostasis in metabolic disorders with an impact on brain function.

In addition to taurine, the amino acids methionine and cysteine from which taurine can be produced (see Section 2.3) have been associated with obesity and metabolic syndrome [207,221,222], and the modulation of the bioavailability of sulphur-containing amino acids might provide further benefits, e.g., by stimulating the synthesis of the antioxidant glutathione (discussed in [203]).

**Funding:** The authors' research is supported by the Swedish foundation for International Cooperation in Research and Higher education (BR2019-8508), the Swedish Research council (2019-01130), the Diabetesfonden (Dia2019-440), the Direktör Albert Påhlssons Foundation, the Crafoord Foundation, the Tage Blücher Foundation, the Dementiafonden, and the Royal Physiographic Society of Lund. J.M.N.D. acknowledges generous financial support from The Knut and Alice Wallenberg foundation, the Faculty of Medicine at Lund University and Region Skåne. The authors acknowledge support from the Lund University Diabetes Centre, which is funded by the Swedish Research Council (Strategic Research Area EXODIAB, grant 2009-1039) and the Swedish Foundation for Strategic Research (grant IRC15-0067).

**Institutional Review Board Statement:** Not applicable.

**Informed Consent Statement:** Not applicable.

**Data Availability Statement:** Not applicable.

**Conflicts of Interest:** The authors have no relationships or activities that might constitute potential conflicts of interest with respect to the research, authorship, and publication of this article.

**Abbreviations**

| | |
|---|---|
| AD | Alzheimer's disease |
| AMPA | α-amino-3-hydroxy-5-methyl-4-isoxazole propionic acid |
| CNS | central nervous system |
| CSF | cerebrospinal fluid |
| GAT-2 | GABA transporter (SLC6A13) |
| MRS | Magnetic resonance spectroscopy |
| NMDA | N-methyl-D-aspartate |
| TauT | taurine transporter (SLC6A6) |
| VRAC | volume-regulated anion channel |

**References**

1. Russell, D.W. The Enzymes, Regulation, and Genetics of Bile Acid Synthesis. *Annu. Rev. Biochem.* **2003**, *72*, 137–174. [CrossRef] [PubMed]
2. Sun, Q.; Wang, B.; Li, Y.; Sun, F.; Li, P.; Xia, W.; Zhou, X.; Li, Q.; Wang, X.; Chen, J.; et al. Taurine Supplementation Lowers Blood Pressure and Improves Vascular Function in Prehypertension. *Hypertension* **2016**, *67*, 541–549. [CrossRef] [PubMed]
3. Azuma, J. Heart Failure Research with Taurine Group Long-Term Effect of Taurine in Congestive Heart Failure: Preliminary Report. *Adv. Exp. Med. Biol.* **1994**, *359*, 425–433. [CrossRef] [PubMed]
4. Milei, J.; Ferreira, R.; Llesuy, S.F.; Forcada, P.; Covarrubias, J.; Boveris, A. Reduction of reperfusion injury with preoperative rapid intravenous infusion of taurine during myocardial revascularization. *Am. Hear. J.* **1992**, *123*, 339–345. [CrossRef]
5. Zhao, H.; Qu, J.; Li, Q.; Cui, M.; Wang, J.; Zhang, K.; Liu, X.; Feng, H.; Chen, Y. Taurine supplementation reduces neuroinflammation and protects against white matter injury after intracerebral hemorrhage in rats. *Amino Acids* **2017**, *50*, 439–451. [CrossRef] [PubMed]
6. Giri, S.N.; Wang, Q. Taurine and Niacin Offer a Novel Therapeutic Modality in Prevention of Chemically-Induced Pulmonary Fibrosis in Hamsters. *Adv. Exp. Med. Biol.* **1992**, *315*, 329–340. [CrossRef]
7. De Carvalho, F.G.; Brandao, C.F.C.; Muñoz, V.R.; Batitucci, G.; Tavares, M.E.D.A.; Teixeira, G.R.; Pauli, J.R.; De Moura, L.P.; Ropelle, E.R.; Cintra, D.E.; et al. Taurine supplementation in conjunction with exercise modulated cytokines and improved subcutaneous white adipose tissue plasticity in obese women. *Amino Acids* **2021**, *53*, 1391–1403. [CrossRef]
8. Jakaria, M.; Azam, S.; Haque, M.E.; Jo, S.-H.; Uddin, M.S.; Kim, I.-S.; Choi, D.-K. Taurine and its analogs in neurological disorders: Focus on therapeutic potential and molecular mechanisms. *Redox Biol.* **2019**, *24*, 101223. [CrossRef]
9. Yeon, J.-A.; Kim, S.-J. Neuroprotective Effect of Taurine against Oxidative Stress-Induced Damages in Neuronal Cells. *Biomol. Ther.* **2010**, *18*, 24–31. [CrossRef]
10. Rezaee-Tazangi, F.; Zeidooni, L.; Rafiee, Z.; Fakhredini, F.; Kalantari, H.; Alidadi, H.; Khorsandi, L. Taurine effects on Bisphenol A-induced oxidative stress in the mouse testicular mitochondria and sperm motility. *JBRA Assist. Reprod.* **2020**, *24*, 428–435. [CrossRef]
11. Nakajima, Y.; Osuka, K.; Seki, Y.; Gupta, R.C.; Hara, M.; Takayasu, M.; Wakabayashi, T. Taurine Reduces Inflammatory Responses after Spinal Cord Injury. *J. Neurotrauma* **2010**, *27*, 403–410. [CrossRef]
12. Albrecht, J.; Schousboe, A. Taurine Interaction with Neurotransmitter Receptors in the CNS: An Update. *Neurochem. Res.* **2005**, *30*, 1615–1621. [CrossRef]
13. Oja, S.S.; Saransaari, P. Significance of Taurine in the Brain. *Adv. Exp. Med. Biol.* **2017**, *1*, 89–94. [CrossRef]
14. Huxtable, R.J. Physiological actions of taurine. *Physiol. Rev.* **1992**, *72*, 101–163. [CrossRef]
15. Jong, C.J.; Sandal, P.; Schaffer, S.W. The Role of Taurine in Mitochondria Health: More Than Just an Antioxidant. *Molecules* **2021**, *26*, 4913. [CrossRef]
16. Wharton, B.; Morley, R.; Isaacs, E.B.; Cole, T.J.; Lucas, A. Low plasma taurine and later neurodevelopment. *Arch. Dis. Child.-Fetal Neonatal Ed.* **2004**, *89*, F497–F498. [CrossRef]
17. Sturman, J.; Moretz, R.; French, J.; Wisniewski, H. Taurine deficiency in the developing cat: Persistence of the cerebellar external granule cell layer. *J. Neurosci. Res.* **1985**, *13*, 405–416. [CrossRef]
18. Rak, K.; Völker, J.; Jürgens, L.; Scherzad, A.; Schendzielorz, P.; Radeloff, A.; Jablonka, S.; Mlynski, R.; Hagen, R. Neurotrophic effects of taurine on spiral ganglion neurons in vitro. *NeuroReport* **2014**, *25*, 1250–1254. [CrossRef]
19. Mersman, B.; Zaidi, W.; Syed, N.I.; Xu, F. Taurine Promotes Neurite Outgrowth and Synapse Development of Both Vertebrate and Invertebrate Central Neurons. *Front. Synaptic Neurosci.* **2020**, *12*, 29. [CrossRef]
20. Zhou, Y.; Qiu, L.; Xiao, Q.; Wang, Y.; Meng, X.; Xu, R.; Wang, S.; Na, R. Obesity and diabetes related plasma amino acid alterations. *Clin. Biochem.* **2013**, *46*, 1447–1452. [CrossRef]
21. De Luca, G.; Calpona, P.; Caponetti, A.; Romano, G.; Di Benedetto, A.; Cucinotta, D.; Di Giorgio, R. Taurine and osmoregulation: Platelet taurine content, uptake, and release in type 2 diabetic patients. *Metabolism* **2001**, *50*, 60–64. [CrossRef] [PubMed]
22. Elshorbagy, A.K.; Valdivia-Garcia, M.; Graham, I.M.; Reis, R.P.; Luis, A.S.; Smith, A.D.; Refsum, H. The association of fasting plasma sulfur-containing compounds with BMI, serum lipids and apolipoproteins. *Nutr. Metab. Cardiovasc. Dis.* **2012**, *22*, 1031–1038. [CrossRef]

23. Tessari, P.; Kiwanuka, E.; Coracina, A.; Zaramella, M.; Vettore, M.; Valerio, A.; Garibotto, G. Insulin in methionine and homocysteine kinetics in healthy humans: Plasma vs. intracellular models. *Am. J. Physiol. Metab.* **2005**, *288*, E1270–E1276. [CrossRef] [PubMed]
24. Berson, E.L.; Schmidt, S.Y.; Rabin, A.R. Plasma amino-acids in hereditary retinal disease. Ornithine, lysine, and taurine. *Br. J. Ophthalmol.* **1976**, *60*, 142–147. [CrossRef] [PubMed]
25. Chiarla, C.; Giovannini, I.; Siegel, J.H.; Boldrini, G.; Castagneto, M. The Relationship between Plasma Taurine and Other Amino Acid Levels in Human Sepsis. *J. Nutr.* **2000**, *130*, 2222–2227. [CrossRef] [PubMed]
26. Engel, J.M.; Mühling, J.; Weiss, S.; Kärcher, B.; Lohr, T.; Menges, T.; Little, S.; Hempelmann, G. Relationship of taurine and other amino acids in plasma and in neutrophils of septic trauma patients. *Amino Acids* **2005**, *30*, 87–94. [CrossRef] [PubMed]
27. Rana, S.K.; Sanders, T.A.B. Taurine concentrations in the diet, plasma, urine and breast milk of vegans compared with omnivores. *Br. J. Nutr.* **1986**, *56*, 17–27. [CrossRef]
28. Suleiman, M.-S.; Rodrigo, G.C.; Chapman, R. Interdependence of intracellular taurine and sodium in guinea pig heart. *Cardiovasc. Res.* **1992**, *26*, 897–905. [CrossRef]
29. Schønheyder, F.; Lyngbye, J. Influence of partial starvation and of acute scurvy on the free amino acids in blood plasma and muscle in the guinea-pig. *Br. J. Nutr.* **1962**, *16*, 75–82. [CrossRef]
30. Lerma, J.; Herranz, A.; Herreras, O.; Abraira, V.; del Rio, R.M. In vivo determination of extracellular concentration of amino acids in the rat hippocampus. A method based on brain dialysis and computerized analysis. *Brain Res.* **1986**, *384*, 145–155. [CrossRef]
31. Trachtman, H.; Futterweit, S.; Sturman, J.A. Cerebral Taurine Transport Is Increased During Streptozocin-Induced Diabetes in Rats. *Diabetes* **1992**, *41*, 1130–1140. [CrossRef]
32. Brand, H.S.; Chamuleau, R.A.F.M.; Jörning, G.G. Changes in urinary taurine and hypotaurine excretion after two-thirds hepatectomy in the rat. *Amino Acids* **1998**, *15*, 373–383. [CrossRef]
33. Larsen, L.H.; Ørstrup, L.K.H.; Hansen, S.H.; Grunnet, N.; Quistorff, B.; Mortensen, O.H. Fructose Feeding Changes Taurine Homeostasis in Wistar Rats. *Adv. Exp. Med. Biol.* **2015**, *803*, 695–706. [CrossRef]
34. Cardoso, S.; Carvalho, C.; Santos, R.; Correia, S.; Santos, M.S.; Seiça, R.; Oliveira, C.R.; Moreira, P.I. Impact of STZ-induced hyperglycemia and insulin-induced hypoglycemia in plasma amino acids and cortical synaptosomal neurotransmitters. *Synapse* **2010**, *65*, 457–466. [CrossRef]
35. Ma, Y.; Maruta, H.; Sun, B.; Wang, C.; Isono, C.; Yamashita, H. Effects of long-term taurine supplementation on age-related changes in skeletal muscle function of Sprague–Dawley rats. *Amino Acids* **2021**, *53*, 159–170. [CrossRef]
36. Chesney, R.W.; Jax, D.K. Developmental Aspects of Renal beta-Amino Acid Transport, I. Ontogeny of Taurine Reabsorption and Accumulation in Rat Renal Cortex. *Pediatr. Res.* **1979**, *13*, 854–860. [CrossRef]
37. Warskulat, U.; Borsch, E.; Reinehr, R.; Heller-Stilb, B.; Mönnighoff, I.; Buchczyk, D.; Donner, M.; Flögel, U.; Kappert, G.; Soboll, S.; et al. Chronic liver disease is triggered by taurine transporter knockout in the mouse. *FASEB J.* **2006**, *20*, 574–576. [CrossRef]
38. Garcia-Serrano, A.M.; Mohr, A.A.; Philippe, J.; Skoug, C.; Spégel, P.; Duarte, J.M.N. Cognitive Impairment and Metabolite Profile Alterations in the Hippocampus and Cortex of Male and Female Mice Exposed to a Fat and Sugar-Rich Diet are Normalized by Diet Reversal. *Aging Dis.* **2022**, *13*, 267. [CrossRef]
39. Tao, Y.; He, M.; Yang, Q.; Ma, Z.; Qu, Y.; Chen, W.; Peng, G.; Teng, D. Systemic taurine treatment provides neuroprotection against retinal photoreceptor degeneration and visual function impairments. *Drug Des. Dev. Ther.* **2019**, *13*, 2689–2702. [CrossRef]
40. Taranukhin, A.G.; Taranukhina, E.Y.; Saransaari, P.; Podkletnova, I.M.; Pelto-Huikko, M.; Oja, S.S. Neuroprotection by taurine in ethanol-induced apoptosis in the developing cerebellum. *J. Biomed. Sci.* **2010**, *17*, S12. [CrossRef]
41. Hadj-Saïd, W.; Froger, N.; Ivkovic, I.; Jiménez-López, M.; Dubus, É.; Dégardin-Chicaud, J.; Simonutti, M.; Quénol, C.; Neveux, N.; Villegas-Pérez, M.P.; et al. Quantitative and Topographical Analysis of the Losses of Cone Photoreceptors and Retinal Ganglion Cells Under Taurine Depletion. *Investig. Opthalmol. Vis. Sci.* **2016**, *57*, 4692–4703. [CrossRef] [PubMed]
42. Gambarota, G.; Mekle, R.; Xin, L.; Hergt, M.; Van Der Zwaag, W.; Krueger, G.; Gruetter, R. In vivo measurement of glycine with short echo-time 1H MRS in human brain at 7 T. *Magn. Reson. Mater. Phys. Biol. Med.* **2008**, *22*, 1–4. [CrossRef]
43. Mekle, R.; Mlynarik, V.; Gambarota, G.; Hergt, M.; Krueger, G.; Gruetter, R. MR spectroscopy of the human brain with enhanced signal intensity at ultrashort echo times on a clinical platform at 3T and 7T. *Magn. Reson. Med.* **2009**, *61*, 1279–1285. [CrossRef] [PubMed]
44. Deelchand, D.K.; Van de Moortele, P.-F.; Adriany, G.; Iltis, I.; Andersen, P.; Strupp, J.P.; Vaughan, J.T.; Uğurbil, K.; Henry, P.-G. In vivo1H NMR spectroscopy of the human brain at 9.4T: Initial results. *J. Magn. Reson.* **2010**, *206*, 74–80. [CrossRef] [PubMed]
45. Schaller, B.; Mekle, R.; Xin, L.; Kunz, N.; Gruetter, R. Net increase of lactate and glutamate concentration in activated human visual cortex detected with magnetic resonance spectroscopy at 7 tesla. *J. Neurosci. Res.* **2013**, *91*, 1076–1083. [CrossRef] [PubMed]
46. Marjańska, M.; Auerbach, E.J.; Valabrègue, R.; Van de Moortele, P.-F.; Adriany, G.; Garwood, M. Localized1H NMR spectroscopy in different regions of human brainin vivoat 7 T:T2relaxation times and concentrations of cerebral metabolites. *NMR Biomed.* **2011**, *25*, 332–339. [CrossRef]
47. Marjańska, M.; McCarten, J.R.; Hodges, J.; Hemmy, L.S.; Grant, A.; Deelchand, D.K.; Terpstra, M. Region-specific aging of the human brain as evidenced by neurochemical profiles measured noninvasively in the posterior cingulate cortex and the occipital lobe using 1 H magnetic resonance spectroscopy at 7 T. *Neuroscience* **2017**, *354*, 168–177. [CrossRef]

48. Ueki, I.; Roman, H.B.; Valli, A.; Fieselmann, K.; Lam, J.; Peters, R.; Hirschberger, L.L.; Stipanuk, M.H. Knockout of the murine cysteine dioxygenase gene results in severe impairment in ability to synthesize taurine and an increased catabolism of cysteine to hydrogen sulfide. *Am. J. Physiol. Metab.* **2011**, *301*, E668–E684. [CrossRef]
49. Wang, W.-T.; Lee, P.; Dong, Y.; Yeh, H.-W.; Kim, J.; Weiner, C.P.; Brooks, W.M.; Choi, I.-Y. In Vivo Neurochemical Characterization of Developing Guinea Pigs and the Effect of Chronic Fetal Hypoxia. *Neurochem. Res.* **2016**, *41*, 1831–1843. [CrossRef]
50. Lei, H.; Berthet, C.; Hirt, L.; Gruetter, R. Evolution of the Neurochemical Profile after Transient Focal Cerebral Ischemia in the Mouse Brain. *J. Cereb. Blood Flow Metab.* **2009**, *29*, 811–819. [CrossRef]
51. Lei, H.; Duarte, J.M.; Mlynarik, V.; Python, A.; Gruetter, R. Deep thiopental anesthesia alters steady-state glucose homeostasis but not the neurochemical profile of rat cortex. *J. Neurosci. Res.* **2009**, *88*, 413–419. [CrossRef] [PubMed]
52. Xin, L.; Gambarota, G.; Duarte, J.M.N.; Mlynárik, V.; Gruetter, R. Direct in vivo measurement of glycine and the neurochemical profile in the rat medulla oblongata. *NMR Biomed.* **2010**, *23*, 1097–1102. [CrossRef]
53. Harris, J.L.; Yeh, H.-W.; Swerdlow, R.H.; Choi, I.-Y.; Lee, P.; Brooks, W.M. High-field proton magnetic resonance spectroscopy reveals metabolic effects of normal brain aging. *Neurobiol. Aging* **2014**, *35*, 1686–1694. [CrossRef]
54. Sonnay, S.; Duarte, J.M.; Just, N.; Gruetter, R. Compartmentalised energy metabolism supporting glutamatergic neurotransmission in response to increased activity in the rat cerebral cortex: A 13C MRS study in vivo at 14.1 T. *J. Cereb. Blood Flow Metab.* **2016**, *36*, 928–940. [CrossRef] [PubMed]
55. Cuellar-Baena, S.; Landeck, N.; Sonnay, S.; Buck, K.; Mlynarik, V.; Zandt, R.I.; Kirik, D. Assessment of brain metabolite correlates of adeno-associated virus-mediated over-expression of human alpha-synuclein in cortical neurons by in vivo 1 H-MR spectroscopy at 9.4 T. *J. Neurochem.* **2016**, *137*, 806–819. [CrossRef] [PubMed]
56. Kulak, A.; Duarte, J.M.N.; Do, K.Q.; Gruetter, R. Neurochemical profile of the developing mouse cortex determined by in vivo1H NMR spectroscopy at 14.1 T and the effect of recurrent anaesthesia. *J. Neurochem.* **2010**, *115*, 1466–1477. [CrossRef]
57. Das Neves Duarte, J.M.; Kulak, A.; Gholam-Razaee, M.M.; Cuenod, M.; Gruetter, R.; Do, K.Q. N-Acetylcysteine Normalizes Neurochemical Changes in the Glutathione-Deficient Schizophrenia Mouse Model During Development. *Biol. Psychiatry* **2012**, *71*, 1006–1014. [CrossRef] [PubMed]
58. Duarte, J.M.; Do, K.Q.; Gruetter, R. Longitudinal neurochemical modifications in the aging mouse brain measured in vivo by 1H magnetic resonance spectroscopy. *Neurobiol. Aging* **2014**, *35*, 1660–1668. [CrossRef]
59. Corcoba, A.; Steullet, P.; Duarte, J.; van de Looij, Y.; Monin, A.; Cuenod, M.; Gruetter, R.; Do, K.Q. Glutathione Deficit Affects the Integrity and Function of the Fimbria/Fornix and Anterior Commissure in Mice: Relevance for Schizophrenia. *Int. J. Neuropsychopharmacol.* **2016**, *19*, pyv110. [CrossRef]
60. Gapp, K.; Corcoba, A.; Van Steenwyk, G.; Mansuy, I.M.; Duarte, J.M. Brain metabolic alterations in mice subjected to postnatal traumatic stress and in their offspring. *J. Cereb. Blood Flow Metab.* **2016**, *37*, 2423–2432. [CrossRef]
61. Roig-Pérez, S.; Moretó, M.; Ferrer, R. Transepithelial Taurine Transport in Caco-2 Cell Monolayers. *J. Membr. Biol.* **2005**, *204*, 85–92. [CrossRef] [PubMed]
62. Jacobsen, J.G.; Smith, L.H. Biochemistry and physiology of taurine and taurine derivatives. *Physiol. Rev.* **1968**, *48*, 424–511. [CrossRef] [PubMed]
63. Chesney, R.W.; Lippincott, S.; Gusowski, N.; Padilla, M.; Zelikovic, I. Studies on Renal Adaptation to Altered Dietary Amino Acid Intake: Tissue Taurine Responses in Nursing and Adult Rats. *J. Nutr.* **1986**, *116*, 1965–1976. [CrossRef] [PubMed]
64. Thaeomor, A.; Wyss, J.M.; Jirakulsomchok, D.; Roysommuti, S. High sugar intake via the renin-angiotensin system blunts the baroreceptor reflex in adult rats that were perinatally depleted of taurine. *J. Biomed. Sci.* **2010**, *17*, S30. [CrossRef] [PubMed]
65. Wójcik, O.P.; Koenig, K.L.; Zeleniuch-Jacquotte, A.; Costa, M.; Chen, Y. The potential protective effects of taurine on coronary heart disease. *Atherosclerosis* **2010**, *208*, 19–25. [CrossRef]
66. Rasgado-Flores, H.; Mokashi, A.; Hawkins, R.A. Na+-dependent transport of taurine is found only on the abluminal membrane of the blood–brain barrier. *Exp. Neurol.* **2012**, *233*, 457–462. [CrossRef] [PubMed]
67. Tamai, I.; Senmaru, M.; Terasaki, T.; Tsuji, A. Na+- and Cl−-Dependent transport of taurine at the blood-brain barrier. *Biochem. Pharmacol.* **1995**, *50*, 1783–1793. [CrossRef]
68. Lee, N.-Y.; Kang, Y.-S. The brain-to-blood efflux transport of taurine and changes in the blood–brain barrier transport system by tumor necrosis factor-α. *Brain Res.* **2004**, *1023*, 141–147. [CrossRef]
69. Zhou, Y.; Holmseth, S.; Guo, C.; Hassel, B.; Höfner, G.; Huitfeldt, H.S.; Wanner, K.; Danbolt, N.C. Deletion of the γ-Aminobutyric Acid Transporter 2 (GAT2 and SLC6A13) Gene in Mice Leads to Changes in Liver and Brain Taurine Contents. *J. Biol. Chem.* **2012**, *287*, 35733–35746. [CrossRef]
70. Geier, E.G.; Chen, E.C.; Webb, A.; Papp, A.C.; Yee, S.W.; Sadee, W.; Giacomini, K.M. Profiling Solute Carrier Transporters in the Human Blood–Brain Barrier. *Clin. Pharmacol. Ther.* **2013**, *94*, 636–639. [CrossRef]
71. Nishimura, T.; Higuchi, K.; Yoshida, Y.; Sugita-Fujisawa, Y.; Kojima, K.; Sugimoto, M.; Santo, M.; Tomi, M.; Nakashima, E. Hypotaurine Is a Substrate of GABA Transporter Family Members GAT2/Slc6a13 and TAUT/Slc6a. *Biol. Pharm. Bull.* **2018**, *41*, 1523–1529. [CrossRef] [PubMed]
72. Pow, D.V.; Sullivan, R.; Reye, P.; Hermanussen, S. Localization of taurine transporters, taurine, and3H taurine accumulation in the rat retina, pituitary, and brain. *Glia* **2002**, *37*, 153–168. [CrossRef] [PubMed]
73. Fujita, T.; Shimada, A.; Wada, M.; Miyakawa, S.; Yamamoto, A. Functional Expression of Taurine Transporter and its Up-Regulation in Developing Neurons from Mouse Cerebral Cortex. *Pharm. Res.* **2006**, *23*, 689–696. [CrossRef] [PubMed]

74. Durkin, M.M.; Smith, K.E.; Borden, L.A.; Weinshank, R.L.; Branchek, T.A.; Gustafson, E.L. Localization of messenger RNAs encoding three GABA transporters in rat brain: An in situ hybridization study. *Mol. Brain Res.* **1995**, *33*, 7–21. [CrossRef]
75. Mongin, A.A. Volume-regulated anion channel—A frenemy within the brain. *Pflügers Arch. Eur. J. Physiol.* **2016**, *468*, 421–441. [CrossRef]
76. Furukawa, T.; Yamada, J.; Akita, T.; Matsushima, Y.; Yanagawa, Y.; Fukuda, A. Roles of taurine-mediated tonic GABAA receptor activation in the radial migration of neurons in the fetal mouse cerebral cortex. *Front. Cell. Neurosci.* **2014**, *8*, 88. [CrossRef]
77. Brand, A.; Leibfritz, D.; Hamprecht, B.; Dringen, R. Metabolism of Cysteine in Astroglial Cells: Synthesis of Hypotaurine and Taurine. *J. Neurochem.* **2002**, *71*, 827–832. [CrossRef]
78. Vitvitsky, V.; Garg, S.K.; Banerjee, R. Taurine Biosynthesis by Neurons and Astrocytes. *J. Biol. Chem.* **2011**, *286*, 32002–32010. [CrossRef]
79. Park, E.; Park, S.Y.; Dobkin, C.; Schuller-Levis, G. Development of a Novel Cysteine Sulfinic Acid Decarboxylase Knockout Mouse: Dietary Taurine Reduces Neonatal Mortality. *J. Amino Acids* **2014**, *2014*, 1–12. [CrossRef] [PubMed]
80. Veeravalli, S.; Phillips, I.R.; Freire, R.T.; Varshavi, D.; Everett, J.R.; Shephard, E.A. Flavin-Containing Monooxygenase 1 Catalyzes the Production of Taurine from Hypotaurine. *Drug Metab. Dispos.* **2020**, *48*, 378–385. [CrossRef]
81. Janmohamed, A.; Hernandez, D.; Phillips, I.R.; Shephard, E. Cell-, tissue-, sex- and developmental stage-specific expression of mouse flavin-containing monooxygenases (Fmos). *Biochem. Pharmacol.* **2004**, *68*, 73–83. [CrossRef] [PubMed]
82. Junyent, F.; De Lemos, L.; Utrera, J.; Paco, S.; Aguado, F.; Camins, A.; Pallàs, M.; Romero, R.; Auladell, C. Content and traffic of taurine in hippocampal reactive astrocytes. *Hippocampus* **2011**, *21*, 185–197. [CrossRef] [PubMed]
83. Banerjee, R.; Vitvitsky, V.; Garg, S.K. The undertow of sulfur metabolism on glutamatergic neurotransmission. *Trends Biochem. Sci.* **2008**, *33*, 413–419. [CrossRef] [PubMed]
84. Brosnan, J.T.; Brosnan, M.E. The Sulfur-Containing Amino Acids: An Overview. *J. Nutr.* **2006**, *136*, 1636S–1640S. [CrossRef] [PubMed]
85. Ouyang, Y.; Wu, Q.; Li, J.; Sun, S.; Sun, S. S-adenosylmethionine: A metabolite critical to the regulation of autophagy. *Cell Prolif.* **2020**, *53*, e12891. [CrossRef] [PubMed]
86. Kvetnansky, R.; Sabban, E.L.; Palkovits, M. Catecholaminergic Systems in Stress: Structural and Molecular Genetic Approaches. *Physiol. Rev.* **2009**, *89*, 535–606. [CrossRef] [PubMed]
87. Sbodio, J.I.; Snyder, S.H.; Paul, B.D. Regulators of the transsulfuration pathway. *Br. J. Pharmacol.* **2019**, *176*, 583–593. [CrossRef]
88. Stipanuk, M.H.; Ueki, I. Dealing with methionine/homocysteine sulfur: Cysteine metabolism to taurine and inorganic sulfur. *J. Inherit. Metab. Dis.* **2011**, *34*, 17–32. [CrossRef] [PubMed]
89. Churchwell, K.B.; Wright, S.H.; Emma, F.; Rosenberg, P.; Strange, K. NMDA Receptor Activation Inhibits Neuronal Volume Regulation after Swelling Induced by Veratridine-Stimulated Na+Influx in Rat Cortical Cultures. *J. Neurosci.* **1996**, *16*, 7447–7457. [CrossRef]
90. Murphy, T.R.; Davila, D.; Cuvelier, N.; Young, L.R.; Lauderdale, K.; Binder, D.K.; Fiacco, T.A. Hippocampal and Cortical Pyramidal Neurons Swell in Parallel with Astrocytes during Acute Hypoosmolar Stress. *Front. Cell. Neurosci.* **2017**, *11*, 275. [CrossRef]
91. Lambert, I.H. Regulation of the cellular content of the organic osmolyte taurine in mammalian cells. *Neurochem. Res.* **2004**, *29*, 27–63. [CrossRef] [PubMed]
92. Walz, W.; Allen, A.F. Evaluation of the osmoregulatory function of taurine in brain cells. *Exp. Brain Res.* **1987**, *68*, 290–298. [CrossRef]
93. Oja, S. Chloride ions, potassium stimulation and release of endogenous taurine from cerebral cortical slices from 3 day old and 3 month old mice. *Neurochem. Int.* **1995**, *27*, 313–318. [CrossRef]
94. Verbalis, J.; Gullans, S. Hyponatremia causes large sustained reductions in brain content of multiple organic osmolytes in rats. *Brain Res.* **1991**, *567*, 274–282. [CrossRef]
95. Lien, Y.H.; Shapiro, J.; Chan, L. Effects of hypernatremia on organic brain osmoles. *J. Clin. Investig.* **1990**, *85*, 1427–1435. [CrossRef] [PubMed]
96. Olson, J.E.; Goldfinger, M.D. Amino acid content of rat cerebral astrocytes adapted to hyperosmotic medium in vitro. *J. Neurosci. Res.* **1990**, *27*, 241–246. [CrossRef] [PubMed]
97. Sánchez-Olea, R.; Morán, J.; Pasantes-Morales, H. Changes in taurine transport evoked by hyperosmolarity in cultured astrocytes. *J. Neurosci. Res.* **1992**, *32*, 86–92. [CrossRef]
98. Bitoun, M.; Tappaz, M. Taurine Down-Regulates Basal and Osmolarity-Induced Gene Expression of Its Transporter, but Not the Gene Expression of Its Biosynthetic Enzymes, in Astrocyte Primary Cultures. *J. Neurochem.* **2002**, *75*, 919–924. [CrossRef] [PubMed]
99. Kimelberg, H.; Goderie, S.; Higman, S.; Pang, S.; Waniewski, R. Swelling-induced release of glutamate, aspartate, and taurine from astrocyte cultures. *J. Neurosci.* **1990**, *10*, 1583–1591. [CrossRef]
100. Qiu, Z.; Dubin, A.E.; Mathur, J.; Tu, B.; Reddy, K.; Miraglia, L.J.; Reinhardt, J.; Orth, A.P.; Patapoutian, A. SWELL1, a Plasma Membrane Protein, Is an Essential Component of Volume-Regulated Anion Channel. *Cell* **2014**, *157*, 447–458. [CrossRef]
101. Schmid, R.; Sieghart, W.; Karobath, M. Taurine Uptake in Synaptosomal Fractions of Rat Cerebral Cortex. *J. Neurochem.* **1975**, *25*, 5–9. [CrossRef]
102. Lähdesmäki, P.; Pasula, M.; Oja, S.S. Effect of electrical stimulation and chlorpromazine on the uptake and release of taurine, γ-aminobutyric acid and glutamic acid in mouse brain synaptosomes. *J. Neurochem.* **1975**, *25*, 675–680. [CrossRef] [PubMed]

103. Kontro, P.; Oja, S.S. Sodium-independent taurine binding to brain synaptic membranes. *Cell. Mol. Neurobiol.* **1983**, *3*, 183–187. [CrossRef] [PubMed]
104. Huxtable, R.; Peterson, A. Sodium-dependent and sodium-independent binding of taurine to rat brain synaptosomes. *Neurochem. Int.* **1989**, *14*, 79–84. [CrossRef]
105. Lynch, J.W. Molecular Structure and Function of the Glycine Receptor Chloride Channel. *Physiol. Rev.* **2004**, *84*, 1051–1095. [CrossRef]
106. Shibanoki, S.; Kogure, M.; Sugahara, M.; Ishikawa, K. Effect of Systemic Administration of N-Methyl-d-Aspartic Acid on Extracellular Taurine Level Measured by Microdialysis in the Hippocampal CA1 Field and Striatum of Rats. *J. Neurochem.* **1993**, *61*, 1698–1704. [CrossRef] [PubMed]
107. Segovia, G.; Del Arco, A.; Mora, F. Endogenous Glutamate Increases Extracellular Concentrations of Dopamine, GABA, and Taurine Through NMDA and AMPA/Kainate Receptors in Striatum of the Freely Moving Rat: A Microdialysis Study. *J. Neurochem.* **1997**, *69*, 1476–1483. [CrossRef] [PubMed]
108. Holopainen, I.; Kontro, P.; Oja, S.S. Release of preloaded taurine and hypotaurine from astrocytes in primary culture: Stimulation by calcium-free media. *Neurochem. Res.* **1985**, *10*, 123–131. [CrossRef] [PubMed]
109. Shain, W.G.; Martin, D.L. Activation of beta-adrenergic receptors stimulates taurine release from glial cells. *Cell. Mol. Neurobiol.* **1984**, *4*, 191–196. [CrossRef]
110. Philibert, R.A.; Rogers, K.L.; Allen, A.J.; Dutton, G.R. Dose-Dependent, K+-Stimulated Efflux of Endogenous Taurine from Primary Astrocyte Cultures Is Ca2+-Dependent. *J. Neurochem.* **1988**, *51*, 122–126. [CrossRef]
111. Philibert, R.; Rogers, K.L.; Dutton, G.R. K+-evoked taurine efflux from cerebellar astrocytes: On the roles of Ca2+ and Na+. *Neurochem. Research* **1989**, *14*, 43–48. [CrossRef] [PubMed]
112. Barakat, L.; Wang, D.; Bordey, A. Carrier-mediated uptake and release of taurine from Bergmann glia in rat cerebellar slices. *J. Physiol.* **2002**, *541*, 753–767. [CrossRef]
113. Choe, K.; Olson, J.E.; Bourque, C.W. Taurine Release by Astrocytes Modulates Osmosensitive Glycine Receptor Tone and Excitability in the Adult Supraoptic Nucleus. *J. Neurosci.* **2012**, *32*, 12518–12527. [CrossRef] [PubMed]
114. McCool, B.; Botting, S.K. Characterization of strychnine-sensitive glycine receptors in acutely isolated adult rat basolateral amygdala neurons. *Brain Res.* **2000**, *859*, 341–351. [CrossRef]
115. Hussy, N.; Brès, V.; Rochette, M.; Duvoid, A.; Alonso, G.; Dayanithi, G.; Moos, F.C. Osmoregulation of Vasopressin Secretion via Activation of Neurohypophysial Nerve Terminals Glycine Receptors by Glial Taurine. *J. Neurosci.* **2001**, *21*, 7110–7116. [CrossRef]
116. Wu, Z.-Y.; Xu, T.-L. Taurine-evoked chloride current and its potentiation by intracellular Ca2+ in immature rat hippocampal CA1 neurons. *Amino Acids* **2003**, *24*, 155–161. [CrossRef] [PubMed]
117. Jiang, Z.; Krnjević, K.; Wang, F.; Ye, J.H. Taurine Activates Strychnine-Sensitive Glycine Receptors in Neurons Freshly Isolated from Nucleus Accumbens of Young Rats. *J. Neurophysiol.* **2004**, *91*, 248–257. [CrossRef]
118. Xu, H.; Zhou, K.-Q.; Huang, Y.-N.; Chen, L.; Xu, T.-L. Taurine activates strychnine-sensitive glycine receptors in neurons of the rat inferior colliculus. *Brain Res.* **2004**, *1021*, 232–240. [CrossRef]
119. Jiang, Z.; Yue, M.; Chandra, D.; Keramidas, A.; Goldstein, P.; Homanics, G.; Harrison, N.L. Taurine Is a Potent Activator of Extrasynaptic GABAA Receptors in the Thalamus. *J. Neurosci.* **2008**, *28*, 106–115. [CrossRef]
120. El Idrissi, A.; Trenkner, E. Growth Factors and Taurine Protect against Excitotoxicity by Stabilizing Calcium Homeostasis and Energy Metabolism. *J. Neurosci.* **1999**, *19*, 9459–9468. [CrossRef]
121. Louzada, P.R.; Lima, A.C.P.; Mendonca-Silva, D.L.; Noël, F.; De Mello, F.G.; Ferreira, S.T. Taurine prevents the neurotoxicity of beta-amyloid and glutamate receptor agonists: Activation of GABA receptors and possible implications for Alzheimer's disease and other neurological disorders. *FASEB J.* **2004**, *18*, 511–518. [CrossRef]
122. Bulley, S.; Shen, W. Reciprocal regulation between taurine and glutamate response via Ca2+- dependent pathways in retinal third-order neurons. *J. Biomed. Sci.* **2010**, *17*, S5. [CrossRef] [PubMed]
123. El Idrissi, A.; Trenkner, E. Taurine as a Modulator of Excitatory and Inhibitory Neurotransmission. *Neurochem. Res.* **2004**, *29*, 189–197. [CrossRef] [PubMed]
124. Saransaari, P.; Oja, S. Excitatory amino acids evoke taurine release from cerebral cortex slices from adult and developing mice. *Neuroscience* **1991**, *45*, 451–459. [CrossRef]
125. Saransaari, P. Taurine release from the developing and ageing hippocampus: Stimulation by agonists of ionotropic glutamate receptors. *Mech. Ageing Dev.* **1997**, *99*, 219–232. [CrossRef]
126. Saransaari, P.; Oja, S. Modulation of the ischemia-induced taurine release by adenosine receptors in the developing and adult mouse hippocampus. *Neuroscience* **2000**, *97*, 425–430. [CrossRef]
127. Saransaari, P.P.; Oja, S.S. Involvement of metabotropic glutamate receptors in taurine release in the adult and developing mouse hippocampus. *Amino Acids* **1999**, *16*, 165–179. [CrossRef]
128. Li, G.; Olson, J.E. Purinergic activation of anion conductance and osmolyte efflux in cultured rat hippocampal neurons. *Am. J. Physiol. Physiol.* **2008**, *295*, C1550–C1560. [CrossRef]
129. Bonhaus, D.W.; Lippincott, S.E.; Huxtable, R.J.; Sanchez, A.P.; Scheffner, D. Subcellular Distribution of Neuroactive Amino Acids in Brains of Genetically Epileptic Rats. *Epilepsia* **1984**, *25*, 564–568. [CrossRef]
130. Chen, W.; Freinkman, E.; Wang, T.; Birsoy, K.; Sabatini, D.M. Absolute Quantification of Matrix Metabolites Reveals the Dynamics of Mitochondrial Metabolism. *Cell* **2016**, *166*, 1324–1337.e11. [CrossRef]

131. Hansen, S.H.; Andersen, M.L.; Cornett, C.; Gradinaru, R.; Grunnet, N. A role for taurine in mitochondrial function. *J. Biomed. Sci.* **2010**, *17*, S23. [CrossRef] [PubMed]
132. Sonnay, S.; Poirot, J.; Just, N.; Clerc, A.-C.; Gruetter, R.; Rainer, G.; Duarte, J.M.N. Astrocytic and neuronal oxidative metabolism are coupled to the rate of glutamate-glutamine cycle in the tree shrew visual cortex. *Glia* **2017**, *66*, 477–491. [CrossRef] [PubMed]
133. Cano-Abad, M.F.; Di Benedetto, G.; Magalhães, P.J.; Filippin, L.; Pozzan, T. Mitochondrial pH Monitored by a New Engineered Green Fluorescent Protein Mutant. *J. Biol. Chem.* **2004**, *279*, 11521–11529. [CrossRef] [PubMed]
134. Azarias, G.; Perreten, H.; Lengacher, S.; Poburko, D.; Demaurex, N.; Magistretti, P.J.; Chatton, J.-Y. Glutamate Transport Decreases Mitochondrial pH and Modulates Oxidative Metabolism in Astrocytes. *J. Neurosci.* **2011**, *31*, 3550–3559. [CrossRef]
135. Poburko, D.; Domingo, J.S.; Demaurex, N. Dynamic Regulation of the Mitochondrial Proton Gradient during Cytosolic Calcium Elevations. *J. Biol. Chem.* **2011**, *286*, 11672–11684. [CrossRef]
136. Thevenet, J.; De Marchi, U.; Domingo, J.S.; Christinat, N.; Bultot, L.; Lefebvre, G.; Sakamoto, K.; Descombes, P.; Masoodi, M.; Wiederkehr, A. Medium-chain fatty acids inhibit mitochondrial metabolism in astrocytes promoting astrocyte-neuron lactate and ketone body shuttle systems. *FASEB J.* **2016**, *30*, 1913–1926. [CrossRef]
137. Mohammadi, H.; Ommati, M.M.; Farshad, O.; Jamshidzadeh, A.; Nikbakht, M.R.; Niknahad, H.; Heidari, R. Taurine and isolated mitochondria: A concentration-response study. *Trends Pharm. Sci.* **2019**, *5*, 197–206.
138. Niknahad, H.; Jamshidzadeh, A.; Heidari, R.; Zarei, M.; Ommati, M.M. Ammonia-induced mitochondrial dysfunction and energy metabolism disturbances in isolated brain and liver mitochondria, and the effect of taurine administration: Relevance to hepatic encephalopathy treatment. *Clin. Exp. Hepatol.* **2017**, *3*, 141–151. [CrossRef]
139. Aruoma, O.I.; Halliwell, B.; Hoey, B.M.; Butler, J. The antioxidant action of taurine, hypotaurine and their metabolic precursors. *Biochem. J.* **1988**, *256*, 251–255. [CrossRef]
140. Parvez, S.; Tabassum, H.; Banerjee, B.D.; Raisuddin, S. Taurine Prevents Tamoxifen-Induced Mitochondrial Oxidative Damage in Mice. *Basic Clin. Pharmacol. Toxicol.* **2008**, *102*, 382–387. [CrossRef] [PubMed]
141. Suzuki, T.; Wada, T.; Saigo, K.; Watanabe, K. Taurine as a constituent of mitochondrial tRNAs: New insights into the functions of taurine and human mitochondrial diseases. *EMBO J.* **2002**, *21*, 6581–6589. [CrossRef] [PubMed]
142. Yasukawa, T.; Kirino, Y.; Ishii, N.; Holt, I.; Jacobs, H.T.; Makifuchi, T.; Fukuhara, N.; Ohta, S.; Suzuki, T.; Watanabe, K. Wobble modification deficiency in mutant tRNAs in patients with mitochondrial diseases. *FEBS Lett.* **2005**, *579*, 2948–2952. [CrossRef] [PubMed]
143. Fakruddin; Wei, F.-Y.; Suzuki, T.; Asano, K.; Kaieda, T.; Omori, A.; Izumi, R.; Fujimura, A.; Kaitsuka, T.; Miyata, K.; et al. Defective Mitochondrial tRNA Taurine Modification Activates Global Proteostress and Leads to Mitochondrial Disease. *Cell Rep.* **2018**, *22*, 482–496. [CrossRef] [PubMed]
144. Schaffer, S.W.; Jong, C.J.; Ito, T.; Azuma, J. Role of taurine in the pathologies of MELAS and MERRF. *Amino Acids* **2012**, *46*, 47–56. [CrossRef]
145. Ohsawa, Y.; Hagiwara, H.; Nishimatsu, S.-I.; Hirakawa, A.; Kamimura, N.; Ohtsubo, H.; Fukai, Y.; Murakami, T.; Koga, Y.; Goto, Y.-I.; et al. Taurine supplementation for prevention of stroke-like episodes in MELAS: A multicentre, open-label, 52-week phase III trial. *J. Neurol. Neurosurg. Psychiatry* **2019**, *90*, 529–536. [CrossRef]
146. Zhang, Y.; Li, D.; Li, H.; Hou, D.; Hou, J. Taurine Pretreatment Prevents Isoflurane-Induced Cognitive Impairment by Inhibiting ER Stress-Mediated Activation of Apoptosis Pathways in the Hippocampus in Aged Rats. *Neurochem. Res.* **2016**, *41*, 2517–2525. [CrossRef]
147. Li, S.; Yang, L.; Zhang, Y.; Zhang, C.; Shao, J.; Liu, X.; Li, Y.; Piao, F. Taurine Ameliorates Arsenic-Induced Apoptosis in the Hippocampus of Mice Through Intrinsic Pathway. *Adv. Exp. Med. Biol.* **2017**, *975*, 183–192. [CrossRef]
148. Agarwal, R.; Arfuzir, N.N.N.; Iezhitsa, I.; Agarwal, P.; Sidek, S.; Ismail, N.M. Taurine protects against retinal and optic nerve damage induced by endothelin-1 in rats via antioxidant effects. *Neural Regen. Res.* **2018**, *13*, 2014. [CrossRef]
149. Sun, M.; Xu, C. Neuroprotective Mechanism of Taurine due to Up-regulating Calpastatin and Down-regulating Calpain and Caspase-3 during Focal Cerebral Ischemia. *Cell. Mol. Neurobiol.* **2007**, *28*, 593–611. [CrossRef]
150. Sun, M.; Gu, Y.; Zhao, Y.; Xu, C. Protective functions of taurine against experimental stroke through depressing mitochondria-mediated cell death in rats. *Amino Acids* **2011**, *40*, 1419–1429. [CrossRef]
151. Zhu, X.-Y.; Ma, P.-S.; Wu, W.; Zhou, R.; Hao, Y.-J.; Niu, Y.; Sun, T.; Li, Y.-X.; Yu, J.-Q. Neuroprotective actions of taurine on hypoxic-ischemic brain damage in neonatal rats. *Brain Res. Bull.* **2016**, *124*, 295–305. [CrossRef]
152. Gharibani, P.M.; Modi, J.; Pan, C.; Menzie, J.; Ma, Z.; Chen, P.-C.; Tao, R.; Prentice, H.; Wu, J.-Y. The Mechanism of Taurine Protection Against Endoplasmic Reticulum Stress in an Animal Stroke Model of Cerebral Artery Occlusion and Stroke-Related Conditions in Primary Neuronal Cell Culture. *Adv. Exp. Med. Biol.* **2013**, *776*, 241–258. [CrossRef]
153. Gharibani, P.; Modi, J.; Menzie, J.; Alexandrescu, A.; Ma, Z.; Tao, R.; Prentice, H.; Wu, J.-Y. Comparison between single and combined post-treatment with S-Methyl-N,N-diethylthiolcarbamate sulfoxide and taurine following transient focal cerebral ischemia in rat brain. *Neuroscience* **2015**, *300*, 460–473. [CrossRef]
154. Duarte, J.M.N. Metabolic Alterations Associated to Brain Dysfunction in Diabetes. *Aging Dis.* **2014**, *6*, 304–321. [CrossRef]
155. Garcia-Serrano, A.M.; Duarte, J.M.N. Brain Metabolism Alterations in Type 2 Diabetes: What Did We Learn from Diet-Induced Diabetes Models? *Front. Neurosci.* **2020**, *14*, 229. [CrossRef]
156. Duarte, J.M.N.; Carvalho, R.; Cunha, R.; Gruetter, R. Caffeine consumption attenuates neurochemical modifications in the hippocampus of streptozotocin-induced diabetic rats. *J. Neurochem.* **2009**, *111*, 368–379. [CrossRef]

157. Wang, W.-T.; Lee, P.; Yeh, H.-W.; Smirnova, I.V.; Choi, I.-Y. Effects of acute and chronic hyperglycemia on the neurochemical profiles in the rat brain with streptozotocin-induced diabetes detected using in vivo1H MR spectroscopy at 9.4 T. *J. Neurochem.* **2012**, *121*, 407–417. [CrossRef]
158. Duarte, J.M.N.; Skoug, C.; Silva, H.B.; Carvalho, R.; Gruetter, R.; Cunha, R. Impact of Caffeine Consumption on Type 2 Diabetes-Induced Spatial Memory Impairment and Neurochemical Alterations in the Hippocampus. *Front. Neurosci.* **2019**, *12*, 1015. [CrossRef]
159. Lizarbe, B.; Soares, A.F.; Larsson, S.; Duarte, J.M.N. Neurochemical Modifications in the Hippocampus, Cortex and Hypothalamus of Mice Exposed to Long-Term High-Fat Diet. *Front. Neurosci.* **2019**, *12*, 985. [CrossRef]
160. Duarte, J.M.N. Metabolism in the Diabetic Brain: Neurochemical Profiling by 1H Magnetic Resonance Spectroscopy. *Diabetes Metab. Disord.* **2016**, *3*, 1–6. [CrossRef]
161. Duarte, J.M.N.; Lei, H.; Mlynárik, V.; Gruetter, R. The neurochemical profile quantified by in vivo1H NMR spectroscopy. *NeuroImage* **2012**, *61*, 342–362. [CrossRef]
162. De La Monte, S.M. Insulin Resistance and Neurodegeneration: Progress Towards the Development of New Therapeutics for Alzheimer's Disease. *Drugs* **2017**, *77*, 47–65. [CrossRef]
163. Barone, E.; Di Domenico, F.; Perluigi, M.; Butterfield, D.A. The interplay among oxidative stress, brain insulin resistance and AMPK dysfunction contribute to neurodegeneration in type 2 diabetes and Alzheimer disease. *Free Radic. Biol. Med.* **2021**, *176*, 16–33. [CrossRef]
164. Liu, H.; Zhang, D.; Lin, H.; Zhang, Q.; Zheng, L.; Zheng, Y.; Yin, X.; Li, Z.; Liang, S.; Huang, S. Meta-Analysis of Neurochemical Changes Estimated via Magnetic Resonance Spectroscopy in Mild Cognitive Impairment and Alzheimer's Disease. *Front. Aging Neurosci.* **2021**, *13*, 606. [CrossRef]
165. Song, T.; Song, X.; Zhu, C.; Patrick, R.; Skurla, M.; Santangelo, I.; Green, M.; Harper, D.; Ren, B.; Forester, B.P.; et al. Mitochondrial dysfunction, oxidative stress, neuroinflammation, and metabolic alterations in the progression of Alzheimer's disease: A meta-analysis of in vivo magnetic resonance spectroscopy studies. *Ageing Res. Rev.* **2021**, *72*, 101503. [CrossRef]
166. Marjańska, M.; McCarten, J.R.; Hodges, J.S.; Hemmy, L.S.; Terpstra, M. Distinctive Neurochemistry in Alzheimer's Disease via 7 T In Vivo Magnetic Resonance Spectroscopy. *J. Alzheimer's Dis.* **2019**, *68*, 559–569. [CrossRef]
167. Degrell, I.; Hellsing, K.; Nagy, E.; Niklasson, F. Amino acid concentrations in cerebrospinal fluid in presenile and senile dementia of Alzheimer type and multi-infarct dementia. *Arch. Gerontol. Geriatr.* **1989**, *9*, 123–135. [CrossRef]
168. Vermeiren, Y.; Le Bastard, N.; Van Hemelrijck, A.; Drinkenburg, W.H.; Engelborghs, S.; De Deyn, P.P. Behavioral correlates of cerebrospinal fluid amino acid and biogenic amine neurotransmitter alterations in dementia. *Alzheimer's Dement.* **2013**, *9*, 488–498. [CrossRef]
169. Mb, D.W.E.; Beal, M.F.; Mazurek, M.F.; Bird, E.D.; Martin, J.B. A postmortem study of amino acid neurotransmitters in Alzheimer's disease. *Ann. Neurol.* **1986**, *20*, 616–621. [CrossRef]
170. Perry, T.L.; Yong, V.W.; Bergeron, C.; Ba, S.H.; Jones, K. Amino acids, glutathione, and glutathione transferase activity in the brains of patients with Alzheimer's disease. *Ann. Neurol.* **1987**, *21*, 331–336. [CrossRef]
171. Pomara, N.; Singh, R.; Deptula, D.; Chou, J.C.; Schwartz, M.B.; LeWitt, P.A. Glutamate and other CSF amino acids in Alzheimer's disease. *Am. J. Psychiatry* **1992**, *149*, 251–254. [CrossRef]
172. Csernansky, J.G.; Bardgett, M.E.; Sheline, Y.I.; Morris, J.C.; Olney, J.W. CSF excitatory amino acids and severity of illness in Alzheimer's disease. *Neurology* **1996**, *46*, 1715–1720. [CrossRef]
173. Aquilani, R.; Costa, A.; Maestri, R.; Ramusino, M.C.; Pierobon, A.; Dossena, M.; Solerte, S.B.; Condino, A.M.; Torlaschi, V.; Bini, P.; et al. Mini Nutritional Assessment May Identify a Dual Pattern of Perturbed Plasma Amino Acids in Patients with Alzheimer's Disease: A Window to Metabolic and Physical Rehabilitation? *Nutrients* **2020**, *12*, 1845. [CrossRef]
174. Chouraki, V.; Preis, S.R.; Yang, Q.; Beiser, A.; Li, S.; Larson, M.G.; Weinstein, G.; Wang, T.J.; Gerszten, R.E.; Vasan, R.S.; et al. Association of amine biomarkers with incident dementia and Alzheimer's disease in the Framingham Study. *Alzheimer's Dement.* **2017**, *13*, 1327–1336. [CrossRef]
175. Roysommuti, S.; Wyss, J.M. Perinatal taurine exposure affects adult arterial pressure control. *Amino Acids* **2014**, *46*, 57–72. [CrossRef]
176. Wang, G.; Jiang, Z.-L.; Fan, X.-J.; Zhang, L.; Li, X.; Ke, K.-F. Neuroprotective effect of taurine against focal cerebral ischemia in rats possibly mediated by activation of both GABAA and glycine receptors. *Neuropharmacology* **2007**, *52*, 1199–1209. [CrossRef]
177. Ravaglia, G.; Forti, P.; Maioli, F.; Bianchi, G.; Martelli, M.; Talerico, T.; Servadei, L.; Zoli, M.; Mariani, E. Plasma amino acid concentrations in patients with amnestic mild cognitive impairment or Alzheimer disease. *Am. J. Clin. Nutr.* **2004**, *80*, 483–488. [CrossRef]
178. Chaney, A.M.; Lopez-Picon, F.R.; Serrière, S.; Wang, R.; Bochicchio, D.; Webb, S.D.; Vandesquille, M.; Harte, M.K.; Georgiadou, C.; Lawrence, C.; et al. Prodromal neuroinflammatory, cholinergic and metabolite dysfunction detected by PET and MRS in the TgF344-AD transgenic rat model of AD: A collaborative multi-modal study. *Theranostics* **2021**, *11*, 6644–6667. [CrossRef]
179. Nilsen, L.H.; Melø, T.M.; Saether, O.; Witter, M.P.; Sonnewald, U.; Sæther, O. Altered neurochemical profile in the McGill-R-Thy1-APP rat model of Alzheimer's disease: A longitudinalin vivo1H MRS study. *J. Neurochem.* **2012**, *123*, 532–541. [CrossRef]
180. Dedeoglu, A.; Choi, J.-K.; Cormier, K.; Kowall, N.W.; Jenkins, B.G. Magnetic resonance spectroscopic analysis of Alzheimer's disease mouse brain that express mutant human APP shows altered neurochemical profile. *Brain Res.* **2004**, *1012*, 60–65. [CrossRef]

181. Mlynarik, V.; Cacquevel, M.; Sun-Reimer, L.; Janssens, S.; Cudalbu, C.; Lei, H.; Schneider, B.L.; Aebischer, P.; Gruetter, R. Proton and phosphorus magnetic resonance spectroscopy of a mouse model of Alzheimer's disease. *J. Alzheimer's Dis.* **2012**, *31* (Suppl. S3), S87–S99. [CrossRef] [PubMed]
182. Forster, D.; Davies, K.; Williams, S. Magnetic resonance spectroscopy in vivo of neurochemicals in a transgenic model of Alzheimer's disease: A longitudinal study of metabolites, relaxation time, and behavioral analysis in TASTPM and wild-type mice. *Magn. Reson. Med.* **2013**, *69*, 944–955. [CrossRef]
183. Chaney, A.; Bauer, M.; Bochicchio, D.; Smigova, A.; Kassiou, M.; Davies, K.E.; Williams, S.R.; Boutin, H. Longitudinal investigation of neuroinflammation and metabolite profiles in the APPswe × PS 1Δe9 transgenic mouse model of Alzheimer's disease. *J. Neurochem.* **2017**, *144*, 318–335. [CrossRef]
184. Su, Y.; Fan, W.; Ma, Z.; Wen, X.; Wang, W.; Wu, Q.; Huang, H. Taurine improves functional and histological outcomes and reduces inflammation in traumatic brain injury. *Neuroscience* **2014**, *266*, 56–65. [CrossRef] [PubMed]
185. Wang, Q.; Fan, W.; Cai, Y.; Wu, Q.; Mo, L.; Huang, Z.; Huang, H. Protective effects of taurine in traumatic brain injury via mitochondria and cerebral blood flow. *Amino Acids* **2016**, *48*, 2169–2177. [CrossRef] [PubMed]
186. Sun, M.; Zhao, Y.; Gu, Y.; Xu, C. Anti-inflammatory mechanism of taurine against ischemic stroke is related to down-regulation of PARP and NF-κB. *Amino Acids* **2011**, *42*, 1735–1747. [CrossRef]
187. Junyent, F.; Utrera, J.; Romero, R.; Pallàs, M.; Camins, A.; Duque, D.; Auladell, C. Prevention of epilepsy by taurine treatments in mice experimental model. *J. Neurosci. Res.* **2009**, *87*, 1500–1508. [CrossRef] [PubMed]
188. Che, Y.; Hou, L.; Sun, F.; Zhang, C.; Liu, X.; Piao, F.; Zhang, D.; Li, H.; Wang, Q. Taurine protects dopaminergic neurons in a mouse Parkinson's disease model through inhibition of microglial M1 polarization. *Cell Death Dis.* **2018**, *9*, 435. [CrossRef]
189. Abuirmeileh, A.N.; Abuhamdah, S.M.; Ashraf, A.; Alzoubi, K.H. Protective effect of caffeine and/or taurine on the 6-hydroxydopamine-induced rat model of Parkinson's disease: Behavioral and neurochemical evidence. *Restor. Neurol. Neurosci.* **2021**, *39*, 149–157. [CrossRef]
190. Haider, S.; Sajid, I.; Batool, Z.; Madiha, S.; Sadir, S.; Kamil, N.; Liaquat, L.; Ahmad, S.; Tabassum, S.; Khaliq, S. Supplementation of Taurine Insulates Against Oxidative Stress, Confers Neuroprotection and Attenuates Memory Impairment in Noise Stress Exposed Male Wistar Rats. *Neurochem. Res.* **2020**, *45*, 2762–2774. [CrossRef]
191. Jangra, A.; Rajput, P.; Dwivedi, D.; Lahkar, M. Amelioration of Repeated Restraint Stress-Induced Behavioral Deficits and Hippocampal Anomalies with Taurine Treatment in Mice. *Neurochem. Res.* **2020**, *45*, 731–740. [CrossRef]
192. Silva, S.P.; Zago, A.M.; Carvalho, F.B.; Germann, L.; Colombo, G.D.M.; Rahmeier, F.L.; Gutierres, J.M.; Reschke, C.R.; Bagatini, M.D.; Assmann, C.E.; et al. Neuroprotective Effect of Taurine against Cell Death, Glial Changes, and Neuronal Loss in the Cerebellum of Rats Exposed to Chronic-Recurrent Neuroinflammation Induced by LPS. *J. Immunol. Res.* **2021**, *2021*, 1–10. [CrossRef] [PubMed]
193. Gebara, E.; Udry, F.; Sultan, S.; Toni, N. Taurine increases hippocampal neurogenesis in aging mice. *Stem Cell Res.* **2015**, *14*, 369–379. [CrossRef] [PubMed]
194. Paula-Lima, A.C.; De Felice, F.G.; Brito-Moreira, J.; Ferreira, S.T. Activation of GABAA receptors by taurine and muscimol blocks the neurotoxicity of beta-amyloid in rat hippocampal and cortical neurons. *Neuropharmacology* **2005**, *49*, 1140–1148. [CrossRef] [PubMed]
195. Kim, H.Y.; Kim, H.V.; Yoon, J.H.; Kang, B.R.; Cho, S.M.; Lee, S.; Kim, J.Y.; Kim, J.W.; Cho, Y.; Woo, J.; et al. Taurine in drinking water recovers learning and memory in the adult APP/PS1 mouse model of Alzheimer's disease. *Sci. Rep.* **2014**, *4*, 7467. [CrossRef] [PubMed]
196. Oh, S.J.; Lee, H.-J.; Jeong, Y.J.; Nam, K.R.; Kang, K.J.; Han, S.J.; Lee, K.C.; Lee, Y.J.; Choi, J.Y. Evaluation of the neuroprotective effect of taurine in Alzheimer's disease using functional molecular imaging. *Sci. Rep.* **2020**, *10*, 1–9. [CrossRef]
197. Santa-María, I.; Hernández, F.; Moreno, F.J.; Avila, J. Taurine, an inducer for tau polymerization and a weak inhibitor for amyloid-beta-peptide aggregation. *Neurosci. Lett.* **2007**, *429*, 91–94. [CrossRef]
198. Caletti, G.; Almeida, F.B.; Agnes, G.; Nin, M.S.; Barros, H.M.T.; Gomez, R. Antidepressant dose of taurine increases mRNA expression of GABAA receptor α2 subunit and BDNF in the hippocampus of diabetic rats. *Behav. Brain Res.* **2015**, *283*, 11–15. [CrossRef]
199. Caletti, G.; Herrmann, A.P.; Pulcinelli, R.R.; Steffens, L.; Morás, A.M.; Vianna, P.; Chies, J.; Moura, D.J.; Barros, H.M.T.; Gomez, R. Taurine counteracts the neurotoxic effects of streptozotocin-induced diabetes in rats. *Amino Acids* **2017**, *50*, 95–104. [CrossRef]
200. Agca, C.A.; Tuzcu, M.; Hayirli, A.; Sahin, K. Taurine ameliorates neuropathy via regulating NF-κB and Nrf2/HO-1 signaling cascades in diabetic rats. *Food Chem. Toxicol.* **2014**, *71*, 116–121. [CrossRef]
201. Rahmeier, F.L.; Zavalhia, L.S.; Tortorelli, L.S.; Huf, F.; Géa, L.P.; Meurer, R.T.; Machado, A.C.; Gomez, R.; Fernandes, M.D.C. The effect of taurine and enriched environment on behaviour, memory and hippocampus of diabetic rats. *Neurosci. Lett.* **2016**, *630*, 84–92. [CrossRef] [PubMed]
202. Li, K.; Shi, X.; Luo, M.; Llah, I.-U.; Wu, P.; Zhang, M.; Zhang, C.; Li, Q.; Wang, Y.; Piao, F. Taurine protects against myelin damage of sciatic nerve in diabetic peripheral neuropathy rats by controlling apoptosis of schwann cells via NGF/Akt/GSK3β pathway. *Exp. Cell Res.* **2019**, *383*, 111557. [CrossRef] [PubMed]
203. Garcia-Serrano, A.M.; Vieira, J.P.P.; Fleischhart, V.; Duarte, J.M.N. Taurine or N-acetylcysteine treatments prevent memory impairment and metabolite profile alterations in the hippocampus of high-fat diet-fed female mice. *bioRxiv* **2022**. [CrossRef]

204. El Idrissi, A.; El Hilali, F.; Rotondo, S.; Sidime, F. Effects of Taurine Supplementation on Neuronal Excitability and Glucose Homeostasis. *Adv. Exp. Med. Biol.* **2017**, *975*, 271–279. [CrossRef] [PubMed]
205. Ribeiro, R.A.; Santos-Silva, J.C.; Vettorazzi, J.F.; Cotrim, B.B.; Mobiolli, D.D.M.; Boschero, A.C.; Carneiro, E.M. Taurine supplementation prevents morpho-physiological alterations in high-fat diet mice pancreatic beta-cells. *Amino Acids* **2012**, *43*, 1791–1801. [CrossRef]
206. Drabkova, P.; Sanderova, J.; Kovarik, J.; Kandar, R. An Assay of Selected Serum Amino Acids in Patients with Type 2 Diabetes Mellitus. *Adv. Clin. Exp. Med.* **2015**, *24*, 447–451. [CrossRef]
207. Lee, S.; Olsen, T.; Vinknes, K.J.; Refsum, H.; Gulseth, H.L.; Birkeland, K.I.; Drevon, C.A. Plasma Sulphur-Containing Amino Acids, Physical Exercise and Insulin Sensitivity in Overweight Dysglycemic and Normal Weight Normoglycemic Men. *Nutrients* **2018**, *11*, 10. [CrossRef]
208. Anuradha, C.V.; Balakrishnan, S.D. Taurine attenuates hypertension and improves insulin sensitivity in the fructose-fed rat, an animal model of insulin resistance. *Can. J. Physiol. Pharmacol.* **1999**, *77*, 10588478. [CrossRef]
209. Nakaya, Y.; Minami, A.; Harada, N.; Sakamoto, S.; Niwa, Y.; Ohnaka, M. Taurine improves insulin sensitivity in the Otsuka Long-Evans Tokushima Fatty rat, a model of spontaneous type 2 diabetes. *Am. J. Clin. Nutr.* **2000**, *71*, 54–58. [CrossRef]
210. Nandhini, A.T.A.; Anuradha, C.V. Taurine modulates kallikrein activity and glucose metabolism in insulin resistant rats. *Amino Acids* **2002**, *22*, 27–38. [CrossRef]
211. Camargo, R.L.; Branco, R.C.S.; De Rezende, L.F.; Vettorazzi, J.F.; Borck, P.C.; Boschero, A.C.; Carneiro, E.M. The Effect of Taurine Supplementation on Glucose Homeostasis: The Role of Insulin-Degrading Enzyme. *Adv. Exp. Med. Biol.* **2015**, *803*, 715–724. [CrossRef] [PubMed]
212. Borck, P.C.; Vettorazzi, J.F.; Branco, R.C.S.; Batista, T.M.; Santos-Silva, J.C.; Nakanishi, V.Y.; Boschero, A.C.; Ribeiro, R.A.; Carneiro, E.M. Taurine supplementation induces long-term beneficial effects on glucose homeostasis in ob/ob mice. *Amino Acids* **2018**, *50*, 765–774. [CrossRef] [PubMed]
213. Vettorazzi, J.F.; Ribeiro, R.A.; Borck, P.C.; Branco, R.C.S.; Soriano, S.; Merino, B.; Boschero, A.C.; Nadal, A.; Quesada, I.; Carneiro, E.M. The bile acid TUDCA increases glucose-induced insulin secretion via the cAMP/PKA pathway in pancreatic beta cells. *Metabolism* **2016**, *65*, 54–63. [CrossRef] [PubMed]
214. Ito, T.; Schaffer, S.W.; Azuma, J. The potential usefulness of taurine on diabetes mellitus and its complications. *Amino Acids* **2011**, *42*, 1529–1539. [CrossRef] [PubMed]
215. Brøns, C.; Spohr, C.; Storgaard, H.; Dyerberg, J.; Vaag, A.A. Effect of taurine treatment on insulin secretion and action, and on serum lipid levels in overweight men with a genetic predisposition for type II diabetes mellitus. *Eur. J. Clin. Nutr.* **2004**, *58*, 1239–1247. [CrossRef]
216. Schlesinger, S.; Neuenschwander, M.; Barbaresko, J.; Lang, A.; Maalmi, H.; Rathmann, W.; Roden, M.; Herder, C. Prediabetes and risk of mortality, diabetes-related complications and comorbidities: Umbrella review of meta-analyses of prospective studies. *Diabetology* **2021**, *65*, 275–285. [CrossRef]
217. Livingston, G.; Huntley, J.; Sommerlad, A.; Ames, D.; Ballard, C.; Banerjee, S.; Brayne, C.; Burns, A.; Cohen-Mansfield, J.; Cooper, C.; et al. Dementia prevention, intervention, and care: 2020 report of the Lancet Commission. *Lancet* **2020**, *396*, 413–446. [CrossRef]
218. Guerreiro, R.J.; Gustafson, D.R.; Hardy, J. The genetic architecture of Alzheimer's disease: Beyond APP, PSENs and APOE. *Neurobiol. Aging* **2012**, *33*, 437–456. [CrossRef]
219. Albanese, E.; Launer, L.J.; Egger, M.; Prince, M.; Giannakopoulos, P.; Wolters, F.J.; Egan, K. Body mass index in midlife and dementia: Systematic review and meta-regression analysis of 589,649 men and women followed in longitudinal studies. *Alzheimer's Dementia Diagn. Assess. Dis. Monit.* **2017**, *8*, 165–178. [CrossRef]
220. Qizilbash, N.; Gregson, J.; Johnson, M.; Pearce, N.; Douglas, I.; Wing, K.; Evans, S.; Pocock, S.J. BMI and risk of dementia in two million people over two decades: A retrospective cohort study. *Lancet Diabetes Endocrinol.* **2015**, *3*, 431–436. [CrossRef]
221. Sun, S.; He, D.; Luo, C.; Lin, X.; Wu, J.; Yin, X.; Jia, C.; Pan, Q.; Dong, X.; Zheng, F.; et al. Metabolic Syndrome and Its Components Are Associated with Altered Amino Acid Profile in Chinese Han Population. *Front. Endocrinol.* **2022**, *12*, 795044. [CrossRef] [PubMed]
222. Li, Y.-C.; Li, Y.-Z.; Li, R.; Lan, L.; Li, C.-L.; Huang, M.; Shi, D.; Feng, R.-N.; Sun, C.-H. Dietary Sulfur-Containing Amino Acids Are Associated with Higher Prevalence of Overweight/Obesity in Northern Chinese Adults, an Internet-Based Cross-Sectional Study. *Ann. Nutr. Metab.* **2018**, *73*, 44–53. [CrossRef] [PubMed]

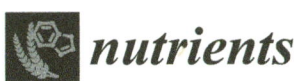

Article

# Dysmetabolism and Sleep Fragmentation in Obstructive Sleep Apnea Patients Run Independently of High Caffeine Consumption

Sílvia V. Conde [1,*], Fátima O. Martins [1], Sara S. Dias [2,3], Paula Pinto [4], Cristina Bárbara [4] and Emília C. Monteiro [1]

1. CEDOC, NOVA Medical School, Faculdade de Ciências Médicas, Universidade Nova de Lisboa, Rua Câmara Pestana 6, Edifício 2, piso 3, 1150-082 Lisboa, Portugal; fatima.martins@nms.unl.pt (F.O.M.); emilia.monteiro@nms.unl.pt (E.C.M.)
2. ciTechCare—Center for Innovative Care and Health Technology, Polytechnic of Leiria, 2411-901 Leiria, Portugal; sara.dias@ipleiria.pt
3. School of Health Sciences, Polytechnic of Leiria, 2411-901 Leiria, Portugal
4. Pneumology Department, Centro Hospitalar de Lisboa Norte, Hospital Pulido Valente, 1649-028 Lisboa, Portugal; paulagpinto@gmail.com (P.P.); cristina.barbara@chln.min-saude.pt (C.B.)
* Correspondence: silvia.conde@nms.unl.pt

**Abstract:** Daytime hypersomnolence, the prime feature of obstructive sleep apnea (OSA), frequently leads to high coffee consumption. Nevertheless, some clinicians ask for patients' caffeine avoidance. Caffeinated drinks are sometimes associated with more severe OSA. However, these effects are not consensual. Here we investigated the effect of caffeine consumption on sleep architecture and apnea/hypopnea index in OSA. Also, the impact of caffeine on variables related with dysmetabolism, dyslipidemia, and sympathetic nervous system (SNS) dysfunction were investigated. A total of 65 patients diagnosed with OSA and 32 without OSA were included after given written informed consent. Polysomnographic studies were performed. Blood was collected to quantify caffeine and its metabolites in plasma and biochemical parameters. 24 h urine samples were collected for catecholamines measurement. Statistical analyses were performed by SPSS: (1) non-parametric Mann-Whitney test to compare variables between controls and OSA; (2) multivariate logistic regression testing the effect of caffeine on sets of variables in the 2 groups; and (3) Spearmans' correlation between caffeine levels and comorbidities in patients with OSA. As expected OSA development is associated with dyslipidemia, dysmetabolism, SNS dysfunction, and sleep fragmentation. There was also a significant increase in plasma caffeine levels in the OSA group. However, the higher consumption of caffeine by OSA patients do not alter any of these associations. These results showed that there is no apparent rationale for caffeine avoidance in chronic consumers with OSA.

**Keywords:** caffeine; obstructive sleep apnea; apnea/hipopnea index; sleep architecture catecholamines; dysmetabolism

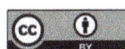

## 1. Introduction

Obstructive sleep apnea (OSA), the most common sleep-disordered breathing, is a highly prevalent disease [1] characterized by repetitive episodes of airflow cessation (apnea) or airflow reduction (hypopnea) during the sleep. These obstructive apneas during sleep result into recurrent arousals during sleep and in repetitive episodes of hypoxia, hypercapnia and apneas, which result in chemoreflex activation and consequent activation of the sympathetic nervous system (SNS) [2,3]. Frequent arousal can cause relevant changes on sleep architecture, namely sleep fragmentation, and may be responsible for diurnal hypersomnolence [3], as well as several adverse safety and health consequences including diurnal hypertension [4], cardiovascular disease, stroke, motor vehicle accidents, and diminished cognitive capacities and quality of life [5].

Daytime hypersomnolence and fatigue are regular symptoms in OSA, being frequently considered the main responsible for the high coffee consumption. It was previously described that OSA patients drink, on average, nearly three times more coffee than control subjects [6]. However, a recent meta-analysis did not show enough evidence to confirm the association between OSA and caffeine consumption [7]. Also, caffeinated drinks have been associated with more severe OSA [8] and some physicians ask for its avoidance, however these effects are not consensual as it has been found that coffee or tea do not seem to impact on OSA severity [8] and that caffeine seemed to improve cognitive function in people with OSA [9].

Several authors have correlated high caffeine consumption with an elevated blood pressure (BP) [10], suggesting that caffeine augments BP and total peripheral resistance in response to stressors [11–13]. Additionally, it has been previously described that caffeine increases SNS activity by increasing catecholamine levels, down-regulating beta-receptors [14] and blocking adenosine receptors [15]. In contrast, several studies have showed beneficial effects of long-term coffee intake on glucose metabolism and insulin action [16,17]. Moreover, some studies have associated coffee chronic consumption with a slower cognitive decline and with a reduced risk of cognitive dysfunction, dementia, and Alzheimer disease [18,19]. In particular, in moderate and severe OSA patient's, daily caffeine intake was associated with less cognitive impairment [9]. However, despite these positive impacts of caffeine on glucose homeostasis in metabolic disease patients and on cognitive dysfunction in OSA patients [9] most of the clinicians remain asking for patient caffeine avoidance.

Besides, all of the literature that can be found regarding the association of OSA and sympathetic activity and BP, the effect of caffeine consumption in other variables closely associated with OSA, such as sleep parameters (e.g., rapid eye movement (REM) sleep, non-REM sleep and arousals), dyslipidemia (e.g., triglycerides (TGs), cholesterol, high-density lipoproteins (HDL) and low-density lipoproteins (LDL) and dysmetabolism (e.g., body mass index (BMI) and glycemia), has not been evaluated so far. Thus, the aim of the present study was to investigate if caffeine plasma levels affect OSA severity and OSA association with dysmetabolism and sympathetic nervous system dysfunction.

## 2. Materials and Methods

### 2.1. Patients and Ethics

Eligible male patients with or without OSA (65 vs. 32) were recruited from the Respiratory Diseases Service of Hospital Pulido Valente (Lisbon). The diagnosis of OSA was established by the presence of typical clinical features of this disorder and confirmed by overnight polysomnography. Patients were included independently of their hypertension condition, hypertension ongoing medication and body mass index (BMI) and excluded if they had any psychiatric disorder, smoking habits, or inability to understand the information required for an informed consent. The study was approved by the Centro Hospitalar Lisboa Norte's Ethics Committee (Ethical approval: 11st November 2009) and by the Ethics Committee of the NOVA Medical School and registered at ClinicalTrials.gov accessed on 17 February 2022 (NCT01803815). It was performed in accordance with the Helsinki Declaration. All volunteers gave their written informed consent.

### 2.2. Study Design

Sociodemographic and anthropometric data, comorbidities and ongoing medication profile were documented. Weight, and abdominal circumference using standardized protocols were assessed.

Polysomnographic studies were performed using a polysomnographer (Medcare, Somnologica, Portugal). Polysomnography report included sleep parameters (e.g., sleep staging, sleep time, sleep latency, sleep efficiency, REM and non-REM sleep and arousals), respiratory events such as number and duration of apneas and hypopneas (apnea is the cessation of airflow at the nose and mouth for more than 10 s associated with oxygen desaturation of 3% and hypopnea is a discernible reduction in respiratory effort accompanied by a decrease of more than 4% of oxygen saturation) and apnea/hypopnea index (AHI). OSA was categorized according to current AHI cut-offs of less than 5 (nondiagnostic), 5≥ and <15 (mild), 15≥ and <30 (moderate), and at least 30 (severe).

In all patients, blood and 24 h urine samples were collected, before and after polysomnographic studies and stored at −80° until analyzed. Xanthine's concentrations, including caffeine, theobromine, theophylline and paraxanthine, glycemia total cholesterol, triglycerides (TG), HDL and LDL were measured in blood and epinephrine (E), norepinephrine (NE) and dopamine were measured in the 24 h urine. Quantifications of xanthines and catecholamines were carried by HPLC with UV and electrochemical detection, respectively, as previously described [20,21].

### 2.3. Statistical Analysis

Data were presented as median (interquartile range) with nonparametric Mann-Whitney test between two independent samples. Spearman correlations were performed between caffeine concentrations and sleep-related parameters in all subjects or in OSA patients and it was considered significantly correlated at $p < 0.05$. We have used nonparametric tests since variables did not follow a normal distribution.

Exploring the OSA patients we have performed an exploratory data analysis by binary logistic regression for each measured parameter for the dependent variable OSA and data were presented as odds ratio (OR), interval of confidence of 95% (IC95%) and correspondent value of p, with $p < 0.05$ being considered statistically significant. Afterwards we have grouped the significantly different variables between the 2 groups in 4 different models [dysmetabolism (glycemia and BMI), dyslipidemia (TGs, HDL and LDL), SNS (dopamine and NE) and sleep (arousals)] and tested its association with OSA when caffeine concentration in blood is present in each model. Each logistic regression was tested for goodness of fit by the Hosmer and Lemeshow test. Statistical analyses were performed using SPSS statistical software (vs 26.0 for Mac) (IBM, NY, US).

## 3. Results

Male patients diagnosed with OSA (65) and male patients without OSA (32) were recruited. The study and the control groups included volunteers aged 50 ± 8 and 34 ± 7 years, respectively.

Table 1 summarizes findings regarding metabolic and sympathetic nervous system variables studied in OSA patients and control subjects. OSA patients showed significantly higher BMI, glycemia, total cholesterol, LDL, TG and dopamine and NE levels in comparison to control patients. OSA patients also showed a significantly lower HDL levels than control subjects (Table 1).

**Table 1.** Comparison between metabolic and sympathetic nervous system variables in patients with and without obstructive sleep apnea (OSA).

| Variables Assessed | Patients without OSA (n = 32) Median (Q$_1$–Q$_3$) | Patients with OSA (n = 65) Median (Q$_1$–Q$_3$) |
|---|---|---|
| BMI (kg m$^{-2}$) | 25.15 (20.8–29.1) | 32.30 (25.2–42.6) *** |
| Glycaemia (mg/dL) | 77.00 (62.0–88.0) | 88.00 (63.0–128.0) *** |
| Total cholesterol (mg/dL) | 171.0 (118.0–237.0) | 191.00 (124.0–275.0) *** |
| LDL (mg/dL) | 98.00 (62.0–169.0) | 125.00 (61.0–188.0) *** |
| HDL (mg/dL) | 51.50 (37.0–57.0) | 43.00 (27.0–61.0) *** |
| TG (mg/dL) | 81.5 (30.0–241.0) | 129.00 (59.0–417.0) * |

Table 1. *Cont.*

| Variables Assessed | Patients without OSA (*n* = 32) Median (Q₁–Q₃) | Patients with OSA (*n* = 65) Median (Q₁–Q₃) |
|---|---|---|
| Dopamine (µg/24 h) | 236.50 (64.0–303.0) | 245.96 (48.0–549.8) ** |
| Epinephrine (µg/24 h) | 4.50 (2.0–11.0) | 6.0 (2.0–29.4) |
| Norepinephrine (µg/24 h) | 30.00 (14.0–56.0) | 58.0 (12.0–149.3) *** |

Data are presented as median (interquartile range). LDL-c, low density lipoproteins; HDL-c, high density lipoproteins; TG, triglycerides; E, epinephrine; NE, norepinephrine (* $p < 0.05$; ** $p < 0.01$; *** $p < 0.001$, median Mann-Whitney statistic test for independent samples, corresponding to the difference between patients with and without OSA).

In Table 2 are summarized the levels of caffeine plasmatic concentrations and sleep parameters for both groups of patients. OSA patients showed significantly higher caffeine plasmatic concentrations than control subjects. As expected, AHI and the number of arousals were also higher for patients included in the study group. As it can be observed in Table 2, no statistical differences between the REM and non-REM sleep period in patients with or without OSA were found.

Table 2. Comparison of caffeine and total xanthine plasmatic concentrations, Apnea-hypopnea index (AHI), sleep architecture (REM and non-REM) and arousals events in patients with or without obstructive sleep apnea (OSA).

| Variables Assessed | Patients without OSA (*n* = 32) Median (Q₁–Q₃) | Patients with OSA (*n* = 65) Median (Q₁–Q₃) |
|---|---|---|
| Caffeine (µg/mL) | 0.18 (0.0–0.77) | 1.25 (0.0–13.4) ** |
| Total xanthine (µg/mL) | 0.93 (0.0–3.6) | 1.91 (0.0–18.5) |
| AHI (events/h) | 1.60 (0.2–4.9) | 26.10 (6.3–137.5) *** |
| NREM (min) | 304.50 (253.0–341.7) | 291.50 (150.5–388.3) |
| REM (min) | 44.25 (16.0–121.0) | 38.50 (5.0–98.5) |
| Arousals (events/h) | 7.00 (4.0–19.5) | 30.60 (10.3–109.1) *** |

Data are presented as median (interquartile range). AHI, apnea-hypopnea index; REM, rapid eye movement sleep; NREM, non-rapid eye movement sleep (** $p < 0.01$; *** $p < 0.001$, median Mann-Whitney statistic test for independent samples, corresponding to the difference between patients with and without OSA).

Aiming to evaluate the impact of caffeine consumption on the prediction of OSA development and on disease severity we correlated caffeine plasma levels and sleep architecture-related parameters for the OSA patients' group. We found that there is no statistically significant correlation for any of the tested parameters, showing that caffeine is not associated with disease severity (Table 3).

To deeply understand if OSA development is associated with dyslipidemia, dysmetabolism, SNS dysfunction and/or sleep fragmentation we performed a binary logistic regression within both groups, OSA and control patients, for all the covariables significantly different in the previous nonparametric test analysis. Blood pressure was not considered as a covariable for the statistical analysis since OSA patients presented normotensive values due to the use of anti-hypertensive medication. Also, apart from this medication no relevant drugs for the present study were taken by patients.

We found that all the tested covariables were associated with the development of OSA, showed by the *p* value in Table 4 for the differences between OR for an interval of confidence of 95% present. The binary logistic regression of each model followed the goodness of the fit by the Hosmer and Lemeshow test.

Table 3. Correlation of caffeine concentration in OSA patients with sleep-related parameters: apnea-hypopnea index (AHI), arousals, rapid-eye movement (REM) and non-rapid eye movement (NREM).

| Variables Correlated with Caffeine | OSA Patients | |
|---|---|---|
| | R (Spearman) | p Value |
| AHI | −0.186 | 0.309 |
| Arousals | −0.164 | 0.370 |
| REM | −0.050 | 0.791 |
| NREM | −0.316 | 0.083 |

Data are presented as Spearman correlation coefficient between caffeine concentrations and sleep-related parameters and correspondent value of $p$, considered significantly correlated at $p < 0.05$; AHI, apnea-hypopnea index; REM, rapid eye movement; NREM, non-rapid eye movement.

Table 4. Binary logistic regression for BMI, glycemia, cholesterol, LDL, HDL, TGs, dopamine, NE, caffeine concentration and arousals with OSA as dependent variable.

| Dependent Variable = OSA Independent Variables | Odds Ratio (OR) | IC$_{95\%}$ | p Value |
|---|---|---|---|
| BMI (kg m$^{-2}$) | 1.93 | 1.44–2.60 | <0.001 |
| Glycaemia (mg/dL) | 1.22 | 1.11–1.34 | <0.001 |
| Total cholesterol (mg/dL) | 1.03 | 1.02–1.05 | <0.001 |
| LDL (mg/dL) | 1.04 | 1.02–1.05 | <0.001 |
| HDL (mg/dL) | 0.92 | 0.87–0.96 | <0.01 |
| TG (mg/dL) | 1.01 | 1.00–1.02 | <0.05 |
| Dopamine (μg/24 h) | 1.01 | 1.00–1.01 | <0.01 |
| Norepinephrine (μg/24 h) | 1.12 | 1.06–1.18 | <0.001 |
| Caffeine (μg/mL) | 3.23 | 1.35–7.74 | <0.01 |
| Arousals (events/h) | 1.31 | 1.17–1.46 | <0.001 |

Data are presented as odds ratio (OR), interval of confidence of 95% (IC95%) and correspondent value of $p$; BMI, body-mass index; LDL, low-density lipoprotein; HDL, high-density lipoprotein; TG, triglycerides.

Coffee and other beverages and foods rich in caffeine consumption has been reported to be increased in OSA condition due to the sleep privation and daily sleepiness, as shown herein in the present study by the higher caffeine concentration in blood in patients diagnosed with OSA. As such, we had interest in investigating if the associations between metabolic and sleep parameters with OSA pathology are influenced by caffeine levels.

Therefore, we performed a multivariate logistic regression with OSA as dependent variable and tested the association of the pathology with dyslipidemia (TG, HDL-c, LDL-c), dysmetabolism (BMI and glycemia), SNS dysregulation (dopamine and norepinephrine) and sleep impairment (arousals) taking in account caffeine concentration in all models. Each model followed the goodness of fit represented by a non-significative Hosmer and Lemeshow test. The results for each model tested are presented in Table 5.

We found that caffeine association with OSA is lost when all the other variables related with OSA comorbidities are taken in account. Moreover, we also observed that all the variables tested maintain their association with OSA even in the presence of caffeine. Regarding the dysmetabolism model we observed that BMI and glycemia associates statistically significantly with OSA independently of the higher caffeine intake in these patients (Table 5a). Similarly, in the dyslipidemia model we found that TGs do not associate with OSA when caffeine factor is present, but HDL and LDL maintains its statistically significantly association with the pathology, with an expected protective association (OR < 1) and risk factor association (OR > 1), respectively (Table 5b). Regarding SNS function association with OSA we found that NE is statistically significantly associated with the pathology and that caffeine levels seem to have a role on SNS association with OSA (Table 5c). Finally, as expected, arousals are positively statistically significantly associated with OSA, but caffeine do not contribute for this association (Table 5d).

**Table 5.** Multivariate logistic regression for four different models with OSA as dependent variable and testing the effect of caffeine on variables association with the development of the pathology. Variables for testing caffeine effect on the association of OSA with: (a) dysmetabolism-related comorbidities; (b) dyslipidaemia; (c) sympathetic nervous system (SNS) dysfunction; and (d) sleep fragmentation.

| (a) Dysmetabolism model: | | | |
|---|---|---|---|
| Dependent Variable = OSA Independent Variables | OR | IC$_{95\%}$ | $p$ Value |
| Caffeine (µg/mL) | 3.05 | 0.587–15.87 | 0.185 |
| BMI (kg m$^{-2}$) | 2.71 | 1.38–5.31 | <0.01 |
| Glycaemia (mg/dL) | 1.234 | 1.03–1.48 | <0.05 |
| (b) Dyslipidaemia model: | | | |
| Dependent Variable = OSA Independent Variables | OR | IC$_{95\%}$ | $p$ Value |
| Caffeine (µg/mL) | 6.93 | 0.79–61.18 | 0.081 |
| TG (mg/dL) | 1.01 | 0.99–1.02 | 0.304 |
| HDL-c (mg/dL) | 0.88 | 0.80–0.97 | <0.01 |
| LDL-c (mg/dL) | 1.03 | 1.00–1.06 | <0.05 |
| (c) SNS model: | | | |
| Dependent Variable = OSA Independent Variables | OR | IC$_{95\%}$ | $p$ Value |
| Caffeine (µg/mL) | 11.28 | 1.29–98.66 | <0.05 |
| Dopamine (µg/24 h) | 1.00 | 0.98–1.01 | 0.263 |
| Norepinephrine (µg/24 h) | 1.14 | 1.06–1.23 | <0.01 |
| (d) Sleep model: | | | |
| Dependent Variable = OSA Independent Variables | OR | IC$_{95\%}$ | $p$ Value |
| Caffeine (µg/mL) | 1.77 | 0.58–5.45 | 0.318 |
| Arousals (events/h) | 1.37 | 1.16–1.61 | <0.001 |

## 4. Discussion

In the present study, we showed that the group of OSA patients studied in the present manuscript exhibit significant dysmetabolic condition with higher BMI and glycemia, dyslipidemia with high total cholesterol, LDL, TG and lower HDL levels and deregulation of the SNS assessed as high dopamine and NE levels. Moreover, we showed, as expected, that OSA patients consume more caffeinated products to compensate daytime sleepiness, this being reflected in the high caffeine plasma levels in these patients. We also found that no correlation exists between caffeine plasma levels and OSA and its severity. Finally, we have shown that metabolic dysfunction, dyslipidemia, and sleep disturbances are associated with OSA independently of caffeine plasma levels.

Caffeine is one of the most widely consumed psychoactive substances in the World and it is known that this xanthine disrupts sleep, diminishing total sleep time and sleep onset in healthy volunteers [15,22]. Apart from some controversy on the effects of caffeine on REM sleep [23,24], it is consensual that caffeine affects arousals [25] and NREM sleep [15,26]. However, our results are not in this line of evidence since we found that caffeine plasma levels lose association with OSA when arousals are taken in account and do not correlate with any sleep-related parameters when this association is analyzed only in OSA group. When subjects from both groups are analyzed for the association of caffeine plasma levels with sleep parameters, both AHI and arousals have a statistically significant correlation, showing that OSA patients indeed drink more caffeine due to sleep fragmentation. Moreover, no correlation has been found between caffeine consumption and the severity of OSA. These results are in line with the findings of the authors in [8], showing that coffee intake is not associated with sleep disorder breathing, a wide spectrum of sleep-related conditions that includes OSA. Interestingly, and in complete contrast with the idea that caffeine may contribute to sleep disruption in OSA or even to its absence of effects, a recent study by Takabayashi et al. [27] showed in a cohort of Japanese men, that individuals who were overweight exhibited a significant inverse association between coffee consumption and oxygen desaturation index, a parameter that correlate with AHI [28,29]. While this study of Takabayashi et al. [27] did not provided causality between coffee consumption and sleep disorder breathing it clearly highlights the importance of further research on the associations between coffee consumption in sleep disorder breathing and especially in OSA. In fact, it was recently emphasized in a meta-analysis that there are insufficient data in the literature to determine whether and how, OSA is associated with caffeine consumption [7].

Some studies in the past have suggested that caffeinated coffee consumption was associated with a lower metabolic control and therefore with an increased risk of type 2 diabetes and metabolic syndrome [17,30], although nowadays is becoming consensual that drinking coffee (whether caffeinated and decaffeinated) may actually decrease the risk of developing metabolic syndrome and type 2 diabetes [16,31]. These results were supported by animal work showing that long-term caffeine intake prevent and reverse fat deposition, insulin resistance and glucose intolerance in hypercaloric animal models [21,32,33]. However, the results for the effect of caffeine on dysmetabolism do not seem to be extrapolated to dyslipidemia as a recent meta-analysis suggested that coffee consumption may be associated with an elevated risk for dyslipidemia [34]. Nevertheless, these results were not supported by previous clinical studies showing that coffee consumption has been positively associated with blood lipid concentration in humans [35,36] and by the findings that caffeine intake in hypercaloric animal models decrease non-esterified fatty acids [21]. Our results show that caffeine-enriched products consumption in OSA patients do not influence OSA metabolic comorbidities. Moreover, we also observed that all of the variables related with dysmetabolism and dyslipidemia tested herein, maintain their association with OSA even in the presence of caffeine, suggesting that caffeine intake in OSA is incapable of prevent or improve dysmetabolic features. Therefore, we can suggest that the mechanisms behind the development of dysmetabolism in OSA might differ from the common dysmetabolic states in where chronic caffeine intake have shown to have beneficial effects [21,32,33].

Regarding SNS-related parameters and following the previous findings of Bardwell et al. [6], where a positive association between NE levels and caffeine consumption in OSA patients was observed, or with the previous observations of Benowitz [14] where an increase in catecholamines circulating levels elicited by caffeine was found, herein we observed that caffeine is directly associated with NE levels in OSA. Therefore, we can suggest that higher caffeine intake in OSA patients can contribute to the overactivity of the SNS activity observed in OSA patients [37] and in here manifested by an increase in NE levels.

In conclusion, caffeine consumption in OSA patients is not associated with OSA severity, as well as with dysmetabolism and sleep fragmentation although we cannot discharge a contribution of high caffeine levels to the overactivation of the SNS observed in OSA patients. While there is no apparent rationale for caffeine avoidance in chronic consumers with OSA, we believe that more studies regarding coffee/caffeine consumption in OSA patients should be performed.

**Author Contributions:** Conceptualization, S.V.C. and E.C.M.; methodology, S.V.C., P.P. and C.B.; formal analysis, S.V.C.; statistical analysis, F.O.M. and S.S.D.; writing—original draft preparation, S.V.C. and F.O.M.; writing—review and editing, S.V.C., F.O.M. and S.S.D.; funding acquisition, E.C.M. All authors have read and agreed to the published version of the manuscript.

**Funding:** This research was funded by the Portuguese Science and Technology Foundation (FCT) with the grant number CEECIND/04266/2017.

**Institutional Review Board Statement:** The study was approved by the Centro Hospitalar Lisboa Norte's Ethics Committee (Ethical approval: 11st November 2009) and by the Ethics Committee of the NOVA Medical School and registered at ClinicalTrials.gov accessed on 17 February 2022

(NCT01803815). It was performed in accordance with the Helsinki Declaration. All volunteers gave their written informed consent.

**Informed Consent Statement:** Informed consent was obtained from all subjects involved in the study.

**Data Availability Statement:** Data available on request due to restrictions (ethical reason). The data presented in this study are available on request from the corresponding author. The data are not publicly available due to ethical concerns.

**Acknowledgments:** The authors would like to thank Eunice Silva for technical support.

**Conflicts of Interest:** The authors declare no conflict of interest.

## References

1. Young, T.; Peppard, P.E.; Gottlieb, D.J. Epidemiology of obstructive sleep apnea: A population health perspective. *Am. J. Respir. Crit. Care Med.* **2002**, *165*, 1217–1239. [CrossRef] [PubMed]
2. Iqbal, M.; Shah, S.; Fernandez, S.; Karam, J.; Jean-Louis, G.; McFarlane, S.I. Obesity, obstructive sleep apnea, and cardiovascular risk. *Curr. Cardiovasc. Risk Rep.* **2008**, *2*, 101–106. [CrossRef]
3. Narkiewicz, K.; Van De Borne, P.J.H.; Montano, N.; Dyken, M.E.; Phillips, B.G.; Somers, V.K. Contribution of tonic chemoreflex activation to sympathetic activity and blood pressure in patients with obstructive sleep apnea. *Circulation* **1998**, *97*, 943–945. [CrossRef] [PubMed]
4. Shamsuzzaman, A.S.M.; Gersh, B.J.; Somers, V.K. Obstructive sleep apnea. *J. Am. Med. Assoc.* **1996**, *290*, 97–100. [CrossRef]
5. Robinson, G.V.; Langford, B.A.; Smith, D.M.; Stradling, J.R. Predictors of blood pressure fall with continuous positive airway pressure (CPAP) treatment of obstructive sleep apnoea (OSA). *Thorax* **2008**, *63*, 855–859. [CrossRef]
6. Bardwell, W.A.; Ziegler, M.G.; Ancoli-Israel, S.; Berry, C.C.; Nelesen, R.A.; Durning, A.; Dimsdale, J.E. Dimsdale Does caffeine confound relationships among adrenergic tone, blood pressure and sleep apnoea? *J. Sleep Res.* **2000**, *9*, 269–272. [CrossRef]
7. Taveira, K.V.M.; Kuntze, M.M.; Berretta, F.; de Souza, B.D.M.; Godolfim, L.R.; Demathe, T.; De Luca Canto, G.; Porporatti, A.L. Association between obstructive sleep apnea and alcohol, caffeine and tobacco: A meta-analysis. *J. Oral Rehabil.* **2018**, *45*, 890–902. [CrossRef]
8. Aurora, R.N.; Crainiceanu, C.; Caffo, B.; Punjabi, N.M. Sleep-disordered breathing and caffeine consumption: Results of a community-based study. *Chest* **2012**, *142*, 631–638. [CrossRef]
9. Norman, D.; Bardwell, W.A.; Loredo, J.S.; Ancoli-Israel, S.; Heaton, R.K.; Dimsdale, J.E. Caffeine intake is independently associated with neuropsychological performance in patients with obstructive sleep apnea. *Sleep Breath.* **2008**, *12*, 199–205. [CrossRef]
10. Riksen, N.P.; Rongen, G.A.; Smits, P. Acute and long-term cardiovascular effects of coffee: Implications for coronary heart disease. *Pharmacol. Ther.* **2009**, *121*, 185–191. [CrossRef]
11. Sung, B.H.; Whitsett, T.L.; Lovallo, W.R.; Al'Absi, M.; Pincomb, G.A.; Wilson, M.F. Prolonged increase in blood pressure by a single oral dose of caffeine in mildly hypertensive men. *Am. J. Hypertens.* **1994**, *7*, 755–758. [CrossRef] [PubMed]
12. Sung, B.H.; Lovallo, W.R.; Whitsett, T.; Wilson, M.F. Caffeine elevates blood pressure response to exercise in mild hypertensive men. *Am. J. Hypertens.* **1995**, *8*, 1184–1188. [CrossRef]
13. Pincomb, A.; Lovallo, W.R.; Mckey, B.S.; Sun, B.H.; Passey, R.B.; Everson, S.A.; Wilson, M.F. Acute Blood Pressure Elevations with Caffeine Systemic HyPertension. *Am. J. Cardiol* **1996**, *77*, 270–274. [CrossRef]
14. Benowitz, N.L. Clinical pharmacology of caffeine. *Annu. Rev. Med.* **1990**, *41*, 277–288. [CrossRef] [PubMed]
15. Fredholm, B.B.; Bättig, K.; Holmén, J.; Nehlig, A.; Zvartau, E.E. Actions of Caffeine in the Brain with Special Reference to Factors That Contribute to Its Widespread Use. *Pharmacol. Rev.* **1999**, *51*, 83–133.
16. Van Dam, R.M.; Feskens, E.J.M. Coffee consumption and risk of type 2 diabetes mellitus. *Lancet* **2002**, *360*, 1477–1478. [CrossRef]
17. Reis, C.E.G.; Dórea, J.G.; da Costa, T.H.M. Effects of coffee consumption on glucose metabolism: A systematic review of clinical trials. *J. Tradit. Complement. Med.* **2019**, *9*, 184–191. [CrossRef]
18. Gardener, S.L.; Rainey-Smith, S.R.; Villemagne, V.L.; Fripp, J.; Doré, V.; Bourgeat, P.; Taddei, K.; Fowler, C.; Masters, C.L.; Maruff, P.; et al. Higher Coffee Consumption Is Associated With Slower Cognitive Decline and Less Cerebral Aβ-Amyloid Accumulation Over 126 Months: Data From the Australian Imaging, Biomarkers, and Lifestyle Study. *Front. Aging Neurosci.* **2021**, *13*, 744872. [CrossRef]
19. Solfrizzi, V.; Panza, F.; Imbimbo, B.P.; D'Introno, A.; Galluzzo, L.; Gandin, C.; Misciagna, G.; Guerra, V.; Osella, A.; Baldereschi, M.; et al. Coffee consumption habits and the risk of mild cognitive impairment: The Italian longitudinal study on aging. *J. Alzheimer's Dis.* **2015**, *47*, 889–899. [CrossRef]
20. Conde, S.V.; Obeso, A.; Rigual, R.; Monteiro, E.C.; Gonzalez, C. Function of the rat carotid body chemoreceptors in ageing. *J. Neurochem.* **2006**, *99*, 711–723. [CrossRef]
21. Conde, S.V.; Nunes Da Silva, T.; Gonzalez, C.; Mota Carmo, M.; Monteiro, E.C.; Guarino, M.P. Chronic caffeine intake decreases circulating catecholamines and prevents diet-induced insulin resistance and hypertension in rats. *Br. J. Nutr.* **2012**. [CrossRef] [PubMed]
22. Roehrs, T.; Roth, T. Caffeine: Sleep and daytime sleepiness. *Sleep Med. Rev.* **2008**, *12*, 153–162. [CrossRef] [PubMed]

23. Carrier, J.; Fernandez-Bolanos, M.; Robillard, R.; Dumont, M.; Paquet, J.; Selmaoui, B.; Filipini, D. Effects of caffeine are more marked on daytime recovery sleep than on nocturnal sleep. *Neuropsychopharmacology* **2007**, *32*, 964–972. [CrossRef] [PubMed]
24. Paterson, L.M.; Nutt, D.J.; Ivarsson, M.; Hutson, P.H.; Wilson, S.J. Effects on sleep stages and microarchitecture of caffeine and its combination with zolpidem or trazodone in healthy volunteers. *J. Psychopharmacol.* **2009**, *23*, 487–494. [CrossRef]
25. Barry, R.J.; Rushby, J.A.; Wallace, M.J.; Clarke, A.R.; Johnstone, S.J.; Zlojutro, I. Caffeine effects on resting-state arousal. *Clin. Neurophysiol.* **2005**, *116*, 2693–2700. [CrossRef]
26. Boutrel, B.; Koob, G.F. What keeps us awake: The neuropharmacology of stimulants and wakefulness-promoting medications. *Sleep* **2004**, *27*, 1181–1194. [CrossRef]
27. Takabayashi, A.; Maruyama, K.; Tanno, Y.; Sakurai, S.; Eguchi, E.; Wada, H.; Shirahama, R.; Saito, I.; Tanigawa, T. The association of coffee consumption and oxygen desaturation index during sleep among Japanese male workers. *Sleep Breath.* **2019**, *23*, 1027–1031. [CrossRef]
28. Chen, L.; Tang, W.; Wang, C.; Chen, D.; Gao, Y.; Ma, W.; Zha, P.; Lei, F.; Tang, X.; Ran, X. Diagnostic Accuracy of Oxygen Desaturation Index for Sleep-Disordered Breathing in Patients With Diabetes. *Front. Endocrinol.* **2021**, *12*, 598470. [CrossRef]
29. Temirbekoy, D.; Gunes, S.; Yazici, Z.M.; Sayin, İ. The Ignored Parameter in the Diagnosis of Obstructive Sleep Apnea Syndrome The Oxygen Desaturation Index. *Turk. Otolarengoloji Arsivi/Turk. Arch. Otolaryngol.* **2018**, *56*, 1–6. [CrossRef]
30. Moisey, L.L.; Kacker, S.; Bickerton, A.C.; Robinson, L.E.; Graham, T.E. Caffeinated coffee consumption impairs blood glucose homeostasis in response to high and low glycemic index meals in healthy men. *Am. J. Clin. Nutr.* **2008**, *87*, 1254–1261. [CrossRef]
31. van Dam, R.M.; Willett, W.C.; Manson, J.E.; Hu, F.B. Coffee, Caffeine, and Risk of Type 2 Diabetes. *Diabetes Care* **2006**, *29*, 398–403. [CrossRef] [PubMed]
32. Coelho, J.C.; Melo, B.F.; Rodrigues, T.; Matafome, P.; Sacramento, J.F.; Guarino, M.P.; Seiça, R.; Conde, S.V. Caffeine Restores Insulin Sensitivity and Glucose tolerance in High-sucrose Diet Rats: Effects on Adipose Tissue. *J. Cardiovasc. Dis.* **2016**, *35*, 440–449.
33. Panchal, S.K.; Wong, W.Y.; Kauter, K.; Ward, L.C.; Brown, L. Caffeine attenuates metabolic syndrome in diet-induced obese rats. *Nutrition* **2012**, *28*, 1055–1062. [CrossRef] [PubMed]
34. Du, Y.; Lv, Y.; Zha, W.; Hong, X.; Luo, Q. Effect of coffee consumption on dyslipidemia: A meta-analysis of randomized controlled trials. *Nutr. Metab. Cardiovasc. Dis.* **2020**, *30*, 2159–2170. [CrossRef]
35. Hartley, T.R.; Lovallo, W.R.; Whitsett, T.L. Cardiovascular effects of caffeine in men and women. *Am. J. Cardiol.* **2004**, *93*, 1022–1026. [CrossRef]
36. Jee, S.H.; He, J.; Appel, L.J.; Whelton, P.K.; Suh, I.; Klag, M.J. Coffee consumption and serum lipids: A meta-analysis of randomized controlled clinical trials. *Am. J. Epidemiol.* **2001**, *153*, 353–362. [CrossRef]
37. Narkiewicz, K.; Somers, V.K. Sympathetic nerve activity in obstructive sleep apnoea. *Acta Physiol. Scand.* **2003**, *177*, 385–390. [CrossRef]

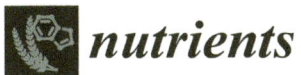

*Review*

# Non-Pharmacological Treatments for Insulin Resistance: Effective Intervention of Plant-Based Diets—A Critical Review

Michalina Banaszak [1], Ilona Górna [2,*] and Juliusz Przysławski [2]

[1] Faculty of Medical Sciences, Poznan University of Medical Sciences, 60-812 Poznan, Poland; mi.banaszak97@gmail.com
[2] Department of Bromatology, Poznan University of Medical Sciences, 60-806 Poznan, Poland; jotespe@ump.edu.pl
* Correspondence: igorna@ump.edu.pl; Tel.: +48-61-641-83-90

**Abstract:** Plant-based diets are becoming increasingly popular. Vegetarian diets are better for the environment and exhibit health benefits. A correctly balanced plant-based diet is appropriate at every stage of life. Compared to omnivores, vegetarians consume more fruits and vegetables, more fibre, vitamins C and E, magnesium and less saturated fats. In general, they have better nutrition knowledge, and they are slimmer, healthier and live longer than omnivores. It also seems that following a plant-based diet prevents the onset of chronic diseases such as cardiovascular diseases, hypertension, type 2 diabetes, obesity and some cancers. Food intake has a key influence on insulin resistance. Consumption of calorie-rich and highly processed foods, meats and sweetened beverages is a characteristic element of Western diets. They promote and elevate insulin resistance and type 2 diabetes. In contrast, intake of pulses and exclusion of meats as well as animal products bring significant benefits to vegetarian diets. According to studies, vegetarians and vegans have better blood parameters, including better glucose, insulin, total cholesterol, and LDL cholesterol levels. Their homeostatic model assessment for insulin resistance (HOMA-IR) test results are also better. More plant-based foods and fewer animal foods in a diet result in lower insulin resistance and a lower risk of prediabetes and type 2 diabetes. The aim of the study was to investigate the effect of plant-based diets on insulin resistance. In this review, we focused on presenting the positive effects of vegetarian and vegan diets on insulin resistance while showing possible clinical applications of plant-based diets in the treatment and prevention of modern-age diseases. Current and reliable publications meeting the requirements of Evidence-Based Medicine (EBM) were taken into account in this review.

**Keywords:** vegetarian diet; vegan diet; insulin resistance; insulin sensitivity

**Citation:** Banaszak, M.; Górna, I.; Przysławski, J. Non-Pharmacological Treatments for Insulin Resistance: Effective Intervention of Plant-Based Diets—A Critical Review. *Nutrients* **2022**, *14*, 1400. https://doi.org/10.3390/nu14071400

Academic Editors: Silvia V. Conde, Fatima O. Martins and Rosa Casas

Received: 23 February 2022
Accepted: 25 March 2022
Published: 27 March 2022

**Publisher's Note:** MDPI stays neutral with regard to jurisdictional claims in published maps and institutional affiliations.

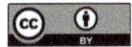

**Copyright:** © 2022 by the authors. Licensee MDPI, Basel, Switzerland. This article is an open access article distributed under the terms and conditions of the Creative Commons Attribution (CC BY) license (https://creativecommons.org/licenses/by/4.0/).

## 1. Introduction

Insulin resistance (IR) is a pathological condition in which cells fail to respond normally to insulin. As a result, glucose remains in the bloodstream. It may be defined as a state where normal or elevated insulin levels result in a poor biological response. Insulin resistance is often accompanied by hyperinsulinemia, a condition where pancreatic β-cells release excessive amounts of insulin to maintain normal glycaemia [1–3]. Unfortunately, over time, the pancreas is unable to secrete adequate amounts of the hormone. This leads to the development of type 2 diabetes. Apart from diabetes, IR is also associated with the development of metabolic syndrome and cardiovascular diseases [4]. It is estimated that insulin resistance precedes the development of diabetes type 2 by 10 to 15 years [5].

The exact causes of insulin resistance have not yet been fully understood. Increased intramuscular fat and fatty acid metabolites are amongst the suspected risk factors. Excess body weight is considered to be the main cause of insulin resistance. It was suggested that IR starts in myocytes due to immune-mediated inflammatory changes and an excess of free fatty acids resulting in ectopic lipid deposition. In the muscles, the process of glucose uptake is disturbed, so that excess glucose returns to the liver, where it increases lipogenesis and the levels of circulating free fatty acids. Increased levels of free fatty acids exacerbate insulin resistance. There are also genetic causes of insulin resistance, including genetic diseases (myotonic dystrophy, Rabson–Mendenhall syndrome, Werner syndrome) and abnormalities in the function of insulin antibodies and insulin receptors. The gold standard for diagnosing insulin resistance is the hyperinsulinemic-euglycemic clamp. This method involves the continuous infusion of insulin at high speed to inhibit the production of glucose by the liver. Simultaneously, 20% dextrose solution is administered at different rates to reduce blood glucose levels in the euglycemic range. Blood glucose is monitored frequently during the test. The amount of glucose required to achieve normoglycemia reflects the excretion of exogenous glucose required to compensate for hyperinsulinemia. However, as this technique is labour-intensive and costly, indices are used to quantify IR. The homeostatic model assessment for insulin resistance (HOMA-IR) is the prevalent method. It is calculated by multiplying fasting insulin and fasting glucose levels and then dividing that figure by 22.5 [4–6].

The primary non-pharmacological treatment for insulin resistance should entail lifestyle approaches. Dietary changes should include a modification of eating habits, reduction in energy intake (for excessive body weight) and avoidance of carbohydrates that excessively stimulate insulin secretion, known as high glycaemic index carbohydrates and high glycaemic load carbohydrates. Regular exercise improves muscle insulin sensitivity [1,5,7,8].

The aim of this review was to show that diets that emphasise whole grains, vegetables, fruits and legumes and exclude animal products are able to reduce insulin resistance and improve tissue insulin sensitivity.

## 2. Materials and Methods

Forty-four publications from the PubMed database, the Web of Science and the Cochrane Library were used for this literature review. The following inclusion criteria were applied for the review: papers in English and only research conducted on adults (over the age of 18). The following keywords were used to search for papers: 'insulin', 'insulin secretion', 'insulin resistance', 'insulin sensitivity', 'vegan diet', 'vegetarian diet', 'plant-based diet', 'vegetarian cuisine', 'vegan cuisine'. The literature included comparative studies, cross-sectional studies and randomised controlled trials (Figure 1).

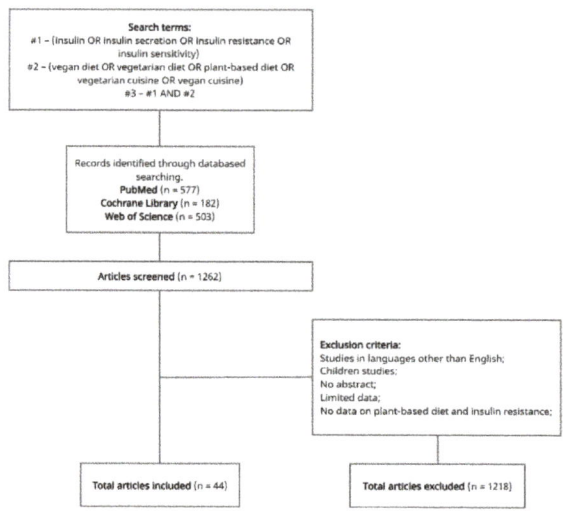

**Figure 1.** Full search strategy.

## 3. Plant-Based Diets

People are showing increasing interest in plant-based diets. Ethical, environmental and social considerations are some of the primary reasons for changing to a plant-based diet. Health issues are also playing an increasingly significant role [9]. Compared to traditional diets, those based on plants are more environmentally friendly. They use fewer natural resources and cause less pollution [10].

A vegetarian diet involves abstaining from meat, poultry, fish and seafood [11]. There are different types of vegetarian diets. Lacto-vegetarians consume dairy products, ovo-vegetarians consume eggs, whereas lacto-ovo-vegetarians consume eggs and dairy products [12]. On the other hand, vegans abstain from all animal products [13]. Such a diet consists exclusively of plant foods such as cereals, vegetables, fruits, legumes, nuts, seeds and vegetable oils [10,14–16]. The most prevalent types of plant-based diets are shown in Table 1.

**Table 1.** Characteristic of plant-based diets.

| Dietary Approach | Type of Diet | Characteristics |
|---|---|---|
| Plant-based diet | Vegetarian | Does not contain meat, fish or seafood. Contains fruit, vegetables, whole grains, pulses, nuts and seeds. May or may not include egg and/or dairy products. |
| | Lacto-ovo-vegetarian | Contains eggs and dairy products. |
| | Lacto-vegetarian | Includes dairy products but excludes eggs. |
| | Ovo-vegetarian | Includes eggs but excludes dairy products. |
| | Vegan | Does not contain any animal products. May exclude honey. |
| | Raw vegan | Includes uncooked vegetables, fruits, nuts, seeds, legumes/beans and whole grains. The amount of uncooked food varies from 75% to 100%. |

There is also a semi-vegetarian diet (flexitarian). This eating pattern limits the consumption of meat or fish to a few portions per week. However, it is not considered vegetarian per se [17].

According to the Academy of Nutrition and Dietetics, well-balanced vegetarian diets, including vegan diets, are suitable at all stages of life, including during pregnancy, lactation, infancy, childhood, adolescence and old age. Such direst is also suitable for athletes [10].

Generally speaking, numerous studies indicate that vegetarians are more aware of the health consequences of poor nutrition that they are slimmer and healthier than people who do not follow such restrictions [11]. Compared to non-vegetarian diets, a plant-based diet may prevent the onset of chronic diseases such as cardiovascular diseases, hypertension, type 2 diabetes, obesity and lower overall cancer risk, especially colorectal cancer, breast cancer and prostate cancer [10]. According to research, for vegans, the risk of hypertension is reduced by 75%, the risk of type 2 diabetes is reduced by 47–78% and the risk of cancer is reduced by 14% [18]. Furthermore, plant-based diets are associated with reduced mortality rates for humans [19,20].

Unfortunately, not every diet based on fruit and vegetables is healthy. A poorly balanced vegetarian diet can be just as harmful as an unbalanced traditional diet. Plant-based diets can be deficient in B vitamins (especially B12), iron, calcium, zinc, omega 3 fatty acids and protein. It is, therefore very important to consume fortified foods and dietary supplements [15,17]. There is some concern as to whether a vegan diet can meet the protein requirements of the human body [21]. A well-balanced vegan diet provides all essential amino acids and an adequate amount of total protein without the need to supplement the diet with special foods [10].

The number of people around the world who follow a vegetarian diet is not precisely known. However, every year that number is growing. It is estimated that there may be 7.3 million vegetarians in the USA, 3.6 million in the UK and 30,000 in Portugal [17]. According to estimates, vegans account for as many as 46% of vegetarians [10].

## 4. Impact of a Vegetarian Diet on Insulin Resistance

The foods we eat have a key impact on insulin resistance. This is especially true for the elderly and those who are not very physically active. The increase in the consumption of highly processed, calorie-rich foods such as fast foods, meats and meat products, refined cereal products and soft drinks is estimated to play an important role in the worldwide growth of type 2 diabetes [22]. Balanced and well-composed diets can play a significant role in reducing insulin resistance and the risk of type 2 diabetes (Table 2) [23].

**Table 2.** The influence of a vegetarian diet on insulin resistance.

| Study | Year | Country | Cohort | Analysed Groups | Time of Intervention | Results |
|---|---|---|---|---|---|---|
| Hosseinpour-Niazi et al. [24] | 2015 | Iran | 31 participants (24 women and 7 men; age: 58.1 ± 6.0 years, with type 2 diabetes) | Legume-based Therapeutic Lifestyle Change (TLC) diet Control diet (legume-free TLC diet) | 8 weeks | Decreased fasting blood glucose ($p = 0.04$), fasting insulin ($p = 0.04$), triglyceride concentrations ($p = 0.04$) and low-density lipoprotein cholesterol ($p = 0.02$) for TLC group. No change in body mass index (BMI), waist circumference. |
| Jenkins et al. [25] | 2012 | Canada | 121 participants with type 2 diabetes (60 women, 61 men, aged 59.5 ± 1 | (1) Low-GI diet (diet rich in legume) (2) High wheat fiber diet (diet rich in high wheat fiber foods) | 3 months | Decreased HbA1c ($p < 0.001$), body weight) ($p = 0.002$), fasting glucose level ($p = 0.001$), systolic BP ($p < 0.001$), diastolic BP ($p < 0.001$), heart rate ($p < 0.001$), absolute CHD risk (10 years) ($p = 0.003$) in both groups. |
| Pittaway et al. [26] | 2008 | Australia | 45 participants (13 premenopausal women, 19 postmenopausal women, 13 men; age: 52.2 ± 6.1 years) | A diet consisting of a minimum of 728 g of chickpeas per week as part of traditional diet for 12 weeks (chickpea phase), followed by 4 weeks of the traditional diet without chickpeas (usual phase). | 20 weeks | Significant decrease in mean serum total cholesterol of 7.7 mg/dL ($p = 0.002$), LDL cholesterol of 7.3 mg/dL ($p = 0.01$), fasting insulin of 0.75 IU/mL ($p = 0.045$) and in HOMA-IR of 0.21 ($p = 0.01$). |
| Tucker et al. [27] | 2015 | USA | 292 participants (nondiabetic women; age: 40.3 ± 3.1 years) | 3 groups: woman with low meat intake ($n = 73$), moderate meat intake ($n = 164$) and high meat intake ($n = 73$) | 7 days | Significantly higher HOMA scores in groups with high and moderate meat consumption ($p = 0.007$). |
| Ley et al. [28] | 2014 | USA | 3690 participants (nondiabetic women from Nurses' Health Study; age 30–55 years) | - | - | Higher red meat consumption was associated with higher plasma CRP, ferritin, fasting insulin, and HbA1c, and lower adiponectin ($p \leq 0.03$ for all). Substituting a serving of total red meat intake with alternative protein food showed improvement in lowering CRP, ferritin, HbA1c and fasting insulin levels ($p \leq 0.02$ for all). |
| Cui et al. [29] | 2019 | China | 558 participants (healthy men and women, age 32–34 years old) | 279 vegetarians (73 vegans, 206 lacto-ovo-vegetarians) and 279 omnivores | 3 months | Vegan diet and lacto-ovo-vegetarian diet were negatively correlated with HOMA-IR after adjusting for BMI. |
| Kim et al. [30] | 2015 | Korea | 102 participants (postmenopausal women, age of 47 to 85 years old) | 54 vegetarian women and 48 non-vegetarian women | - | Significantly lower body weight ($p < 0.01$), body mass index ($p < 0.001$), % of body fat ($p < 0.001$), serum levels of leptin ($p < 0.05$), glucose ($p < 0.001$), insulin ($p < 0.01$) and HOMA-IR ($p < 0.01$) in the vegetarians group. |
| Yang et al. [31] | 2012 | China | 295 participants (men aged 21–76 years) | 169 lacto-vegetarians 126 omnivores | - | Remarkably lower body mass index ($p = 0.049$), triglyceride level ($p = 0.016$), total cholesterol ($p < 0.001$), LDL cholesterol ($p < 0.001$) and fasting blood glucose ($p < 0.001$) in lacto-vegetarians group. Higher homeostasis model assessment β cell function ($p < 0.001$) and insulin secretion index ($p = 0.048$) in lacto-vegetarians. |
| Gammon et al. [32] | 2012 | New Zealand | 124 participants (women at least 20 years old) | 90 non-vegetarians 34 vegetarians | - | Increased body mass index, waist circumference and HOMA2-IR levels in non-vegetarians group. Higher serum vitamin B12 levels in non-vegetarians ($p < 0.001$). |

Table 2. Cont.

| Study | Year | Country | Cohort | Analysed Groups | Time of Intervention | Results |
|---|---|---|---|---|---|---|
| Hung et al. [33] | 2006 | Taiwan | 98 participants (healthy women, age 31–45 years old) | 49 lactovegetarians 49 omnivores | - | Significantly lower levels of fasting insulin ($p < 0.001$), plasma glucose ($p < 0.001$) and i resistance (HOMA-IR) ($p < 0.001$) in lactovegetarians group. No difference in beta-cell function between the two groups ($p = 0.062$). |
| Kuo et al. [34] | 2004 | Taiwan | 36 healthy participants (omnivore—55.7 ± 3.7; vegetarians—58.6 ± 3.6 years old) | 19 vegetarians 17 omnivores | - | Significantly lower levels of steady-state plasma glucose (SSPG) ($p < 0.001$), fasting insulin ($p = 0.004$), HOMA-IR ($p = 0.002$), HOMA %S ($p = 0.018$). |
| Kahleova et al. [35] | 2011 | Czech Republic | 74 participants with type 2 diabetes (experimental group—54.6 ± 7.8, control group—57.7 ± 4.9 years old) | (1) experimental group ($n = 37$; vegetarian diet) (2) the control group ($n = 37$; conventional diet) | 24 weeks | Reduced diabetes medication in the experimental group (43% participants; $p < 0.001$). Decreased body weight ($p = 0.001$) and visceral and subcutaneous fat in the experimental group ($p = 0.007$ and $p = 0.02$, respectively). Increased insulin sensitivity ($p = 0.04$) and plasma adiponectin ($p = 0.02$) in the experimental group. |
| Valachovicová et al. [36] | 2006 | Slovak Republic | 202 participant (healthy adult subjects (age range 19–64 years; BMI 18.6–25.0 kg/m²) | (1) a vegetarian group (95 long-term lacto-ovo-vegetarians) (2) a non-vegetarian control group (107 participants on a traditional western diet) | - | Significantly lower glucose ($p < 0.001$), insulin concentrations ($p < 0.01$) and IR (HOMA) ($p < 0.01$) in the vegetarian group. Significantly higher intake of whole grain products, pulses, products from oat and barley ($p < 0.001$) in the vegetarians group. |
| Chiang et al. [37] | 2013 | Taiwan | 706 female participants (age 56.4 ± 8.4 years old, overall healthy) | 391 vegetarians (~80% lacto-ovo-vegetarians) 315 non-vegetarians | - | Significantly lower body mass index ($p < 0.001$), waist circumference ($p < 0.001$), lower total cholesterol ($p < 0.001$), LDL cholesterol (LDL-C) ($p < 0.001$), glucose ($p < 0.001$), insulin ($p < 0.001$), HOMA-IR ($p < 0.001$) and the risks for the MetS ($p = 0.006$). |
| Vučić Lovrenčić et al. [38] | 2020 | Croatia | 76 participants (healthy non-obese adult, age- and gender matched; BMI < 30 kg/m²; 18–60 years old) | Vegetarians ($n = 40$) Omnivore ($n = 36$) | - | Significantly higher levels of adiponectin in female ($p = 0.03$) and the HOMA2-%B in vegetarians group than omnivore controls ($p = 0.04$). No differences in HOMA2-IRI, inflammatory and metabolic biomarkers. |
| Ellsworth et al. [39] | 2016 | USA | 325 participants (subjects with diagnosed type-2 diabetes, CAD or significant risk factors; average age was 60.3 years (range 40.7–79.8)—intensive lifestyle and 61.5 years (range 33.9–86.2) in moderate lifestyle) | (1) intensive non-randomised program with a strict vegetarian diet ($n = 90$ participants, 90 matched controls) (2) moderate randomised trial following a Mediterranean-style diet ($n = 89$ subjects, 58 controls) | 1 year | Decrease in weight loss (−8.9% (95% CI, −10.3 to −7.4), intensive programme; −2.8% (95% CI, −3.8 to −1.9), moderate programme; adjusted $p < 0.001$) and the LPIR score (−13.3% (95% CI, −18.2 to −8.3), intensive; −8.8% (95% CI, −12.9 to −4.7), moderate; adjusted $p < 0.01$) in both intervention with an advantage in the vegetarian diet. |
| Garousi et al. [40] | 2021 | Iran | 75 participants (overweight/obese adults with NAFLD, aged between 20 and 55 years) | (1) lacto-ovo-vegetarian diet (LOV-D) ($n = 37$) (2) a standard weight-loss diet (SWL-D) ($n = 38$) | 3 months | Decreased levels of alanine aminotransferase (ALT) ($p < 0.001$), body weight ($p < 0.001$), waist circumference ($p < 0.001$), BMI ($p < 0.001$), fasting blood sugar ($p < 0.001$), insulin ($p < 0.001$), HOMA-IR ($p < 0.001$), triacylglycerol (TG) ($p = 0.001$), cholesterol ($p < 0.001$), LDL cholesterol ($p < 0.001$), and systolic blood pressure ($p = 0.001$) in LOV-D group. |
| Chen et al. [41] | 2018 | The Netherlands | 6798 participants (age 62.0 ± 7.8) | (1) 6514 participants for plant-based diet with insulin resistance (2) 5768 participants for a plant-based diet with prediabetes risk (3) 6770 participants for a plant-based diet with T2D risk | - | Higher score on the plant-based dietary index was associated with lower insulin resistance (per 10 units higher score: β = −0.09; 95% CI: −0.10; −0.08), lower prediabetes risk (HR = 0.89; 95% CI: 0.81; 0.98) and lower T2D risk (HR = 0.82 (0.73; 0.92)). |

Those following vegetarian diets consume more monounsaturated fatty acids (MUFA), more polyunsaturated fatty acids (PUFA) and less saturated fatty acids (SFA) as compared to non-vegetarians [42]. Saturated fatty acids and palmitic acid, in particular, interfere with insulin signalling in muscle cells due to the accumulation of free fatty acid intermediates, ceramides and diacylglycerol [43,44]. Diets that include animal products contain much more SFAs than plant-based diets. This means that vegetarians and vegans have less insulin resistance [41]. In addition, replacing SFAs in a diet with MUFAs and PUFAs has anti-inflammatory effects and improves insulin sensitivity [45].

Studies have shown that legumes, which are an important source of protein in a vegetarian diet, reduce insulin resistance, which is associated with protection against the onset of metabolic syndrome [24,25,46,47]. Pittaway et al. [26] demonstrated an improvement in tested blood parameters after 12 weeks of consuming chickpeas (minimum 728 g per week). In addition to a reduction in total cholesterol, there was a 0.75 µIU/mL decrease in fasting insulin ($p = 0.045$), and the HOMA-IR insulin resistance index fell by 0.21 compared with the start of the study ($p = 0.01$).

Animal products, in particular red meat, show a tendency to elevate insulin resistance [27,28,48–51]. A study by Tucker et al. [27] on a group of 292 females without diabetes found that women who consumed large and moderate amounts of meat had significantly higher HOMA-IR insulin resistance index scores than those with a lower meat intake (F = 7.4; $p = 0.0070$). They put forward the idea that meat consumption could lead to insulin resistance. This is associated with a reduced risk of type 2 diabetes for vegetarians compared to omnivores.

Numerous studies show a positive effect of a vegetarian diet on insulin resistance compared to traditional, non-vegetarian diets [29–38].

In their study, Kahleova et al. [35] compared a vegetarian diet (~60% energy from carbohydrates, 15% proteins and 25% fats) with a conventional diabetic diet (50% energy from carbohydrates, 20% proteins and <30% fats). A group of 74 patients with type 2 diabetes was randomly assigned to 2 groups: an experimental group ($n = 37$) that followed a vegetarian diet and a control group ($n = 37$) that followed a conventional diabetic diet. The results from the experimental group showed that as many as 43% of those on a vegetarian diet were able to reduce the doses of their diabetes medication (compared with 5% in the control group; $p < 0.001$). Bodyweight also decreased more for those in the experimental group than in the control group (−6.2 kg (95% CI −6.6 to −5.3) vs. −3.2 kg (95% CI −3.7 to −2.5)). Furthermore, there was a significant increase in insulin sensitivity in the experimental group (30%; 95% CI 24.5–39) compared to the control group (20%; 95% CI 14–25) ($p = 0.04$). A vegetarian diet was also shown to reduce visceral adipose tissue volume and positively affect adiponectin and oxidative stress markers. The results indicate that a vegetarian diet alone or in combination with exercise is more effective in reducing insulin resistance than a conventional diabetic diet.

Metabolic abnormalities are a factor that can trigger age-related diseases. This may be more intense for obese individuals. With that in mind, Valachovicová et al. [36] evaluated insulin resistance in relation to diet. Fasting glucose and fasting insulin concentrations, as well as insulin resistance (HOMA) values, were analysed in normal-weight adults. The group included 95 vegetarians and 107 non-vegetarians on a Western diet. The results were significantly lower in the vegetarian group (glucose concentration $4.47 \pm 0.05$ vs. $4.71 \pm 0.07$ mmol/L; insulin concentration $4.96 \pm 0.23$ vs. $7.32 \pm 0.41$ mU/L; HOMA-IR index $0.99 \pm 0.05$ vs. $1.59 \pm 0.10$). Vegetarians were significantly more likely to consume whole grain products, pulses, oat and barley products, as well as fruit and vegetables. Studies show the beneficial effects of long-term use of a plant-based diet in the prevention of metabolic syndrome, diabetes and cardiovascular disease.

On the other hand, Chiang et al. [37] found that vegetarianism was associated with better lipid profiles, insulin resistance and lower risks of metabolic syndrome. The study comprised 391 female vegetarians (80% lacto-vegetarians) and 315 non-vegetarian Buddhist women from Taiwan. The vegetarians had a lower BMI ($22.9 \pm 2.7$ vs. $23.8 \pm 3.2$ kg/m$^2$), smaller waist circumference (72.9 ± 6.9 vs. 75.3 ± 7.6 cm), lower fasting glucose (4.98 ± 0.89 vs. 5.15 ± 0.97 mmol/L) and fasting insulin (41.67 ± 37.50 vs. 52.09 ± 41.67 pmol/L) levels, lower total cholesterol (4.68 ± 0.83 vs. 5.21 ± 0.90 mmol/L) and lower LDL cholesterol (3.01 ± 0.74 vs. 3.43 ± 0.81 mmol/L) compared to non-vegetarians ($p < 0.001$). These vegetarians also had better insulin sensitivity, which was associated with lower HOMA levels (vegetarians 1.3 ± 1.2 vs. non-vegetarians 1.7 ± 1.5; $p < 0.001$). According to the study, a lacto-vegetarian diet was associated with reduced insulin resistance and risk of metabolic syndrome.

Vučić Lovrenčić et al. [38] reached similar conclusions. Female vegetarians had significantly lower fasting insulin levels (38.4 (35.1–46.4) vs. 49.9 (37.7–63.8) pmol/L) and lower HOMA index values (0.80 (0.75–0.95) vs. 1.10 (0.80–1.30)) than omnivorous women ($p = 0.02$) Additionally, pancreatic β-cell function as estimated by HOMA2 (HOMA2%B) was significantly higher in subjects on a plant-based diet than in those consuming meat products (115.5 ± 42.9 vs. 91.0 ± 35.0, $p = 0.04$), indicating that a vegetarian diet had a positive effect on improving β-cell function.

Ellsworth et al. [39] focused on verifying whether lifestyle changes would improve IR in individuals with different severities of metabolic dysfunction. Participants with type 2 diabetes, ischaemic heart disease or at risk from these diseases were allocated to two groups: an intensive non-randomised programme with a strict vegetarian diet (90 participants in the study group, 90 in the control group) or a moderately randomised trial on a Mediterranean diet (89 participants in the study group, 58 in the control group). The research carried out over one year showed that both interventions resulted in weight loss (−8.9% (95% CI, −10.3 to −7.4)—intensive programme; −2.8% (95% CI, −3.8 to −1.9)—moderate programme; $p < 0.001$). Insulin resistance was measured using the Lipoprotein IR Index (LPIR) score. LPIR are six lipoprotein parameters that exhibit the strongest association with insulin resistance. This index may be useful for identifying patients at risk of developing type 2 diabetes and ischaemic heart disease [52]. Insulin resistance significantly decreased for subjects in both groups (LPIR −13.3% (95% CI, −18.2 to −8.3)—intensive; −8.8% (95% CI, −12.9 to −4.7)—moderate; $p < 0.01$). Based on the results, one may conclude that both a strict change to a vegetarian diet as well as a moderate change to a Mediterranean diet is effective in improving IR as defined by LPIR [39].

On the other hand, Garousi et al. [40] compared the effects of a lacto-vegetarian diet with a standard weight loss diet in a group of 75 adults with nonalcoholic fatty liver disease (NAFLD). The nutritional make-up for both diets was similar: 50–55% carbohydrates, 15–20% protein and 25–30% fats. After 3 months of research, alanine aminotransferase (ALT) levels were significantly lower for the lacto-ovo-vegetarian group (−21.32 ± 19.77 vs. −10.15 ± 20.30 IU/L; $p = 0.04$) as compared with the standard weight loss diet. In addition to improving liver function, the lacto-vegetarian diet resulted in significant reductions in body weight, BMI, waist circumference and lipid profile parameters. Additionally, compared to the group on a weight loss diet, the lacto-vegetarian diet resulted in a significant reduction in insulin (−4.94 ± 5.40 vs. +0.81 ± 8.35 µU/mL; $p = 0.006$) and lower HOMA-IR index values (−1.62 ± 1.48 vs. +0.02 ± 2.14; $p < 0.001$). According to research, following a lacto-vegetarian diet had a more beneficial effect on improving the health of NAFLD patients than following a standard reduction diet.

The association of insulin resistance, prediabetes and type 2 diabetes with vegan and vegetarian diets was also analysed. Chen et al. [41] carried out research on a group of 6798 subjects. They showed that more plant-based foods and fewer animal products in a diet result in lower insulin resistance and a lower risk of prediabetes and type 2 diabetes. This suggests that plant-based products may reduce the risk of insulin resistance and its negative effects.

## 5. Impact of a Vegan Diet on Insulin Resistance

Compared to other vegetarian diets, vegans generally consume less saturated fat, less cholesterol and more fibre. Higher intakes of antioxidants and magnesium also elevate insulin sensitivity (Table 3) [53].

**Table 3.** The influence of a vegan diet on insulin resistance.

| Study | Year | Country | Cohort | Analysed Groups | Time of Intervention | Results |
|---|---|---|---|---|---|---|
| Kahleova et al. [54] | 2018 | USA | 75 participants (healthy overweight or obese adult men and women, BMI between 28 and 40 kg/m$^2$, age 53.2 ± 12.6 years old) | (1) a plant-based diet ($n$ = 38) (2) a control diet (current participant's diet) ($n$ = 37) | 16 weeks | Significant reductions in body weight ($-6.5$ kg; $p < 0.001$), fat mass ($-4.3$ kg; $p < 0.001$) and HOMA-IR ($-1.0$; $p = 0.004$) in the vegan group. |
| Barnard et al. [55] | 2021 | USA | 62 participants (healthy, overweight adults, BMI between 28 and 40 kg/m$^2$, group 1—56.6 ± 10.9 years old, group 2—58.3 ± 8.4 years old) | (1) group on the Mediterranean diet (2) group on a low-fat vegan diet | 16 weeks | Decreased weight ($-6.0$ kg; $p < 0.001$) and HOMA-IR ($-0.7$; $p = 0.21$) in vegan group. Increased oral glucose insulin sensitivity (OGIS) ($+35.8$ mL/min/m$^2$; $p = 0.003$) in vegan group. No significant change in the Mediterranean diet group. |
| Kahleova et al. [56] | 2018 | USA | 75 participants (healthy, overweight adults with a BMI between 28 and 40 kg/m$^2$, age 53.2 ± 12.6 years old) | (1) plant-based high-carbohydrate, low-fat (vegan) diet ($n$ = 38) (2) control group (current participant's diet) ($n$ = 37) | 16 weeks | Significant reduction in body weight ($-6.5$ kg; $p < 0.001$), fat mass ($-4.3$ kg; $p < 0.001$) and HOMA-IR ($-1.0$; $p = 0.004$) in the vegan group. |
| Kahleova et al. [57] | 2020 | USA | 168 participants (overweight, but otherwise healthy adult men and women with a BMI between 28 and 40 kg/m$^2$; vegan group—52.9 ± 11.7 years old, control group—57.5 ± 10.2 years old) | (1) vegan group ($n$ = 84) (2) control group (current participant's diet) ($n$ = 84) | 16 weeks | Decreased body weight ($-5.9$ kg; $p < 0.001$), fat mass ($-3.9$ kg; $p < 0.001$) and visceral fat ($-240$ cm$^3$; $p < 0.001$) in the vegan group. Increased PREDIcted M, insulin sensitivity index (PREDIM) in the vegan group ($+0.83$; $p < 0.001$). Significant changes in gut microbiota ($p < 0.001$) due to the low-fat vegan diet. |
| Kahleova et al. [58] | 2019 | USA | 75 participants (healthy, overweight adults with a BMI between 28 and 40 kg/m$^2$, age 53.2 ± 12.6 years old) | (1) low-fat vegan diet ($n$ = 38) (2) control diet (current participant's diet) ($n$ = 37) | 16 weeks | Decreased intakes of C18:0 ($p = 0.004$) and CLA-trans-10-cis12 ($p = 0.002$) in the vegan group. Increased intake of C18:2 ($p = 0.002$) and C18:3 ($p = 0.006$). Changes in the consumption of fatty acids have caused a decrease in HOMA-IR ($p = 0.02$) in the vegan group. The main fatty acids associated with changes in fasting insulin secretion were C12:0 ($p = 0.03$) and TRANS 16:1 ($p = 0.02$). |
| Kahleova et al. [59] | 2018 | USA | 75 participants (healthy, overweight adults with a BMI between 28 and 40 kg/m$^2$, age 53.2 ± 12.6 years old) | (1) vegan group (low-fat plant-based diet) ($n$ = 38) (2) control group (current participant's diet) ($n$ = 37) | 16 weeks | Decreased significantly HOMA-IR in the vegan group ($-1.0$; $p = 0.004$). Changes in HOMA-IR correlated positively with changes in body mass index ($p = 0.009$) and visceral fat volume ($p = 0.001$). |
| Kahleova et al. [60] | 2021 | USA | 244 healthy participants (intervention group—52.6 ± 14.7 years old, control group—54.3 ± 9.9 years old) | (1) intervention group (vegan) ($n$ = 122) (2) control group (current participant's diet)($n$ = 122) | 16 weeks | Reduction in Potential Renal Acid Load (PRAL) ($-24.7$ mEq/day; $p < 0.001$) and Net Endogenous Acid Production (NEAP) ($-23.8$ mEq/day; $p < 0.001$), body weight ($-5.9$ kg; $p < 0.001$) and HOMA-IR ($p = 0.008$) in vegan group. Increased PREDIM in the vegan group ($p < 0.001$). |
| Kahleova et al. [61] | 2020 | USA | 244 healthy participants (BMI between 28 and 40 kg/m$^2$, age 25 to 75 years) | (1) intervention group(low-fat vegan diet) ($n$ = 122) (2) control group (current participant's diet) ($n$ = 122) | 16 weeks | Decreased body weight ($-5.9$ kg; $p < 0.001$), HOMA ($-1.3$; $p < 0.001$), hepatocellular lipid levels ($-34.4$%; $p = 0.002$) and intramyocellular lipid levels ($-10.4$%; $p = 0.03$) in the intervention group. Increased thermic effect of food ($+14.1$%; $p < 0.001$) and PREDIM ($+0.9$; $p < 0.001$) in the intervention group. No significant changes in the control group. |

Table 3. *Cont.*

| Study | Year | Country | Cohort | Analysed Groups | Time of Intervention | Results |
|---|---|---|---|---|---|---|
| Barnard et al. [62] | 2005 | USA | 64 participants (overweight or obese, postmenopausal women; mean age for intervention group—57.4 y, for control group—55.6 y) | (1) intervention group (low-fat, vegan diet) (2) control group (control diet based on National Cholesterol Education Program guidelines) | 14 weeks | Decreased body weight ($-5.8 \pm 3.2$ kg in the intervention group; $-3.8 \pm 2.8$ kg in the control group; $p = 0.012$). Increased index of insulin sensitivity (from $4.6 \pm 2.9$ to $5.7 \pm 3.9$; $p = 0.017$) in the intervention group. |
| Śliż et al. [63] | 2021 | Poland | 98 participants (healthy Polish males, athletes, aged 20–39 years) | (1) vegan group (VEG; $n = 44$) (2) omnivore group (OMN; $n = 54$) | - | Higher intake of carbohydrate ($p < 0.01$), unsaturated fatty acids ($p < 0.01$) in the VEG group. Lover intake of protein ($p < 0.01$), fat ($p < 0.01$), saturated fatty acids ($p < 0.01$) and EPA + DHA ($p < 0.01$) in the VEG group. Significantly better outcomes in $n$-6/$n$-3 fatty acid ratio ($6.5\% \pm 2.3\%$ vs. $5.0\% \pm 2.1\%$; $p < 0.01$) insulin sensitivity (HOMA-IR), C-peptide and total blood cholesterol levels ($p < 0.01$) in the VEG group. |

The composition of dietary proteins influences glucagon and insulin activity in the body [64], which in turn affects body composition and insulin resistance [65]. It was found that a high intake of branched-chain amino acids (leucine, isoleucine and valine) can increase insulin resistance. Kahleova et al. [54] conducted a study to determine the effects of plant protein on body weight, body composition and insulin resistance in overweight individuals. A group of 75 participants with excessive body weight was randomly assigned to a group on a plant-based diet ($n = 38$) or following a control diet ($n = 37$). The vegan group achieved significant reductions in body weight ($-6.5$ kg (95% CI $-8.9$ to $-4.1$ kg); $p < 0.001$), fat mass ($-4.3$ kg (95% CI $-5.4$ to $-3.2$ kg); $p < 0.001$) and HOMA-IR (treatment effect $-1.0$ (95% CI $-1.2$ to $-0.8$); $p = 0.004$). Interestingly, it was noted that a decrease in fat mass was associated with an increase in plant protein intake and a decrease in animal protein intake (r = $-0.30$, $p = 0.011$; r = $+0.39$, $p = 0.001$, respectively). Proportionally reduced dietary leucine intake was positively correlated with decreased fat mass (r = $+0.40$; $p < 0.001$), and proportionally reduced histidine intake was associated with decreased insulin resistance (r = $+0.38$; $p = 0.003$). To conclude, plant protein as a component of a plant-based diet was associated with improved body composition, reduced body weight and reduced insulin resistance.

The positive effects of a low-fat vegan diet on insulin resistance and insulin sensitivity index (PREDIM) were shown by numerous studies [55–60]. Kahleova et al. [61] used a randomised controlled trial to examine the effects of a low-fat vegan diet on body weight, insulin resistance as well as hepatic and intracellular lipid levels in overweight adults. The study group comprised 244 people, 122 of whom were allocated to an intervention group on a low-fat vegan diet (approximately 75% energy from carbohydrates, 15% from proteins and 10% from fats), with the remaining 122 eating as before during the 16-week study period. Based on the results, participants in the intervention group recorded a weight reduction of 5.9 kg (95% CI, 5.0–6.7 kg; $p < 0.001$). The HOMA insulin resistance index was also lower ($-1.3$; 95% CI, $-2.2$ to $-0.3$; $p < 0.001$) and the predicted insulin sensitivity index (PREDIM) increased (0.9; 95% CI, 0.5–1.2; $p < 0.001$) for the vegan group. The low-fat vegan diet also had a positive effect on lipid levels, with hepatic cell lipid amounts down by 34.4% and intracellular lipids down by 10.4%. The above variables did not change significantly for the control group. The results confirm the positive effects of a plant-based diet on both body weight, insulin resistance and body lipid levels.

Barnard et al. [62] carried out a similar study. A group of 64 postmenopausal women with excessive body weight were randomly assigned to a group on a low-fat vegan diet (10% energy from fats, 15% from protein, 75% from carbohydrates) or a control diet (fat 30%, protein about 15%, carbohydrate 55%). An analysis of these results showed that mean body weight in the intervention group decreased by 5.8 ± 3.2 kg as compared with 3.8 ± 2.8 kg in the control group ($p$ = 0.012). On the other hand, the insulin sensitivity index, calculated using a quotient of fasting blood glucose and fasting insulin, mean blood glucose and mean insulin concentration, increased from 4.6 ± 2.9 to 5.7 ± 3.9 ($p$ = 0.017) in the intervention group; however, differences between groups were not significant ($p$ = 0.17). Studies have shown that despite not specifying recommended portion sizes or amounts of food, women switching to a low-fat vegan diet lost significant amounts of weight.

Śliż et al. [63] compared a vegan diet ($n$ = 44) to an omnivorous diet ($n$ = 54) among Polish athletes. The vegan group had significantly better HOMA-IR (0.96 ± 0.49 vs. 1.17 ± 0.44; $p$ < 0.01), fasting glucose (4.3 ± 0.6 vs. 4.8 ± 0.5 mmol/L; $p$ = 0.01) and C-peptide (1.2 ± 0.4 vs. 1.5 ± 0.35 ng/mL; $p$ < 0.01) results than the group consuming animal products. Vegan athletes who consumed sufficient macronutrients with their diet had better insulin sensitivity and lower cholesterol levels than omnivorous athletes. However, the content of dietary protein, EPA and DHA may have been insufficient, and supplementation should be considered for vegan athletes.

## 6. Discussion

Research indicates that people decide to change to a plant-based diet mainly for health reasons, then for satisfaction and well-being. The environmental and ethical factors were reported less frequently [66,67]. In addition to many positive effects on human health, plant diets can also show negative features. It was suggested that plant-based diets are suitable for people at all stages of life, as long as they are well-balanced and planned [68]. One of the main objections to using plant-based diets is that they are deficient in protein. Research shows that currently, there are no significant differences in covering protein requirements, provided that plant sources of protein are used: legumes, soy products, nuts and seeds [10,67,69,70]. The nutritional value of legume protein is slightly lower than that of meat. Due to the limiting amino acids in plant protein sources, it is necessary to combine the legumes with cereal products, which supplement the missing amino acids [71,72]. Incorrect selection of plant foods may result in deficiencies of micronutrients, in particular B vitamins (B2 and B12), vitamin D, iron, zinc and calcium. Vitamin B12 is present mainly in animal products (liver, meat, milk, dairy products, eggs); therefore, it is essential to choose products enriched with this vitamin or take dietary supplements [68,73]. It is important to seek health and dietary advice based on scientific evidence [74].

Some people cannot decide to exclude animal products from the diet completely, and therefore they limit their consumption [68]. The maintenance of plant-based diet habits is influenced by many factors, including personal factors, friends and family and the availability of vegetarian and vegan products [68,75]. Questionnaire research indicates that the main barrier to changing eating habits is the pleasure of eating meat and the difficulty in giving up eating it [67,76]. For many people, the difficulty adapting plant diets is the complicated process of preparing meals, the availability of ready-made products and dishes, high prices, lack of variety and unpalatable meals [67,77–80]. Research shows that replacing animal proteins with legumes is difficult. The respondents indicate that dishes based on legumes are unattractive and unpalatable, which is a severe barrier to plant-based diets [71,81–84].

In addition, vegetarians can experience discrimination and social constraints. Individuals may feel rejected and judged by other family members due to plant-based diets. Moreover, established eating habits and attitudes constitute a barrier to changing the diet to a plant-based, mainly for the elderly [67,68].

The main limitations of our study include the extensive literature on plant-based diets. Unfortunately, among many articles, few of them focused on the impact of plant-based diets on insulin resistance, which makes the presented results favourable and unambiguous. We did not find any study showing a negative effect of plant-based diets on insulin resistance. Many of the 44 references used for the review were comparative studies. Few randomised controlled trials limit the possibility of unequivocally establishing the effect of plant-based diets on insulin resistance. We believe that more research of this type is needed, setting future research directions. Thanks to the PRISMA diagram, we were able to conduct the above literature review. It made our work easier and systematised the analysis of the topic of the influence of plant-based diets on insulin resistance.

## 7. Conclusions

Vegetarian diets show beneficial effects not only on insulin resistance but also on other health parameters, including body weight, body fat, BMI and lipid profile parameters. Meat-free diets are suitable for everyone, regardless of age or health. Unfortunately, improperly balanced plant-based diets may carry a risk of nutritional deficiencies, in particular deficiencies in protein, B vitamins, iron, zinc and omega 3 fatty acids.

This review has such limitations as studies in languages other than English, children studies, no abstract, limited data and no data on plant-based diet and insulin resistance. However, more research is needed to determine whether plant-based diets can be used to treat diseases.

Based on available research, it may be concluded that vegetarian diets deliver good results, that more plant-based foods and fewer animal products in a diet result in lower insulin resistance and a lower risk of prediabetes and type 2 diabetes.

**Author Contributions:** Conceptualisation, M.B. and I.G.; formal analysis, M.B.; writing—original draft preparation, M.B.; writing—review and editing, M.B., I.G. and J.P.; supervision, I.G and J.P. All authors have read and agreed to the published version of the manuscript.

**Funding:** This research received no external funding.

**Conflicts of Interest:** The authors declare no conflict of interest.

## References

1. Wilcox, G. Insulin and Insulin Resistance. *Clin. Biochem. Rev.* **2005**, *26*, 19–39. [PubMed]
2. Reaven, G. The Metabolic Syndrome or the Insulin Resistance Syndrome? Different Names, Different Concepts, and Different Goals. *Endocrinol. Metab. Clin. N. Am.* **2004**, *33*, 283–303. [CrossRef] [PubMed]
3. Cefalu, W.T. Insulin Resistance: Cellular and Clinical Concepts. *Exp. Biol. Med.* **2001**, *226*, 13–26. [CrossRef] [PubMed]
4. Brown, A.E.; Walker, M. Genetics of Insulin Resistance and the Metabolic Syndrome. *Curr. Cardiol. Rep.* **2016**, *18*, 1–8. [CrossRef]
5. Freeman, A.M.; Pennings, N. *Insulin Resistance*; StatPearls: Treasure Island, FL, USA, 2021.
6. Pacini, G.; Mari, A. Methods for Clinical Assessment of Insulin Sensitivity and Beta-Cell Function. *Best Pract. Res. Clin. Endocrinol. Metab.* **2003**, *17*, 305–322. [CrossRef]
7. Gołąbek, K.; Regulska-Ilow, B. Dietary Support in Insulin Resistance: An Overview of Current Scientific Reports. *Adv. Clin. Exp. Med.* **2019**, *28*, 1577–1585. [CrossRef]
8. Mirabelli, M.; Russo, D.; Brunetti, A. The Role of Diet on Insulin Sensitivity. *Nutrients* **2020**, *12*, 3042. [CrossRef]
9. Leitzmann, C. Vegetarian Nutrition: Past, Present, Future. *Am. J. Clin. Nutr.* **2014**, *100* (Suppl. 1), 496S–502S. [CrossRef]
10. Melina, V.; Craig, W.; Levin, S. Position of the Academy of Nutrition and Dietetics: Vegetarian Diets. *J. Acad. Nutr. Diet.* **2016**, *116*, 1970–1980. [CrossRef]
11. Dinu, M.; Abbate, R.; Gensini, G.F.; Casini, A.; Sofi, F. Vegetarian, Vegan Diets and Multiple Health Outcomes: A Systematic Review with Meta-Analysis of Observational Studies. *Crit. Rev. Food Sci. Nutr.* **2017**, *57*, 3640–3649. [CrossRef]
12. Bradbury, K.E.; Crowe, F.L.; Appleby, P.N.; Schmidt, J.A.; Travis, R.C.; Key, T.J. Serum Concentrations of Cholesterol, Apolipoprotein A-I and Apolipoprotein B in a Total of 1694 Meat-Eaters, Fish-Eaters, Vegetarians and Vegans. *Eur. J. Clin. Nutr.* **2014**, *68*, 178–183. [CrossRef] [PubMed]
13. Robberecht, H.; De Bruyne, T.; Hermans, N. Effect of Various Diets on Biomarkers of the Metabolic Syndrome. *Int. J. Food Sci. Nutr.* **2017**, *68*, 627–641. [CrossRef] [PubMed]
14. Veronese, N.; Reginster, J.-Y. The Effects of Calorie Restriction, Intermittent Fasting and Vegetarian Diets on Bone Health. *Aging Clin. Exp. Res.* **2019**, *31*, 753–758. [CrossRef] [PubMed]
15. Sakkas, H.; Bozidis, P.; Touzios, C.; Kolios, D.; Athanasiou, G.; Athanasopoulou, E.; Gerou, I.; Gartzonika, C. Nutritional Status and the Influence of the Vegan Diet on the Gut Microbiota and Human Health. *Medicina* **2020**, *56*, 88. [CrossRef] [PubMed]
16. Marrone, G.; Guerriero, C.; Palazzetti, D.; Lido, P.; Marolla, A.; Di Daniele, F.; Noce, A. Vegan Diet Health Benefits in Metabolic Syndrome. *Nutrients* **2021**, *13*, 817. [CrossRef] [PubMed]
17. Silva, S.; Pinho, J.; Borges, C.; Teixeira Santos, M.; Santos, A.; Graça, P. *Guidelines for a Healthy Vegetarian Diet*; National Programme for the Promotion of Healthy Eating: Lisbon, Portugal, 2015.

18. Le, L.T.; Sabaté, J. Beyond Meatless, the Health Effects of Vegan Diets: Findings from the Adventist Cohorts. *Nutrients* **2014**, *6*, 2131–2147. [CrossRef]
19. Orlich, M.J.; Singh, P.N.; Sabaté, J.; Jaceldo-Siegl, K.; Fan, J.; Knutsen, S.; Beeson, W.L.; Fraser, G.E. Vegetarian Dietary Patterns and Mortality in Adventist Health Study 2. *JAMA Intern. Med.* **2013**, *173*, 1230–1238. [CrossRef]
20. Orlich, M.J.; Fraser, G.E. Vegetarian Diets in the Adventist Health Study 2: A Review of Initial Published Findings1234. *Am. J. Clin. Nutr.* **2014**, *100*, 353S–358S. [CrossRef]
21. Mariotti, F. *Vegetarian and Plant-Based Diets in Health and Disease Prevention*; Elsevier/Academic Press: London, UK, 2017.
22. Ley, S.H.; Hamdy, O.; Mohan, V.; Hu, F.B. Prevention and Management of Type 2 Diabetes: Dietary Components and Nutritional Strategies. *Lancet* **2014**, *383*, 1999–2007. [CrossRef]
23. Mann, J.I. Nutrition Recommendations for the Treatment and Prevention of Type 2 Diabetes and the Metabolic Syndrome: An Evidenced-Based Review. *Nutr. Rev.* **2006**, *64*, 422–427. [CrossRef]
24. Hosseinpour-Niazi, S.; Mirmiran, P.; Hedayati, M.; Azizi, F. Substitution of Red Meat with Legumes in the Therapeutic Lifestyle Change Diet based on Dietary Advice Improves Cardiometabolic Risk Factors in Overweight Type 2 Diabetes Patients: A Crossover Randomized Clinical Trial. *Eur. J. Clin. Nutr.* **2015**, *69*, 592–597. [CrossRef] [PubMed]
25. Jenkins, D.J.A.; Kendall, C.W.C.; Augustin, L.S.A.; Mitchell, S.; Sahye-Pudaruth, S.; Blanco Mejia, S.; Chiavaroli, L.; Mirrahimi, A.; Ireland, C.; Bashyam, B.; et al. Effect of Legumes as Part of a Low Glycemic Index Diet on Glycemic Control and Cardiovascular Risk Factors in Type 2 Diabetes Mellitus: A Randomized Controlled Trial. *Arch. Intern. Med.* **2012**, *172*, 1653–1660. [CrossRef] [PubMed]
26. Pittaway, J.K.; Robertson, I.K.; Ball, M.J. Chickpeas May Influence Fatty Acid and Fiber Intake in an Ad Libitum Diet, Leading to Small Improvements in Serum Lipid Profile and Glycemic Control. *J. Am. Diet. Assoc.* **2008**, *108*, 1009–1013. [CrossRef] [PubMed]
27. Tucker, L.A.; LeCheminant, J.D.; Bailey, B.W. Meat Intake and Insulin Resistance in Women without Type 2 Diabetes. *J. Diabetes Res.* **2015**, *2015*, 174742. [CrossRef] [PubMed]
28. Ley, S.H.; Sun, Q.; Willett, W.C.; Eliassen, A.H.; Wu, K.; Pan, A.; Grodstein, F.; Hu, F.B. Associations between Red Meat Intake and Biomarkers of Inflammation and Glucose Metabolism in Women. *Am. J. Clin. Nutr.* **2014**, *99*, 352–360. [CrossRef]
29. Cui, X.; Wang, B.; Wu, Y.; Xie, L.; Xun, P.; Tang, Q.; Cai, W.; Shen, X. Vegetarians Have a Lower Fasting Insulin Level and Higher Insulin Sensitivity than Matched Omnivores: A Cross-Sectional Study. *Nutr. Metab. Cardiovasc. Dis.* **2019**, *29*, 467–473. [CrossRef]
30. Kim, M.-H.; Bae, Y.-J. Comparative Study of Serum Leptin and Insulin Resistance Levels between Korean Postmenopausal Vegetarian and Non-Vegetarian Women. *Clin. Nutr. Res.* **2015**, *4*, 175–181. [CrossRef]
31. Yang, S.-Y.; Li, X.-J.; Zhang, W.; Liu, C.-Q.; Zhang, H.-J.; Lin, J.-R.; Yan, B.; Yu, Y.-X.; Shi, X.-L.; Li, C.-D.; et al. Chinese Lacto-Vegetarian Diet Exerts Favorable Effects on Metabolic Parameters, Intima-Media Thickness, and Cardiovascular Risks in Healthy Men. *Nutr. Clin. Pract.* **2012**, *27*, 392–398. [CrossRef]
32. Gammon, C.S.; von Hurst, P.R.; Coad, J.; Kruger, R.; Stonehouse, W. Vegetarianism, Vitamin B12 Status, and Insulin Resistance in a Group of Predominantly Overweight/Obese South Asian Women. *Nutrition* **2012**, *28*, 20–24. [CrossRef]
33. Hung, C.-J.; Huang, P.-C.; Li, Y.-H.; Lu, S.-C.; Ho, L.-T.; Chou, H.-F. Taiwanese Vegetarians Have Higher Insulin Sensitivity than Omnivores. *Br. J. Nutr.* **2006**, *95*, 129–135. [CrossRef]
34. Kuo, C.-S.; Lai, N.-S.; Ho, L.-T.; Lin, C.-L. Insulin Sensitivity in Chinese Ovo-Lactovegetarians Compared with Omnivores. *Eur. J. Clin. Nutr.* **2004**, *58*, 312–316. [CrossRef] [PubMed]
35. Kahleova, H.; Matoulek, M.; Malinska, H.; Oliyarnik, O.; Kazdova, L.; Neskudla, T.; Skoch, A.; Hajek, M.; Hill, M.; Kahle, M.; et al. Vegetarian Diet Improves Insulin Resistance and Oxidative Stress Markers More than Conventional Diet in Subjects with Type 2 Diabetes. *Diabet. Med.* **2011**, *28*, 549–559. [CrossRef]
36. Valachovicová, M.; Krajcovicová-Kudláčková, M.; Blazícek, P.; Babinská, K. No Evidence of Insulin Resistance in Normal Weight Vegetarians. A Case Control Study. *Eur. J. Nutr.* **2006**, *45*, 52–54. [CrossRef]
37. Chiang, J.-K.; Lin, Y.-L.; Chen, C.-L.; Ouyang, C.-M.; Wu, Y.-T.; Chi, Y.-C.; Huang, K.-C.; Yang, W.-S. Reduced Risk for Metabolic Syndrome and Insulin Resistance Associated with Ovo-Lacto-Vegetarian Behavior in Female Buddhists: A Case-Control Study. *PLoS ONE* **2013**, *8*, e71799. [CrossRef] [PubMed]
38. Vučić Lovrenčić, M.; Gerić, M.; Košuta, I.; Dragičević, M.; Garaj-Vrhovac, V.; Gajski, G. Sex-Specific Effects of Vegetarian Diet on Adiponectin Levels and Insulin Sensitivity in Healthy Non-Obese Individuals. *Nutrition* **2020**, *79*, 110862. [CrossRef] [PubMed]
39. Ellsworth, D.L.; Costantino, N.S.; Blackburn, H.L.; Engler, R.J.M.; Kashani, E.; Vernalis, M.N. Lifestyle Modification Interventions Differing in Intensity and Dietary Stringency Improve Insulin Resistance through Changes in Lipoprotein Profiles. *Obes. Sci. Pract.* **2016**, *2*, 282–292. [CrossRef] [PubMed]
40. Garousi, N.; Tamizifar, B.; Pourmasoumi, M.; Feizi, A.; Askari, G.; Clark, C.C.T.; Entezari, M.H. Effects of Lacto-Ovo-Vegetarian Diet vs. Standard-Weight-Loss Diet on Obese and Overweight Adults with Non-Alcoholic Fatty Liver Disease: A Randomised Clinical Trial. *Arch. Physiol. Biochem.* **2021**, 1–9. [CrossRef]
41. Chen, Z.; Zuurmond, M.G.; van der Schaft, N.; Nano, J.; Wijnhoven, H.A.H.; Ikram, M.A.; Franco, O.H.; Voortman, T. Plant versus Animal based Diets and Insulin Resistance, Prediabetes and Type 2 Diabetes: The Rotterdam Study. *Eur. J. Epidemiol.* **2018**, *33*, 883–893. [CrossRef]
42. Satija, A.; Hu, F.B. Plant-Based Diets and Cardiovascular Health. *Trends Cardiovasc. Med.* **2018**, *28*, 437–441. [CrossRef]
43. Nolan, C.J.; Larter, C.Z. Lipotoxicity: Why do Saturated Fatty Acids Cause and Monounsaturates Protect against It? *J. Gastroenterol. Hepatol.* **2009**, *24*, 703–706. [CrossRef]

44. Najjar, R.S.; Feresin, R.G. Plant-Based Diets in the Reduction of Body Fat: Physiological Effects and Biochemical Insights. *Nutrients* **2019**, *11*, 2712. [CrossRef] [PubMed]
45. Risérus, U.; Willett, W.C.; Hu, F.B. Dietary Fats and Prevention of Type 2 Diabetes. *Prog. Lipid Res.* **2009**, *48*, 44–51. [CrossRef] [PubMed]
46. Rizkalla, S.W.; Bellisle, F.; Slama, G. Health Benefits of Low Glycaemic Index Foods, Such as Pulses, in Diabetic Patients and Healthy Individuals. *Br. J. Nutr.* **2002**, *88* (Suppl. 3), 255–262. [CrossRef] [PubMed]
47. Polak, R.; Phillips, E.M.; Campbell, A. Legumes: Health Benefits and Culinary Approaches to Increase Intake. *Clin. Diabetes* **2015**, *33*, 198–205. [CrossRef]
48. Pan, A.; Sun, Q.; Bernstein, A.M.; Schulze, M.B.; Manson, J.E.; Willett, W.C.; Hu, F.B. Red Meat Consumption and Risk of Type 2 Diabetes: 3 Cohorts of US Adults and an Updated Meta-Analysis123. *Am. J. Clin. Nutr.* **2011**, *94*, 1088–1096. [CrossRef]
49. Pan, A.; Sun, Q.; Bernstein, A.M.; Manson, J.E.; Willett, W.C.; Hu, F.B. Changes in Red Meat Consumption and Subsequent Risk of Type 2 Diabetes: Three Cohorts of US Men and Women. *JAMA Intern. Med.* **2013**, *173*, 1328–1335. [CrossRef]
50. Barnard, N.; Levin, S.; Trapp, C. Meat Consumption as a Risk Factor for Type 2 Diabetes. *Nutrients* **2014**, *6*, 897–910. [CrossRef]
51. Fretts, A.M.; Follis, J.L.; Nettleton, J.A.; Lemaitre, R.N.; Ngwa, J.S.; Wojczynski, M.K.; Kalafati, I.P.; Varga, T.V.; Frazier-Wood, A.C.; Houston, D.K.; et al. Consumption of Meat is Associated with Higher Fasting Glucose and Insulin Concentrations Regardless of Glucose and Insulin Genetic Risk Scores: A Meta-Analysis of 50,345 Caucasians. *Am. J. Clin. Nutr.* **2015**, *102*, 1266–1278. [CrossRef]
52. Frazier-Wood, A.C.; Garvey, W.T.; Dall, T.; Honigberg, R.; Pourfarzib, R. Opportunities for Using Lipoprotein Subclass Profile by Nuclear Magnetic Resonance Spectroscopy in Assessing Insulin Resistance and Diabetes Prediction. *Metab. Syndr. Relat. Disord.* **2012**, *10*, 244–251. [CrossRef]
53. Craig, W.J. Health Effects of Vegan Diets. *Am. J. Clin. Nutr.* **2009**, *89*, 1627S–1633S. [CrossRef]
54. Kahleova, H.; Fleeman, R.; Hlozkova, A.; Holubkov, R.; Barnard, N.D. A Plant-Based Diet in Overweight Individuals in a 16-Week Randomized Clinical Trial: Metabolic Benefits of Plant Protein. *Nutr. Diabetes* **2018**, *8*, 58. [CrossRef] [PubMed]
55. Barnard, N.D.; Alwarith, J.; Rembert, E.; Brandon, L.; Nguyen, M.; Goergen, A.; Horne, T.; do Nascimento, G.F.; Lakkadi, K.; Tura, A.; et al. A Mediterranean Diet and Low-Fat Vegan Diet to Improve Body Weight and Cardiometabolic Risk Factors: A Randomized, Cross-over Trial. *J. Am. Coll. Nutr.* **2021**, 1–13. [CrossRef] [PubMed]
56. Kahleova, H.; Dort, S.; Holubkov, R.; Barnard, N.D. A Plant-Based High-Carbohydrate, Low-Fat Diet in Overweight Individuals in a 16-Week Randomized Clinical Trial: The Role of Carbohydrates. *Nutrients* **2018**, *10*, 1302. [CrossRef] [PubMed]
57. Kahleova, H.; Rembert, E.; Alwarith, J.; Yonas, W.N.; Tura, A.; Holubkov, R.; Agnello, M.; Chutkan, R.; Barnard, N.D. Effects of a Low-Fat Vegan Diet on Gut Microbiota in Overweight Individuals and Relationships with Body Weight, Body Composition, and Insulin Sensitivity. A Randomized Clinical Trial. *Nutrients* **2020**, *12*, 2917. [CrossRef]
58. Kahleova, H.; Hlozkova, A.; Fleeman, R.; Fletcher, K.; Holubkov, R.; Barnard, N.D. Fat Quantity and Quality, as Part of a Low-Fat, Vegan Diet, are Associated with Changes in Body Composition, Insulin Resistance, and Insulin Secretion. A 16-Week Randomized Controlled Trial. *Nutrients* **2019**, *11*, 615. [CrossRef]
59. Kahleova, H.; Tura, A.; Hill, M.; Holubkov, R.; Barnard, N.D. A Plant-Based Dietary Intervention Improves Beta-Cell Function and Insulin Resistance in Overweight Adults: A 16-Week Randomized Clinical Trial. *Nutrients* **2018**, *10*, 189. [CrossRef]
60. Kahleova, H.; McCann, J.; Alwarith, J.; Rembert, E.; Tura, A.; Holubkov, R.; Barnard, N.D. A Plant-Based Diet in Overweight Adults in a 16-Week Randomized Clinical Trial: The Role of Dietary Acid Load. *Clin. Nutr. ESPEN* **2021**, *44*, 150–158. [CrossRef]
61. Kahleova, H.; Petersen, K.F.; Shulman, G.I.; Alwarith, J.; Rembert, E.; Tura, A.; Hill, M.; Holubkov, R.; Barnard, N.D. Effect of a Low-Fat Vegan Diet on Body Weight, Insulin Sensitivity, Postprandial Metabolism, and Intramyocellular and Hepatocellular Lipid Levels in Overweight Adults: A Randomized Clinical Trial. *JAMA Netw. Open* **2020**, *3*, 2025454. [CrossRef]
62. Barnard, N.D.; Scialli, A.R.; Turner-McGrievy, G.; Lanou, A.J.; Glass, J. The Effects of a Low-Fat, Plant-Based Dietary Intervention on Body Weight, Metabolism, and Insulin Sensitivity. *Am. J. Med.* **2005**, *118*, 991–997. [CrossRef]
63. Śliż, D.; Parol, D.; Wełnicki, M.; Chomiuk, T.; Grabowska, I.; Dąbrowska, D.; Król, W.; Price, S.; Braksator, W.; Mamcarz, A. Macronutrient Intake, Carbohydrate Metabolism and Cholesterol in Polish Male Amateur Athletes on a Vegan Diet. *Nutr. Bull.* **2021**, *46*, 120–127. [CrossRef]
64. Krajcovicova-Kudlackova, M.; Babinska, K.; Valachovicova, M. Health Benefits and Risks of Plant Proteins. *Bratisl. Lek. Listy* **2005**, *106*, 231–234. [PubMed]
65. McCarty, M.F. Vegan Proteins May Reduce Risk of Cancer, Obesity, and Cardiovascular Disease by Promoting Increased Glucagon Activity. *Med. Hypotheses* **1999**, *53*, 459–485. [CrossRef] [PubMed]
66. Lea, E.J.; Crawford, D.; Worsley, A. Public Views of the Benefits and Barriers to the Consumption of a Plant-Based Diet. *Eur. J. Clin. Nutr.* **2006**, *60*, 828–837. [CrossRef] [PubMed]
67. Lea, E.J.; Crawford, D.; Worsley, A. Consumers' Readiness to Eat a Plant-Based Diet. *Eur. J. Clin. Nutr.* **2006**, *60*, 342–351. [CrossRef]
68. Fehér, A.; Gazdecki, M.; Véha, M.; Szakály, M.; Szakály, Z. A Comprehensive Review of the Benefits of and the Barriers to the Switch to a Plant-Based Diet. *Sustainability* **2020**, *12*, 4136. [CrossRef]
69. Thomas, D.T.; Erdman, K.A.; Burke, L.M. Position of the Academy of Nutrition and Dietetics, Dietitians of Canada, and the American College of Sports Medicine: Nutrition and Athletic Performance. *J. Acad. Nutr. Diet.* **2016**, *116*, 501–528. [CrossRef]
70. Lea, E.; Worsley, A. Influences on Meat Consumption in Australia. *Appetite* **2001**, *36*, 127–136. [CrossRef]

71. Śmiglak-Krajewska, M.; Wojciechowska-Solis, J. Consumption Preferences of Pulses in the Diet of Polish People: Motives and Barriers to Replace Animal Protein with Vegetable Protein. *Nutrients* **2021**, *13*, 454. [CrossRef]
72. Caire-Juvera, G.; Vázquez-Ortiz, F.A.; Grijalva-Haro, M.I. Amino Acid Composition, Score and in Vitro Protein Digestibility of Foods Commonly Consumed in Northwest Mexico. *Nutr. Hosp.* **2013**, *28*, 365–371. [CrossRef]
73. Watanabe, F. Vitamin B12 Sources and Bioavailability. *Exp. Biol. Med.* **2007**, *232*, 1266–1274. [CrossRef]
74. Wickramasinghe, K.; Breda, J.; Berdzuli, N.; Rippin, H.; Farrand, C.; Halloran, A. The Shift to Plant-Based Diets: Are We Missing the Point? *Glob. Food Secur.* **2021**, *29*, 100530. [CrossRef]
75. Jabs, J.; Devine, C.M.; Sobal, J. Model of the Process of Adopting Vegetarian Diets: Health Vegetarians and Ethical Vegetarians. *J. Nutr. Educ.* **1998**, *30*, 196–202. [CrossRef]
76. Graça, J.; Oliveira, A.; Calheiros, M.M. Meat, beyond the Plate. Data-Driven Hypotheses for Understanding Consumer Willingness to Adopt a More Plant-Based Diet. *Appetite* **2015**, *90*, 80–90. [CrossRef] [PubMed]
77. Lea, E.; Worsley, A. Benefits and Barriers to the Consumption of a Vegetarian Diet in Australia. *Public Health Nutr.* **2003**, *6*, 505–511. [CrossRef]
78. Pohjolainen, P.; Vinnari, M.; Jokinen, P. Consumers' Perceived Barriers to following a Plant-Based Diet. *Br. Food J.* **2015**, *117*, 1150–1167. [CrossRef]
79. Vanhonacker, F.; Van Loo, E.J.; Gellynck, X.; Verbeke, W. Flemish Consumer Attitudes towards More Sustainable Food Choices. *Appetite* **2013**, *62*, 7–16. [CrossRef]
80. Mullee, A.; Vermeire, L.; Vanaelst, B.; Mullie, P.; Deriemaeker, P.; Leenaert, T.; De Henauw, S.; Dunne, A.; Gunter, M.J.; Clarys, P.; et al. Vegetarianism and Meat Consumption: A Comparison of Attitudes and Beliefs between Vegetarian, Semi-Vegetarian, and Omnivorous Subjects in Belgium. *Appetite* **2017**, *114*, 299–305. [CrossRef]
81. Vainio, A.; Niva, M.; Jallinoja, P.; Latvala, T. From Beef to Beans: Eating Motives and the Replacement of Animal Proteins with Plant Proteins among Finnish Consumers. *Appetite* **2016**, *106*, 92–100. [CrossRef]
82. Melendrez-Ruiz, J.; Buatois, Q.; Chambaron, S.; Monnery-Patris, S.; Arvisenet, G. French Consumers Know the Benefits of Pulses, but do not Choose Them: An Exploratory Study Combining Indirect and Direct Approaches. *Appetite* **2019**, *141*, 104311. [CrossRef]
83. Havemeier, S.; Erickson, J.; Slavin, J. Dietary Guidance for Pulses: The Challenge and Opportunity to Be Part of Both the Vegetable and Protein Food Groups. *Ann. N. Y. Acad. Sci.* **2017**, *1392*, 58–66. [CrossRef]
84. Figueira, N.; Curtain, F.; Beck, E.; Grafenauer, S. Consumer Understanding and Culinary Use of Legumes in Australia. *Nutrients* **2019**, *11*, 1575. [CrossRef] [PubMed]

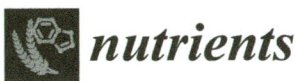

*Review*

# Dysmetabolism and Neurodegeneration: Trick or Treat?

Adriana M. Capucho †, Ana Chegão †, Fátima O. Martins, Hugo Vicente Miranda and Sílvia V. Conde *

CEDOC, NOVA Medical School, Faculdade de Ciências Médicas, Universidade NOVA de Lisboa, 1150-082 Lisboa, Portugal; adriana.capucho@nms.unl.pt (A.M.C.); ana.chegao@nms.unl.pt (A.C.); fatima.martins@nms.unl.pt (F.O.M.); hmvmiranda@nms.unl.pt (H.V.M.)
* Correspondence: silvia.conde@nms.unl.pt
† These authors contributed equally to this work.

**Abstract:** Accumulating evidence suggests the existence of a strong link between metabolic syndrome and neurodegeneration. Indeed, epidemiologic studies have described solid associations between metabolic syndrome and neurodegeneration, whereas animal models contributed for the clarification of the mechanistic underlying the complex relationships between these conditions, having the development of an insulin resistance state a pivotal role in this relationship. Herein, we review in a concise manner the association between metabolic syndrome and neurodegeneration. We start by providing concepts regarding the role of insulin and insulin signaling pathways as well as the pathophysiological mechanisms that are in the genesis of metabolic diseases. Then, we focus on the role of insulin in the brain, with special attention to its function in the regulation of brain glucose metabolism, feeding, and cognition. Moreover, we extensively report on the association between neurodegeneration and metabolic diseases, with a particular emphasis on the evidence observed in animal models of dysmetabolism induced by hypercaloric diets. We also debate on strategies to prevent and/or delay neurodegeneration through the normalization of whole-body glucose homeostasis, particularly via the modulation of the carotid bodies, organs known to be key in connecting the periphery with the brain.

**Keywords:** insulin signaling; metabolic disorders; hypercaloric diets; neurodegeneration

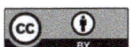

## 1. Introduction

Aging is broadly defined as the time-dependent functional decline that affects most living organisms. It is characterized by a progressive loss of physiological integrity, leading to impaired function and increased vulnerability to death [1]. Aging is pointed as the main risk factor for major human pathologies, including cancer, diabetes mellitus (DM), cardiovascular disorders, and neurodegenerative diseases. The hallmarks of aging are genomic instability, telomere attrition, epigenetic alterations, loss of proteostasis, deregulated nutrient sensing, mitochondrial dysfunction, cellular senescence, stem cell exhaustion, and altered intercellular communication [1]. Aging is therefore accompanied by a variety of physiological changes that make the organisms highly prone to so-called aged-related disorders. On the other hand, several diseases such as cardiometabolic and metabolic disorders can accelerate the aging and senescence process.

The metabolic syndrome is defined as a cluster of disorders including obesity, DM, and cardiovascular disease, and is reaching pandemic levels worldwide. Several studies have shown that the prevalence of metabolic diseases increases up to 50% in people aged over 65 years [2,3]. Consequently, as the global population ages, there will be a higher prevalence of obesity, DM, and cardiovascular disease [4,5].

Additionally, neurodegenerative diseases, which are characterized by the progressive loss of the structure or function of neurons, are classified as an age-related cluster of pathologies that were shown to be increased in the set of metabolic disorders [6,7]. Age and metabolic disorder-related neurodegenerative diseases, such as Alzheimer's (AD) and

Parkinson's (PD), are increasing worldwide, and it is not clear whether metabolic syndrome is the cause or the consequence of these neurodegenerative diseases [7–10].

Changing lifestyles and eating habits opened a door to pronounced alterations in the aging process. In this review, we mainly focus on the relationship between metabolic syndrome and neurodegenerative diseases, exploring the role of hypercaloric diets in brain function and the physiological role of insulin and insulin resistance in the central nervous system (CNS).

## 2. Insulin and Insulin Signaling Pathways

Around one hundred years ago, in 1921, an important hormone—insulin—was discovered by Frederick G. Banting, Charles Best, and John MacLeod in Canada. This event completely changed the lives of mankind, and since then thousands of lives have been saved [11].

Insulin is a 51 amino acids peptide hormone, organized in 2 polypeptides chains, A (21 amino acids) and B (30 amino acids), which are connected by disulfide bonds. Insulin production and release is carried out by pancreatic β-cells. This hormone plays a fundamental role in regulating fat and carbohydrate metabolism, promoting their conversion into storage macromolecules such as glycogen, proteins, and lipids [12–14].

Insulin is the most important anabolic hormone in the organism and plays a critical role in the regulation of different physiological processes, including metabolism, cell growth and differentiation [12,15]. The effects of insulin are highly pleiotropic and differ according to the target tissue. Concerning the peripheral regulation of metabolism, the major insulin-sensitive tissues include the skeletal muscle, adipose tissue, and liver [16]. Insulin stimulates the uptake of glucose in the skeletal muscle and adipose tissue, inhibits hepatic glucose production, and promotes the storage of substrates in the adipose tissue, liver, and muscle by triggering lipogenesis, glycogen, and protein synthesis, and by inhibiting lipolysis, glycogenolysis, and protein breakdown [15–17]. Insulin also plays a role in the CNS, mainly controlling appetite, by acting in the hypothalamus, one of the most important neuronal centers to the control of satiety and feeding through negative feedback to ensure balanced energy homeostasis [18].

Although insulin plays several functions in the organism, it is widely known as a glucose homeostasis regulating hormone. The tight control of the plasma levels of glucose is driven by the balance between glucose absorption from the intestine after feeding, production by the liver and uptake and utilization by peripheral tissues. An increase in the plasma glucose levels after a meal triggers insulin production in the pancreatic islets by β-cells.

Insulin acts by binding to its receptor, the insulin receptor (IR). IR is a glycoprotein that belongs to the tyrosine kinase receptor family, being composed by an α extracellular and β transmembrane subunits. When insulin binds to the α subunit, it triggers the dimerization of the receptor, forming an α2β2 complex, leading to the autophosphorylation of β subunit at Tyr1158, 1162, and 1163, the so-called activation of IR phosphorylation cascade (Figure 1) [15].

Activation of IR signaling pathway leads to the recruitment and phosphorylation of several proteins such as the insulin receptor substrates (IRS 1-4), that will induce the activation of intracellular pathways as phosphatidylinositide-3-kinase (PI3K) and the mitogen-activated protein kinase (MAPK) cascades [15,19]. Insulin-induced activation of Ras-MAPK promotes the regulation of cell growth and mitogenesis, whereas PI3K activation generates phosphatidylinositol (3,4,5)-triphosphate (PIP3) that will activate phosphoinositide dependent protein kinase-1 and -2 (PDK1 and PDK2), which regulate the effect of insulin on metabolism and pro-survival. Also, PDK1 and 2, have an important function in the activation of Protein Kinase B (AKT/ PKB) [15,17,20]. AKT has a key function in phosphorylating several downstream proteins, as glycogen synthase kinase b (Gsk3b), that inhibits glycogen synthesis [20,21]. AKT also phosphorylates other mediators such as the activation of AKT substrate 160 kDa (AS160) and activates Rab10 GTPase that leads to the translocation of the glucose transporter 4 (GLUT4) to the plasma membrane to promote glucose uptake [22]. Phosphodiesterase 3B (PDE3B), an enzyme that catalyzes the degradation of cyclic adenosine monophosphate (cAMP), is also activated by AKT. Additionally, AKT inhibits cAMP response element-binding protein (CREB)-regulated transcription coactivator 2 (CRTC2), important to increase hepatic gluconeogenesis. AKT also triggers liver lipogenesis by phosphorylating sterol regulatory element-binding protein 1 (SREBP1) [23], and phosphorylates Forkhead box protein O1 (Foxo1), inhibiting its transcriptional activity and leading to a suppressed liver glucose production [15,21].

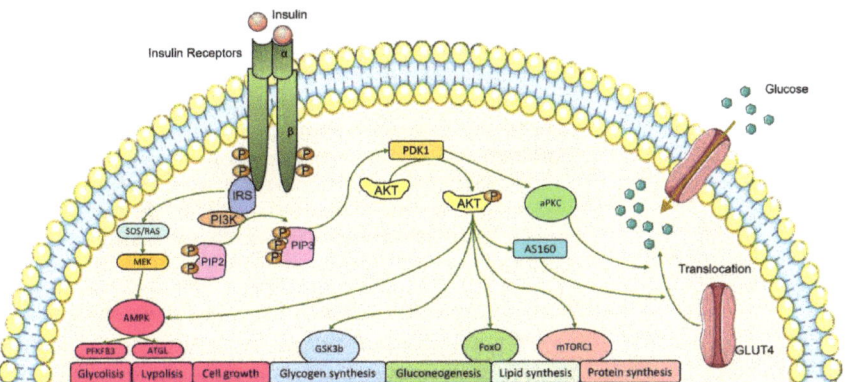

**Figure 1.** Schematic representation of insulin signaling pathways. When insulin binds to its receptor (IR), autophosphorylation of tyrosine kinase residues occurs and various downstream regulatory proteins are recruited. The insulin signal is transduced among the target proteins/enzymes ending with the fusion of the glucose transporter 4 (GLUT4) vesicle with the cell plasma membrane and the placement of GLUT4 transporters in the plasma membrane leading to the uptake of glucose. IRS, insulin receptor substrate; PI3K, phosphatidylinositide-3-kinase; PIP2, phosphatidylinositol (4,5)-biphosphate; PIP3, phosphatidylinositol (3,4,5)-triphosphate; PDK1, phosphoinositide-dependent protein kinase-1; AKT, protein kinase B; AS160, Akt substrate of 160 kDa; aPKC, atypical protein kinase C; SOS/RAS, son of sevenless; MEK, mitogen-activated protein kinase; AMPK, mitogen-activated protein kinase; PFKFB3, 6-phosphofructo-2-kinase/fructose-2,6-biphosphatase 3; ATGL, adipose triglyceride lipase; GSK3b, glycogen synthase kinase b; FoxO, forkhead box protein O1; mTORC1, mammalian target of rapamycin complex 1; GLUT4, glucose transporter type 4.

## 3. Metabolic Syndrome: Insulin Resistance and Diabetes

Failure in insulin production, insulin tissue-sensitivity, and/or insulin signaling is a pathophysiological hallmark of pre-diabetic states, resulting in hyperglycemia due to impaired uptake of glucose by cells and deregulation of hepatic glucose production [24]. Furthermore, insulin resistance together with obesity, hypertension, hyperlipidemia, dyslipidemia and hyperglycemia are key features of metabolic syndrome. DM is one of the most prevalent metabolic disorders, characterized by chronic hyperglycemia.

DM has reached pandemic levels, affecting more than 463 million people and being among the top 10 causes of deaths in adults worldwide [25]. DM is a complex, chronic condition that has a major impact on the lives and well-being of individuals, families, and a vast associated economic burden for societies [26]. DM refers to a group of chronic metabolic diseases characterized by hyperglycemia and dysfunction or destruction of pancreatic β-cells, causing defects in insulin secretion, insulin action, or both [27–29]. The heterogeneous etiopathology mechanisms leading to the decline in function, or the complete destruction of β-cells includes genetic predisposition and abnormalities, epigenetic processes, insulin resistance, autoimmunity, concurrent illnesses, inflammation, and environmental factors [27,30]. Moreover, DM is also associated with disturbances of carbohydrate, fat, and protein metabolism.

The World Health Organization (WHO) has recently proposed the classification of DM into six subtypes: type 1 diabetes mellitus (T1D); type 2 diabetes mellitus (T2D); hybrid forms of DM; other specific types; unclassified DM; hyperglycemia during pregnancy [31]. T1D is characterized by the destruction of pancreatic β-cells, resulting in the inability of the body to produce insulin. Consequently, individuals suffering from T1D are insulin dependent. In contrast, T2D which accounts for 90% of all diabetic cases, is characterized by insulin resistance. The pathogenesis of T2D involves abnormalities in both peripheral insulin action and insulin secretion by pancreatic β-cells, resulting in hyperglycemia. Insulin resistance, in an initial phase called prediabetes, is usually compensated by hyperinsulinemia, that, although it might be tolerated in the short term, will lead to a vicious cycle in which chronic hyperinsulinemia exacerbates insulin resistance and contributes directly to β-cells exhaustion and the definitive settlement of T2D.

DM predisposes to long-term complications including retinopathy, nephropathy, and neuropathy. DM increases the risk for cardiovascular diseases, obesity, cataracts, erectile dysfunction, and non-alcoholic fatty liver disease (NAFLD) [31].

Furthermore, insulin resistance syndrome negatively impacts the CNS function and DM is associated with an increased risk to develop neuropsychiatric conditions and neurodegenerative disorders [6]. As such, the control of peripheral and central insulin levels can be an important approach to prevent the development of those pathologies.

*Impact of Hypercaloric Diets on Insulin Resistance and Metabolic Syndrome*

The consumption of hypercaloric diets and overnutrition is a common trigger for the development of obesity, which is the major driver to insulin resistance, prediabetes and T2D. In recent years, the role of nutrition and lifestyle in the development of metabolic diseases has been extensively explored. Due to the fast-paced and sedentary lifestyles of modern society, the intake of hypercaloric and unhealthy food has risen, increasing the incidence of metabolic diseases in the population, and negatively impacting the aging process, aggravating the aging-associated consequences [25,31].

It is well known that the amount and nature of macro and micronutrient consumption is associated with the development of obesity and T2D, since the dietary composition and volume could be implicated in insulin resistance states, being in the genesis of T2D [32]. More than the hypercaloric composition, overnutrition is also one of the causes to the development of dysmetabolism [33]. Excessive or incorrect nutrients consumption, both carbohydrates or fat, promotes a general state of inflammation, which has an important role in insulin dysfunction as well as in energy production and catabolism of those nutrients [34].

Studies, both in animal models and humans, showed that hypercaloric diets, independently of their composition, lead to dysmetabolic states. For example, diets enriched in fat, free sugars, and fructose lead to whole-body insulin resistance [32,35]. However, different diets composition originates different metabolic features [36]. Melo et al. [36], by submitting different groups of Wistar rats to a high-fat diet (HF), high-fat–high-sucrose diet (HFHSu) and high-sucrose diet (HSu) for different periods of time, showed that the animals submitted to a HF diet for 19 weeks exhibited increased weight gain when compared to the other groups. On the other hand, animals fed with an HSu diet for 16 weeks did not exhibit a significant increase in weight gain, while animals under HFHSu diet showed an intermediate increase in weight gain between the HSu and HF groups. In fact, Melo et al. showed that the HF diet feeding model was the hypercaloric diet model that presented more phenotypic features related to T2D and obesity in humans, since they developed insulin resistance, impaired lipid and glucose metabolism, elevated sympathetic activity, hypertension, hypertriglyceridemia, and increased lipid deposition in the liver resembling NAFLD [37]. In the case of the HFHSu diet, animals exhibit significant alterations in insulin and C-peptide levels, which can be associated with impaired pancreatic insulin secretion and/or impaired insulin clearance. This finding suggests that the combination of sucrose with fat has a greater impact in glucose metabolism and insulin secretion [36,38]. These differences in the effects of diet nutrient composition over metabolism needs more clarification for a full understanding of the mechanisms in physiological and pathophysiological conditions, as well as for developing new therapies for these types of pathologies.

The adipose tissue is the most important organ for fatty acids storage. However, adipocytes have a limited capacity to accumulate fat, and when they over-expand, they create a hypoxic environment. This environment triggers the overactivation of hypoxic inducible factor 1 (HIF-1) protein creating an inflammatory state that leads to insulin resistance in the adipocytes [39–41]. Additionally, insulin has a role as anti-lipolytic hormone, therefore inhibiting the release of adipose tissue fatty acids to the circulation [42]. However, in a state of excessive fat accumulation within the adipose tissue and a state of insulin resistance, the levels of free fatty acids in the circulation increase. This will stimulate the uptake of fatty acids by other tissues, such as the liver, which does not have the capacity to store high amounts of fat. This increased uptake of free fatty acids by the liver contributes to liver insulin resistance and consequent hepatic glucose production and glycogen synthesis deregulation, aggravating the whole-body insulin resistance and glucose homeostasis impairment [43,44]. This event is one of the first consequences of dysmetabolism, leading to the development of NAFLD, which is present in 90% of obese T2D patients [45].

Regarding the role of sugar on metabolism and dysmetabolism, it is known that the different types of sugars are additive, palatable, and rewarding compounds from food [46]. Excessive sugar consumption leads to several metabolic disorders, and some related brain pathologies, impairing reward systems which may lead to compulsive eating [47,48].

Sugar refers to a category of carbohydrates which includes fructose and glucose (monosaccharides), and lactose and sucrose (disaccharides), having different roles in the organism. Many people consider fructose as a healthy sugar because it is naturally present in fruit and other vegetables. However, our body does not respond similarly to the fructose that is present in the fruit and the fructose that is added on the diet [49–51]. In fact, the added fructose, mainly in the form of corn syrup, is one of the major causes of insulin resistance and impaired lipid metabolism associated to T2D and its comorbidities [49–53]. Additionally, recent studies have shown that when fructose is replaced by glucose in starch form in the diet these pathological features were alleviated [54,55]. The differences in the metabolic features promoted by glucose and fructose indicate that the metabolic pathways involved are different. In fact, fructose absorption in the gut promoted by GLUT5 is independent of insulin as well as its usage in the liver. In the liver, fructose is converted into glucose, lactate, and fatty acids, that will be released to the blood, oxidized, and used by other tissues [51,56,57]. Glucose is taken by muscle and the adipose tissue to be used as energy source. In contrast, these tissues do not uptake fructose since this sugar is not a primary source of energy [46]. In opposition to glucose and sucrose, fructose promotes smaller effects in plasma glucose levels, satiety hormones and insulin action, leading to overconsumption of calories to promote satiety [58].

## 4. The Role of Insulin in the Brain

As stated before, insulin acts in insulin-sensitive peripheral tissues such as the liver, the skeletal muscle, the pancreas, and the adipose tissue to regulate glucose homeostasis. However, insulin has been also described to play a key role in the CNS [19,20]. Insulin action in the brain regulates several processes including energy expenditure, glucose homeostasis, feeding behavior and satiety, reward pathways, reproduction, cell proliferation and differentiation. Moreover, insulin has neuroprotective and neuromodulatory properties and plays a crucial role in neuronal transmission and survival, neurogenesis, plasticity, and memory and cognition [19,20,59,60].

Insulin reaches the brain from circulation by crossing the blood–brain barrier (BBB) through a selective, saturable transport [19,61,62]. Although insulin levels in cerebrospinal fluid (CSF) are much lower than in plasma, these levels are correlated, indicating that most insulin in the brain may derive from circulating pancreatic insulin [63,64]. Some authors demonstrated the presence of relatively high concentrations of insulin in brain extracts, suggesting that insulin could also be synthetized in the CNS and released locally, as already established for other hormones [65,66]. In fact, some data supports that neurons and astrocytes may produce insulin in relative higher amounts [67–69]. Insulin synthesis was described to be independent of its peripheral concentrations, since insulin levels in the hypothalamus were not related to pancreatic insulin concentrations during fasting [70]. Additionally, it was found that GABAergic neurons synthetize insulin in the rat cerebral cortex, as well as in the hypothalamus and hippocampus [71]. However, insulin production by neurons and glial cells is still under debate.

Nevertheless, it is widely accepted that most insulin in the brain originates in the pancreas. The rate of insulin transport across the BBB is influenced by physiological factors such as exposure to hypercaloric diets, hyperglycemia, or a diabetic state. These conditions lead to a decreased transport of insulin to the brain, and/or to a disruption of the BBB. Rhea et al., showed that IR inhibition with the selective antagonist S961, does not modify insulin transport across the BBB, suggesting that the hormone is able to cross this barrier in an IR signaling-independent manner [72].

In the brain, two different isoforms of IR can be found: a long isoform, IR-B, and a short predominant isoform [73], IR-A, with insulin having similar affinity and potency for both isoforms [74–76]. IR are expressed at high levels in different brain regions such as the hypothalamus, olfactory bulb, hippocampus, striatum, cerebral cortex, and cerebellum, where they are involved in different functions. The olfactory bulb is the region of the brain that contains the highest amount of IR, although its function in this area is not fully understood. The cortex and the hippocampus also have high levels of IR with very important functions in terms of synaptic plasticity and cognitive processes. The third region that contains the highest levels of this receptor is the hypothalamus with a central role in the regulation of glucose homeostasis and regulation of satiety pathways [77]. Most of these actions seem to be independent of glucose utilization [62,78].

*4.1. Role of Insulin in Brain Glucose Metabolism and Feeding*

Glucose is the main source of energy in the brain, reaching this organ through the GLUTs, which have numerous isoforms [6]. Most glucose uptake to brain and by neuronal and glial cells is insulin-independent and relies on the insulin-insensitive GLUT1 and GLUT3, among other less abundant region-specific GLUTs [79–81]. However, in brain regions related to cognition and metabolic control, such as the basal forebrain, hippocampus, amygdala, cortex, cerebellum, and hypothalamus, the inducible insulin-sensitive GLUT4 is reported to be co-expressed with GLUT3 [82–84]. Activation by insulin induces the translocation of GLUT4 to the membrane and is thought to improve glucose flux into neurons during periods of high metabolic demand, such as learning [85,86]. The effect of insulin and its relevance on glucose uptake in the brain is not consensual and for a long time was thought to be exclusively insulin independent. In fact, several studies from the 80's that focused on the effect of insulin in brain glucose uptake showed that brain glucose metabolism was unaffected by insulin. Goodner et al. measured glucose uptake in fasting rats 30 min after 0.1U insulin administration [87] and observed that the brain did not increase the rate of glucose uptake, concluding that the brain was "insensitive to insulin" [88]. However, subsequent studies using 18-fluorodeoxyglucose positron emission tomography showed that insulin increases brain glucose uptake in humans, mostly marked in cortical areas [89]. In agreement with the role of insulin in regulating glucose uptake in the brain, GLUT4 colocalizes with IR in several brain regions [90].

Another important role of insulin in the indirect control of glucose homeostasis is related with the mesolimbic reward pathways on the dopaminergic neurons [91]. Insulin can alter food choices and preferences, as it increases dopamine release in the reward pathways after food restriction, an effect not seen in animals submitted to hypercaloric diets. Therefore, it has been shown that dopaminergic pathways are negatively regulated by insulin, as insulin causes the desire to consume high-calorie foods rich in sugar and fat, promoting a feeling of satiety and reward [91,92].

Beyond its role on controlling glucose homeostasis, insulin in the brain also impacts insulin sensitivity at the periphery. Heni and colleagues have found in lean men that central insulin action, achieved by an intra-nasal insulin spray application, improved peripheral insulin sensitivity measured by hyperglycemic clamp [93]. When they explored the mechanisms involved, they discovered that the vagus nerve and the parasympathetic system activation is involved in the peripheral insulin sensitivity regulation by CNS insulin. The hypothalamus appears to be one of the most important brain regions in this link [94]. Moreover, they have found an impairment in the central regulation of peripheral insulin signaling in obese people, showing the tight link between brain and peripheral insulin resistance in dysmetabolism conditions [94].

Apart from glucose homeostasis regulation, insulin and its receptors have implications in the regulation of energy balance where the hypothalamus also plays a major role [18]. Together with insulin, leptin, an adipokine produced by the adipose tissue, plays a role in the regulation of feeding behavior. Both hormones act on the hypothalamus affecting the expression of neuropeptides involved in satiety pathways [18,95]. In the hypothalamus, these hormones act in the arcuate nucleus (ARC) which is composed by two antagonistic types of neurons: the anorexigenic neurons or the appetite-suppressing neurons known as proopiomelanocortin-expressing neurons (POMC) neurons, and the orexigenic or appetite-stimulating neurons known as neuropeptide Y (NPY) and agouti-related peptide (AgRP) expressing neurons [18,95] (Figure 2). Both orexigenic and anorexigenic neurons express insulin and leptin receptors.

The POMC neurons project to the second order neurons in the paraventricular nucleus (PVN) but also to the lateral hypothalamus (LH), the ventromedial hypothalamus (VMN) and the dorsomedial hypothalamus (DMH) [96]. The PVN is responsible, in part, for the secretion of a wide range of regulatory neuropeptides and by the control of sympathetic nervous system activity to peripheral organs [18]. After a meal, POMC is cleaved in α-melanocyte- stimulating hormone (α-MSH) that is released by the POMC neurons to activate melanocortin 3 and 4 receptors (MC3/4R) in both hypothalamic and extra-hypothalamic neurons to suppress feeding and food intake and stimulate energy expenditure [97]. In general, insulin and leptin, by acting on POMC neurons, suppress feeding and promote energy expenditure (Figure 2). In fact, these hormones in POMC neurons also have a role in the regulation of peripheral glucose homeostasis, although the mechanisms involved are not so clear. The disruption of hypothalamic insulin and leptin pathways in POMC neurons, driven by insulin and leptin receptors deletion in these neurons, leads to a state of systemic insulin resistance and deterioration of glucose homeostasis [18]. This suggests that intact insulin and leptin hypothalamic pathways are required for a correct peripheral insulin and glucose homeostasis.

In contrast, in AgRP/NPy neurons, insulin regulates hepatic glucose production by inducing hyperpolarization and decreasing firing between AgRP neurons, which leads to reduced gluconeogenesis. Also, leptin directly acts on AgRP neurons at the hypothalamus to exert an inhibitory effect. As such, the crucial effect of leptin in the hypothalamus is to promote energy expenditure and inhibit food intake [18,97].

Apart from the regulation of feeding behavior and glucose homeostasis, insulin has been shown to have other functions in the brain as the regulation of cognitive functions, particularly memory. Notably, defects in insulin signaling in the brain may contribute to neurodegenerative disorders and damage of the cognitive system leading to dementia states.

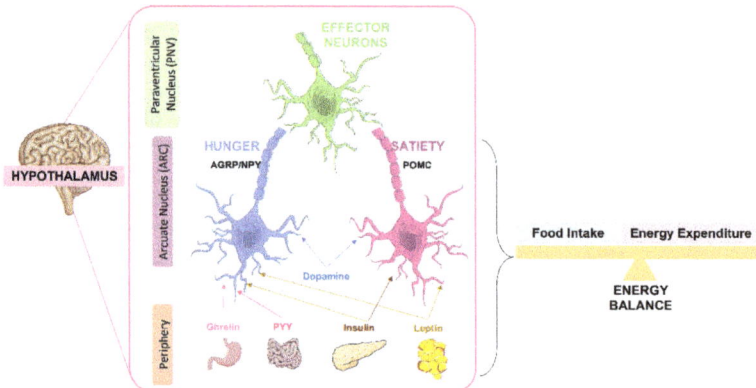

**Figure 2.** Role of the hypothalamus in the regulation of energy balance. Signals as leptin and insulin act antagonistically in the two antagonistic neurons of the arcuate nucleus (ARC): the orexigenic (appetite-stimulating) neuropeptide Y (NPY) and agouti-related peptide (AgRP)-expressing AgRP/NPY neurons and the anorexigenic (appetite-suppressing) proopiomelanocortin (POMC)-expressing POMC neurons. By one way, insulin and leptin stimulate POMC neurons, in another way they inhibit AgRP/NPY neurons. Both AgRP/NPY neurons and POMC neurons project to second-order neurons in the paraventricular nucleus (PVN), leading to an integrated response on energy intake and expenditure. The intestine also secretes peptide YY (PYY) and the stomach ghrelin that act on AgRP/NPY neurons to stimulate hunger. Dopamine modulates both AgRP/NPY and POMC neurons.

*4.2. Insulin and Cognitive Function*

The role of insulin in the brain was first studied in the context of energy homeostasis, a process mainly regulated by the hypothalamus [68]. More recently, the role of insulin in other brain functions such as memory and cognition, neuronal development, and plasticity have been explored [6,98]. Insulin has a key role in the hippocampus, a brain region that expresses high levels of IR and that is involved in learning and memory [99].

The hippocampus is a complex structure in the brain located in the temporal lobe. It forms part of the limbic system, being an extension of the cerebral cortex [100]. The hippocampus is a very plastic region, with a key role in memory formation, organization, and storage [100]. The hippocampus converts short-term memory into long-term memory, solves spatial memory, and recollects the past experiences of places. It also plays a pivotal role in emotions and behavior [101]. Different parts of the hippocampus have distinct functions in certain types of memory: spatial memory, mainly processed by the rear part of the hippocampus; memory consolidation, a process by which the hippocampus organizes the stored information in the neocortex; and memory transfer, since long term memories are not stored in the hippocampus [101]. Information in the hippocampus travels along a unidirectional trisynaptic circuit originating from the entorhinal cortex and projecting to the dentate gyrus (DG), then to area CA3, and finally to area CA1 of the horn of Ammon [102,103]. These areas of the hippocampus have different functions, being composed of different types of neurons: the granular cells in the DG and pyramidal cells in the areas CA1 and CA3 of the horn of Ammon with a vast network of interneurons [102]. Special attention has been paid to the CA3 region for its specific role in memory formation and neurodegeneration [104]. CA3 receive excitatory inputs from the pyramidal cells and then inhibitory feedback that inhibit the pyramidal cells. This recurrent inhibition is a simple feedback circuit that can dampen excitatory responses in the hippocampus, being involved in memory formation processes [105,106].

The hippocampus has also an important role in brain plasticity. Brain plasticity underlies learning and memory and depends both on the activity and the number of synapses.

Synapses may be modulated via potentiation or depression, processes that regulate the formation of new dendritic spines promoting tasks, learning, and consolidating behavioral alterations [6,107]. It has been postulated that insulin may be involved in the regulation of synaptic plasticity mechanisms and memory formation, since the mRNA levels of IR in dendrites and synapses at the hippocampus is high [99,108]. In fact, hippocampal neurons treated with insulin for 48 h show an increase in the frequency of miniature excitatory postsynaptic currents (mEPSCs), whilst downregulation of IR with short hairpin RNAs (ShRNAs) leads to the formation of few dendritic spines and therefore to reduced frequency of mEPSCs [6,109]. Insulin was also shown to regulate neuronal plasticity by controlling long-term potentiation (LTP) and long-term depression (LTD) [110]. Moreover, IR substrate p53 (IRSp53) interacts with the postsynaptic density protein 95 (PSD-95), present at excitatory synapses, therefore regulating a variety of receptors and channels, and increasing dendritic spine formation [6,111]. Insulin further plays a role on glutamatergic response by increasing the recruitment of the N-methyl-D-aspartate receptors (NMDARs) to the membrane and by enhancing the phosphorylation of NR2A and NR2B subunits [112]. In agreement, IRS2 knockout mice showed lower activation of NR2B subunits and a decrease in the LTP at CA3-CA1 synapses, however with higher density of CA1 dendritic spines [112–114]. Additionally, downregulation of a-amino-3-hydroxy-5-methyl-4-isoxazolepropionic acid receptors (AMPARs) activity of CA1 neurons in the hippocampus is crucial to insulin-induced LTD, an important feature to process memory formation [115].

The hippocampus is not the single player in the generation and regulation of memory and cognition. The prefrontal cortex is known to mediate decision making being involved in the retrieval of remote long-term memory and supporting memory and consolidation in a time scale ranging from seconds to days [116]. In fact, the hippocampus and prefrontal cortex work together to support the rapid encoding of new information, consolidation, and organization of memory networks. The cerebral cortex is known to process information about objects and events that we experience, and about the places where they occurred. Additionally, the ventral hippocampus (in the rat) and the anterior hippocampus (in humans) sends information to the medial prefrontal cortex (mPFC), suggesting that the mPFC could accumulate interrelated memories. The information of mPFC is sent back to other cortical regions, however the mPFC may bias or select the retrieval of event information in the 'what' stream. Therefore, interactions between these two brain regions can support the ability to create contextual representations that are associated with recent memories and use them to remember memories that are appropriate within a given context [117].

Considering the key role of the cortex in memory and decision making, it was reported that patients with frontal lobe damage exhibit inappropriate social behaviors and memory decline [89], suggesting that these dysfunctions can result from an impairment of memory storage in the prefrontal cortex. In fact, insulin has also an important role in the cortex, specially the IGFs since they are involved in the process of dendritic elaboration and to the stimulation of neurite outgrowth from dissociated neurons [118].

Therefore, the impairment of insulin signaling in the brain will have a negative impact in some neuronal functions additionally to the ones related with metabolism. These defects in insulin action in the CNS and specially in the hippocampus and prefrontal cortex represent a possible relationship between metabolic and cognitive disorders [119,120].

## 5. Metabolic Syndrome and the Neurodegenerative Process

It is consensual that hypercaloric diet consumption leads to obesity and several comorbidities such as insulin resistance, which can be in the genesis of T2D. The defects in insulin signaling also affects the CNS, since obesity and T2D are clear risk factors for several pathologies related with the CSN, like AD and PD [120]. It was observed that patients with T2D and/or obesity, show decreased concentrations of insulin in the cerebrospinal fluid, despite having high insulin levels in plasma [121,122]. Moreover, obesity and inflammation are reported to decrease the transport of insulin to the brain through the BBB, and T2D patients show a decreased expression of IR in the brain [121].

It was described by García-Cáceres and colleagues that alterations in insulin signaling in the brain promotes several alterations not only in neural but also in glial cell function [123]. In fact, insulin action in the brain has a direct effect on neurodegenerative and psychiatric disorders, which include alterations in dopaminergic signaling, hippocampal synaptic plasticity, expression of some proteins, and BBB function, among others [123,124].

In addition, changes in insulin action at the level of the hippocampus affect molecular mechanisms involved in synaptic formation and plasticity, having a negative impact in the maintenance of mental abilities and being a great risk factor for dementia [125]. In states of insulin resistance, IR-dependent molecular cascades may start to be insensitive to this hormone, leading to brain insulin resistance (BIR), and in this situation, insulin lose its ability to improve plasticity [122]. It is well described by different authors that rodents submitted to HF diet is a well-established animal model to study metabolic disorders since it induces metabolic features that resemble T2D in humans. Moreover, it was also described that HF diet leads to alterations in functional and structural brain plasticity, a characteristic similar to other models of insulin resistance [126]. Insulin signaling impairment promoted by a HF diet leads to the decreased expression of a post-synaptic protein, PSD-95, which has a role in promoting maturation and regulation of synaptic strength and plasticity [127]. Moreover, studies performed in Zucker rats, which are known to be insulin resistant, also showed altered hippocampal insulin signaling that was negatively associated with synaptic activity, since those animals presented impairment of LTP at CA3-CA1 synapses [128].

Several studies explored the relationship between obesity and/or T2D and neurodegenerative disorders such as PD and AD, since it was already established that people who develop T2D at an early age have an increased risk to develop neurodegenerative disorders (Figure 3) [6,122,129–131].

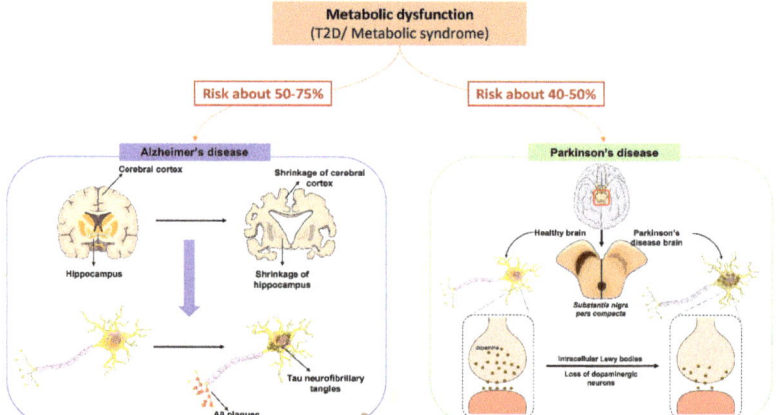

**Figure 3.** Metabolic syndrome increases the risk of developing Alzheimer's and Parkinson's diseases. **Left** and **right** panels show, respectively, the pathophysiology of Alzheimer's (AD) and Parkinson's (PD) diseases. The **left** panel, in violet, shows the physiological structure of a healthy brain and an Alzheimer's disease brain, presenting extracellular accumulation of Aβ plaques and intraneuronal accumulation of neurofibrillary tangles of hyperphosphorylated tau protein. The **right** panel, in green, shows the physiological structure of a healthy substantia nigra versus a substantia nigra of PD patient. In PD there is the aggregation and accumulation of aSyn in Lewy bodies which are toxic leading to dopaminergic neuronal loss.

Neurodegeneration is the progressive loss of structure or function of neurons, which may ultimately involve cell death and is considered an age-related process. Neurogenerative diseases are often associated with the misfolding and aggregation of given proteins. AD is the most common neurodegenerative disease, and its pathological hallmark is the extra-neuronal accumulation of beta-amyloid (Aβ) plaques and intra-neuronal hyperphosphorylation of tau protein and formation of tau neurofibrillary tangles [132,133]. Synucleinopathies comprise a wide group of neurodegenerative disorders with a broader spectrum of clinical presentations, which includes PD, dementia with Lewy bodies, multiple system atrophy, and pure autonomic failure. These disorders are believed to result from the pathological accumulation of neuronal or glial insoluble aggregates of alpha-synuclein (aSyn) [134–139]. Although several genetic mutations and polymorphisms are described to be associated with familiar forms of neurodegenerative diseases, the etiology of these diseases remain largely elusive and molecular mechanisms poorly characterized.

In human studies, AD, cognitive impairment, and other forms of dementia have also been linked to a HF diet, obesity, DM, and metabolic syndrome [7,140–143]. Prospective studies have shown that a diet enriched in saturated fats and refined carbohydrates prime middle-aged and elderly adults to an increased risk for neurological disorders such as AD and to a faster rate of normal age-related cognitive decline [141,144,145]. Additionally, intake of this type of diet in adolescents negatively correlates with visual-spatial learning and memory performance later on and with school performance problems, especially with self-reported difficulties in mathematics [146,147]. Moreover, in children, body mass index negatively correlates with visual-spatial intelligence [148]. Even more, healthy adults exposed to a high saturated fat diet for one week had worse performance on tasks measuring attention and speed of retrieval than they had prior to the diet [149,150]. Epidemiologic reports demonstrate not only an association between obesity caused by dietary fat intake and an increased risk for AD, but also that patients with DM have a 50 to 75% increased risk of developing AD compared to age and gender matched control groups (Figure 4) [151–154]. Furthermore, T2D or impaired fasting blood glucose are reported in 80% of AD patients [155]. Accumulating data suggests that AD is closely related to insulin resistance and the dysfunction of both insulin signaling and glucose metabolism in the brain. The evidence of systemic insulin resistance and defective insulin signaling in the brain being common features of AD transformed T2D as an important risk factor for this neurological disorder. In fact, evidence suggests that insulin resistance and T2D aggravate AD pathology and cognitive deficits [156–159]. Moreover, post-mortem studies have demonstrated central insulin signaling dysregulation in hippocampal and cortical samples from patients with both mild cognitive impairment and early AD [160,161].

The hippocampus and cerebral cortex are the brain regions most vulnerable to aggregation and accumulation of Aβ and Tau, pathological hallmarks of AD. These brain regions express high levels of IRs; however, under AD conditions it has been reported that the levels of insulin mRNA are decreased [162]. In fact, impaired insulin signaling leads to decreased PI3K/AKT signaling, leading to the overactivation of GSK-3β [163]. Consequently, the over-activation of GSK-3β results in the hyperphosphorylation of tau and to a higher production of Aβ peptides, contributing to cognitive impairment (Figure 4) [163–165]. Additionally, insulin deficiency leads to a decrease in GLUTs levels, leading to an impairment in glucose uptake/metabolism in the brain [22]. Decreased intraneuronal glucose uptake causes a reduction of intraneuronal generation of ATP, impairing synaptic activity and cognitive function. It also leads to a decrease in the levels of uridine diphosphate (UDP)- β-N-acetylglucosamine (GlcNAc) via the hexosamine biosynthetic pathway and, consequently, decreasing tau O-GlcNAcylation, a process that inversely regulates tau phosphorylation. An increase of tau phosphorylation induces the formation of tau oligomers, which are neurotoxic, contributing to neuronal loss and degeneration [166].

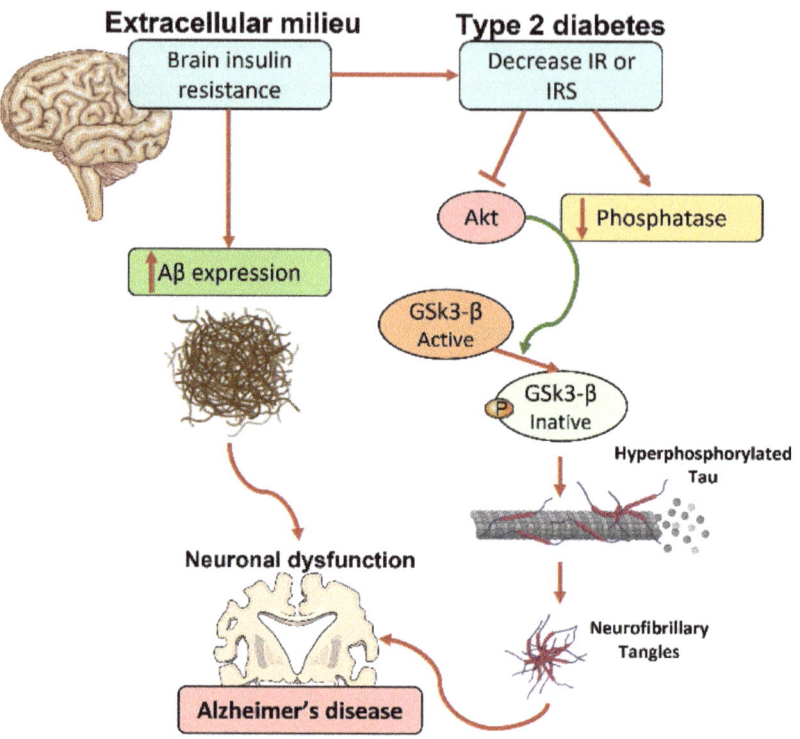

**Figure 4.** Type 2 diabetes accelerates Alzheimer's disease pathology. Brain insulin resistance leads to alterations in the insulin signaling pathway that inactivate AKT triggering the inactivation of GSK3-β leading to tau hyperphosphorylation and higher production of Aβ peptides. AKT, Protein kinase B; GSK-3β, Glycogen synthase kinase 3 beta; IR, insulin receptor; IRS, insulin receptor substrate.

The unequivocal link between AD and T2D prompted the concept of type 3 diabetes or insulin-resistant brain state to refer to AD [142]. Importantly, epidemiologic studies point long-term hyperinsulinemia as a risk factor for dementia, while insulin administration to AD patients improves memory formation, by keeping glucose levels in the brain constant [167].

The risk for PD has been shown to increase in metabolic syndrome, with T2D and obesity being important risk factors for PD [130,168–171]. Epidemiological studies revealed that 80% of PD patients have impaired glucose metabolism. Moreover, T2D can increase the risk of developing PD up to 50% in the general population and significantly accelerates the progression of both motor and cognitive deficits [9,131,172]. Impressively, this risk increases up to 380% for young diabetic individuals [130,131]. Predictably, obesity also affects motor control capabilities, degrading daily functions and health [171]. Children who are obese or overweight are poorer in gross and fine motor control and have delayed motor development [173–179]. PD is characterized by motor and non-motor symptoms, being a disease deeply associated with aSyn aggregation, accumulation and toxicity, and dopaminergic neuronal loss in the substantia nigra pars compacta [180].

Following the strong evidence of a link between metabolic syndrome and neurodegenerative diseases dissected in clinical and epidemiological studies, animal models of human diseases have been largely used to scrutinize the molecular mechanisms and pathways underling this association. An extensive description of these studies will be provided below.

*5.1. The Impact of Diet in Neurodegeneration: Evidence from Animal Models*

Evidence provided by exhaustive research using animal models strongly suggests that diet plays a crucial role in brain physiology and pathology. Currently, the research field is based on both pharmacological and genetic model of AD and PD, both in rats and mice, that have been crucial to disclose molecular mechanisms and dysregulated pathways associated to these neurodegenerative disorders. In the case of metabolic syndrome, as previously described, researchers can also count with diet-induced and genetic models of the disease.

5.1.1. Parkinson's Disease Animal Models

The most accepted and used pharmacological models of PD use 6-hydroxydopamine (6-OHDA) or 1-methyl-4-phenyl-1,2,3,6-tetrahydropyridine (MPTP) to induce dopaminergic degeneration and to induce parkinsonism. Most of the work that aimed to study the impact of diet on neurodegenerative diseases has been performed by submitting these PD models to hypercaloric diets. As it can be seen in Table 1, several studies pointed towards an exacerbation of neurotoxic/neurodegenerative mechanism in the presence of hypercaloric diets, and in particular HF diet.

In pharmacological PD-like models, several studies reported that the HF diet potentiated the decrease of tyrosine hydroxylase (TH) and dopamine depletion in the substantia nigra and/or striatum, suggesting that both MPTP and 6-OHDA exacerbate dopaminergic neurodegeneration. Furthermore, a few studies correlated these alterations with motor abnormalities [181–185]. In transgenic models of PD, the same trend for the impact of HF diet in neurodegeneration features was observed (Table 1). In the transgenic mouse models, HF diet accelerated the onset of aSyn pathology, locomotor impairment, and enhanced dopaminergic degeneration [186,187].

In recent years, more physiological studies, based on challenging the animal models to hypercaloric diets, have been the gold standard in the field. Although beyond insulin resistance, DM, and obesity phenotypes, several studies have been reporting the effects of non-standard diets on brain function and physiology, on motor performance and cognition, and on neurodegenerative-associated processes. In more physiological models using wild type (WT) rats and mice, HF diets reduced the levels of TH in the substantia nigra and striatum and attenuated dopamine release and clearance, accompanied by a decrease in movement together with abnormal motor behavior and other behavior alterations [180,188–190]. In a study where no alterations were observed in the levels of aSyn, the authors claimed that the reduction of TH levels in the nigrostriatal axis occurs through an aSyn-independent pathway and can be attributed to brain inflammation, oxidative stress and metabolic syndrome induced by obesity [180].

However, even if these few studies point towards a link between hypercaloric diets-associated defects in insulin signaling and brain glucose metabolism and the neuropathological features related with PD, the mechanisms by which the hypercaloric diets impact in these neuropathological features deserves further investigation. Also, we would like to highlight, that contrary to what happens for other neurodegenerative diseases as dementia and AD, there are not so many studies evaluating the impact of hypercaloric diets per se and dysmetabolism on the neuronal function and degeneration leading to motor alteration conducting to PD, as well as the impact of different diet composition on these neuropathological features.

**Table 1.** Effects of hypercaloric diets on Parkinson's disease-like and wild-type rodent models.

| Study | Diet Regiment | Rodent Model | Outcomes |
|---|---|---|---|
| Choi et al. [181] | 8 weeks of HF diet | MPTP-lesioned PD-like mice | Severe decrease in the levels of striatal dopamine and of nigral microtubule-associated protein 2, manganese superoxide dismutase, TH. Elevated striatal nNOS phosphorylation and dopamine turnover. |
| Bousquet et al. [182] | 8 weeks of HF diet | MPTP-lesioned PD-like mice | Decreased levels of striatal TH and dopamine, exacerbated MPTP-induced dopaminergic degeneration. |
| Sharma and Taliyan [183] | 8 weeks of HF diet | 6-OHDA-induced PD-like rats | Decreased levels of striatal dopamine, motor abnormalities, exacerbated 6-OHDA mediated neurotoxicity. |
| Morris et al. [184] | 5 weeks of HF diet | 6-OHDA-induced PD-like rats | Peripheral dysmetabolic features, increased dopamine depletion and oxidative stress in the substantia nigra and the striatum, without locomotor dysfunction. |
| Ma et al. [185] | 3 month of HF diet, followed by 3 months of a low-fat diet | 6-OHDA-induced PD-like rats | Reversed peripheral dysmetabolism and mitochondrial and proteasomal function in the striatum, although without altering nigrostriatal vulnerability. |
| Rotermund et al. [191] | HF diet from 5 weeks old onward throughout their lifespan | Mutant A30P aSyn transgenic mice | Accelerated onset of brainstem aSyn pathology and lethal locomotor features. |
| Hong et al. [192] | 2 weeks of HF diet | MitoPark transgenic mice | Increased *SNCA* expression (coding for aSyn) in the dopaminergic neurons of both the WT and MitoPark mice; enhanced dopaminergic degeneration in the MitoPark mice. |
| Morris et al. 2011 [188] | 12 weeks of HF diet | WT rats | Attenuated dopamine release and clearance and increased iron deposition in the substantia nigra. |
| Jang et al. [189] | 13 weeks of HF diet | WT mice | Decreased in movement accompanied by abnormal motor behavior. Decreased levels of TH in the substantia nigra and striatum. |
| Kao et al. [193] | 5 months of HF diet | WT mice | Dopaminergic neurons degeneration and reduced dopaminergic neuroplasticity in the substantia nigra. |
| Bittencourt et al. [180] | 25 weeks of HF diet | WT rats | Reduced levels of TH through metabolic dysfunction, neuroinflammation and oxidative stress, associated with impaired locomotor activity, and anxiety-related behaviors, without changes in motor coordination or memory. No differences in the levels of aSyn. |

6-OHDA, 6-hydroxydopamine; aSyn, alpha-synuclein; HF, high-fat; MPTP, 1-methyl-4-phenyl-1,2,3,6-tetrahydropyridine; PD, Parkinson's disease; TH, tyrosine hydroxylase; WT, ild type.

### 5.1.2. Alzheimer's Disease Animal Models

As stated before, there is an unequivocal link between AD and T2D/impaired insulin signaling, which prompted the concept of type 3 diabetes to refer to AD. This link comes from the extensive literature reporting the deregulation of insulin signaling in AD animal models and patients. Valuable insights on the role of hypercaloric diets in cognitive function were provided by several studies, associating their intake with pathological markers of AD (see Table 2).

**Table 2.** Effects of hypercaloric diets on Alzheimer's disease-like and wild-type rodent models.

| Study | Diet Regiment | Rodent Model | Outcomes |
|---|---|---|---|
| Velazquez et al. [194] | NC diet | Tg2576 and 3xTg-AD transgenic AD-like mice | Central insulin dysregulation and energy dyshomeostasis, developed before peripheral insulin resistance. |
| Sah et al. [195] | 16 weeks of HF diet | 3xTg-AD transgenic AD-like mice | Enhanced memory impairment, without alteration in the levels of Aβ and phosphorylation of tau in the cortical region. Increased neuronal oxidative stress and apoptosis. |
| Thériault et al. [196] | 4 months of a HF diet | APPswe/PS1 transgenic AD-like mice | Accelerated age-associated cognitive decline without affecting parenchymal Aβ. Loss of synaptic plasticity and exacerbated systemic inflammation and oxidative stress. |
| Valladolid-Acebes et al. [197] | 8 weeks of HF diet | WT mice | Spatial memory impairment and changes in hippocampal morphology, accompanied by an increase of dendritic spine density in CA1 pyramidal neurons that correlated with the upregulation of neural cell adhesion molecule (NCAM) in this area and a desensitization of the Akt pathway coupled to hippocampal leptin receptors. |
| Ledreux et al. [198] | 6 months of HF or high cholesterol diet | WT rats | Memory impairment, neurodegeneration in the hippocampus, increased activation of microglia and abnormal phosphorylation of Tau. |
| Busquets et al. [199] | 15 months of a HF diet | WT mice | Long-term exposure to HF diet favors the appearance of Aβ depositions in the brain, thought increased inflammation leading to a decrease in the neuronal precursor cells, and dysregulation in normal autophagy and apoptosis. |
| Tran and Westbrook [200] | HFHSu and NC diets | WT rats | Impairment in place-recognition memory, that is reversible and training-dependent. |
| Spencer et al. [201] | 3 days of HF diet | WT rats | Impaired long-term contextual (hippocampal-dependent) and auditory-cued fear (amygdalar-dependent) memory in aged, but not young adult rats. Increased activation of microglia. |
| Kothari et al. [202] | 14 weeks of HFHSu diet | WT mice | Induced brain insulin resistance, accompanied by inflammatory and stress responses as well as by increased Aβ deposition and neurofibrillary tangle formation, and decreased synaptic plasticity and cognitive impairment. |
| Fu et al. [203] | 6 months of HF diet | WT rats | Induced hippocampal microvascular insulin resistance and cognitive dysfunction. |
| Fazzari et al. [204] | 12 weeks of HF diet | WT hamsters | Reduced locomotor activities such as exploratory bouts, rearing and grooming behaviors, cognitive and memory impairment. |

AD, Alzheimer's disease; HF, high-fat; HFHSu, High-fat–high-sucrose; NC, normal chow; WT, wild-type.

Velazquez and collaborators reported central insulin dysregulation and energy dyshomeostasis in two transgenic mouse models of AD, the Tg2576 and the triple transgenic AD (3xTg-AD) mice [194]. Moreover, HF diet in transgenic AD-like mice enhanced memory impairment and cognitive decline without affecting the levels of Aβ and phospho-tau protein. The exacerbated phenotype seems to be mediated by increased inflammation and oxidative stress [195,196]. Moreover, both HF or HFHSu diets in WT mice and rats are reported to induce significant cognitive alterations, mainly short- and long-term, contextual, and auditory-cued fear memory impairment. These behavioral phenotypes were associated with insulin resistance, increased neuroinflammation, Aβ deposition and neurofibrillary tangle formation, and decreased synaptic plasticity [197–204]. In agreement, Abbott and co-workers conducted a meta-analysis of the results from rodent studies using different diets (HF, HSu, or HFHSu diets) and reported that each type of diet and task adversely affected performance, with the largest effect produced by exposure to a combined HFHSu diet, as assessed by the radial arm maze to evaluate the effect of such diets on cognition [205].

Altogether, hypercaloric diets prompt to neurogenerative processes that are in the basis of cognitive dysfunction and that different diet composition conduce to different pathological mechanisms originating different neuropathological features. Moreover, several mechanisms contribute to these neurogenerative processes, namely insulin signaling dysregulation, altered brain glucose homeostasis, neuroinflammation, and oxidative stress, among others. Therefore, strategies aiming to prevent and regulate the hypercaloric diets—associated pathological mechanisms, namely the control of dysmetabolic states might be extremely useful for the prevention and delay of neurodegenerative processes.

## 5.2. Sex Differences in the Link Dysmetabolism-Neurodegeneration

Gender or sex is a significant variable in the prevalence and incidence of neurodegenerative disorders, such as AD and PD. In fact, sex dimorphisms have a cardinal role in the pathogenesis, progression, age of onset, and treatment response in AD and PD. The prevalence of AD has been reported to be higher in women than in men (1.6–3:1 female/male ratio) [206–213]. Several studies showed that the extent of cognitive deficits is higher in AD females, with enhanced clinical expression of disease pathology due to more neurofibrillary tangles [214]. In contrast, the prevalence of PD is reported to be higher in men than women (1:1.5–3 female/male ratio) [215–218]. Studies reveled that PD symptoms like rigidity, rapid eye movement behavior disorder, sleep disturbances, deficits in verbal communication, and lack of facial emotions are more prevalent in males. On the other hand, the onset of PD is delayed in females, that exhibit a tremor-dominant form of the disease with greater impairment of postural stability, depression, and reduced ability to conduct daily activities, and in which reduction in visuospatial cognition is more frequent [214].

Although the biological factors and molecular mechanisms underlying these gender disparities are still poorly understood, sex steroid hormones, including estrogens, progestogens, and androgens, have been implicated in these sexual dimorphisms. Notably, sexual steroid hormones are known to regulate energy metabolism [219–223] and exert neuroprotective effects on the adult brain, increasing neural function and resilience and promoting neuronal survival [224–227]. The aging process is characterized by a shift in the hormonal profile both in men and women, with an abrupt loss of estrogens during menopause in women and a gradual but significant decline of testosterone during andropause in men [219,224]. Despite the brain levels of steroid hormones depend on both endocrine gland production and on the local synthesis of neurosteroids, the brain also accounts with a decline in the levels of sex steroids [228]. Thus, reproductive senescence has been implicated in metabolic alterations and negatively impacts neural function and represents a significant age-associated risk factor for AD and PD.

## 6. Regulation of Metabolic Function as a Prevention of Neurodegeneration

The existing therapies for neurodegenerative disorders are not disease-modifying. For the case of PD, they are only able to alleviate the symptoms. They are mostly dopamine-replacing therapies (levodopa-carbidopa, dopamine agonists), able to improve PD-motor features in the initial stages of the disease. Tackling non-motor features require non-dopaminergic approaches as for example, the selective serotonin reuptake inhibitors [229]. For the case of AD, current treatments also aim to attenuate symptoms (e.g., NMDA receptor antagonists and drugs that target cholinergic transmission) such as cognitive impairment, aggression, and seizures, and do not target disease pathology [230].

Considering the increased risk for neurodegenerative diseases among patients with T2D and the remarkable pathophysiological mechanisms shared, there is mounting interest in the potential of antidiabetic agents for the treatment of these neurological disorders. Hundreds of pre-clinical and clinical studies have explored the potential of antidiabetic medications both for lowering the risk of and as a novel therapeutic avenue for neurodegenerative diseases such as PD and AD.

In recent years, several anti-diabetic drugs have been investigated in PD and AD patients, including metformin, glucagon like peptide (GLP-1) analogues, dipeptidyl peptidase 4 (DPP-4) inhibitors or gliptins, among others. For example, a study performed in a Taiwanese cohort evaluated the usage of metformin, known to reduce blood glucose levels and to decrease insulin resistance, in PD patients and reported that the combination of metformin with sulfonylurea therapy was able to reduce the risk for PD [231,232]. Indeed, findings from human studies are recapitulated in animal models. Metformin administered to MPTP-induced PD mice was shown to improve locomotor activity in these animals [233]. Metformin was also demonstrated to be able to cross the BBB and to act as a neuroprotective agent by reducing tau phosphorylation in primary cortical neurons of a transgenic mouse with the lack of microtubule-associated protein tau (MAPT), a known mechanism of AD development [234]. Moreover, metformin is also reported to have anti-inflammatory properties, to lower reactive oxygen species (ROS) production, and to act as methylglyoxal scavenger and an advanced glycation end products (AGEs) inhibitor [235–239]. Metformin was shown to prevent amyloid plaque deposition and memory impairment in APP/PS1 mice, to restore neuronal insulin signaling and prevent AD-associated pathological changes in neuronal cultures and to protect against Aβ-induced mitochondrial dysfunction [240–242]. Metformin prevents aSyn accumulation, aggregation, and phosphorylation, and prevents or attenuates dopaminergic neurodegeneration, ameliorates pathology, and improves locomotor activity and coordination in acute MPTP- and 6-hydroxydopamine (6-OHDA)-induced Parkinsonism rodent models [233,243–247]. Additionally, a Singapore longitudinal aging study showed that long-term treatment with metformin is associated with reduced risks of cognitive decline in T2D patients. [248]. Controversially, studies conducted by Imfeld and Moore reported a slightly higher risk of AD and cognitive impairment in patients with T2D under metformin therapy [249,250]. Furthermore, Kuan, Ping, and Qin showed overall lack of correlation between metformin therapy and the prevention of PD and reported that long-term metformin exposure in patients with T2D may increase the risk for PD and dementia [251–253]. These conflicting results may derive from the high heterogeneity among clinical studies in terms of population, treatment plan, and follow-up. Furthermore, the effect of metformin likely depends on complex neurodegeneration-associated pathological processes and may not be beneficial for all patients with PD or AD, rather than for patients with evidence of metabolic disease.

Thiazolidinediones (TZDs) are insulin sensitizers that primarily reduce insulin resistance in insulin-sensitive tissues in the periphery. Promising results from preclinical studies reported that pioglitazone and rosiglitazone are able to ameliorate memory and cognitive impairment and decrease AD-related pathology in several rodent models of AD, including the 3xTg-AD mice and Tg2576 mice, by enhancing AKT signaling and attenuating tau hyperphosphorylation, neuroinflammation, and AD pathology [254–257]. Furthermore, pioglitazone, rosiglitazone and mitoglitazone were also shown to prevent dopaminergic neurodegeneration and locomotor deficits in MPTP-, STZ-, and 6-OHDA-lesioned rodent models of PD, by modulating the neuroinflammatory response in a neuroprotective fashion [258–264]. These findings are consistent with data from clinical studies. TZDs lead to an improvement in memory and selective attention in patients with AD and amnestic mild cognitive impairment [265–267].

Another class of antidiabetic drugs used to manage the neurodegenerative process are the sulfonylureas, which act to increase insulin release from the beta cells in the pancreas. In fact, several studies support the idea that sulfonylureas could be used as therapeutics to AD and PD. For example, the use of glimepiride was shown to protect against Aβ induced synaptic damage in neuronal cultures [268]. Also, T2D patients treated with sulfonylureas exhibit low risk of dementia, and a combination of metformin with sulfonylureas decreased the risk by 35% over 8 years [269].

Sodium-glucose cotransporter 2 (SGLT2) inhibitors, the newest class of anti-diabetic drugs used in T2D treatment, act via the inhibition of renal glucose reabsorption therefore promoting glucose excursion [270]. SGLT2 inhibitors have neuroprotective actions in T2D mouse models, particularly by reducing inflammation and oxidative stress [271–273]. In agreement, empagliflozin reduced cerebral oxidative stress and impairment of cognitive function in db/db animals [271]. Moreover, dapagliflozin improved cognitive decline in HF diet animals [273].

Another class of anti-diabetics are the modulators of incretins, that include GLP-1 receptor agonists and DPP-4 inhibitors (vildagliptin or sitagliptin) used for T2D and obesity (in the case of GLP-1 agonists). Dulaglutide, a GLP-1 receptor agonist, ameliorated STZ-induced AD-like impairment of learning and memory ability by modulating hyperphosphorylation of tau and neurofilaments [274]. Liraglutide, also a GLP-1 receptor agonist, prevented the accumulation of Aβ plaques, decreased tau hyperphosphorylation and neurofilament proteins, prevented the loss of brain IR and synapses, and reversed cognitive and memory impairment in several mouse models of AD-like pathology and in a non-human primate model of AD [275–277]. In relation to PD, a huge amount of evidence supported the repurpose of the use of GLP-1 agonists for the treatment of this pathology [278,279]. Exenatide and Ex4 both in animal models and humans was shown to promote neuroprotection (for a review see [278,279]). For example, these drugs in human trials led to an improvement of motor symptoms, to benefits in cognitive performance, as well as to better results in tremor-dominant phenotype [280–283]. Liraglutide and lixisenatide ameliorated locomotor function and prevented dopaminergic neurons degeneration, by suppressing neuroinflammation in the substantia nigra in the MPTP-induced PD-like mice and rotenone-lesioned PD-like rats [284–286]. Also, semaglutide in chronic MPTP mouse model of PD showed to promote neuroprotection by decreasing aSyn levels and neuroinflammation with consequent improvement in motor function [287,288].

Sitagliptin, saxagliptin and vildagliptin, DPP-4 inhibitors, improves learning and memory deficits through decreasing abnormal phosphorylation of tau and neurofilaments (NFs), reducing intercellular Aβ accumulation in 3xTg-AD and STZ-lesioned mice [289–291]. Sitagliptin reversed nigrostriatal degeneration, improved motor performance, and rescued the memory deficits in rotenone-lesioned PD-like rats [286,292]. The use of DPP4 inhibitors and GLP-1 mimetics is associated with a lower risk for PD and AD among patients with T2D, even compared to the use of other oral antidiabetic drugs [293,294]. All together, these clearly state that the decrease in insulin resistance and the regulation of whole-body glucose homeostasis, and therefore a better metabolic control, is associated with better cognitive function and slower deterioration of brain capacities related to the neurodegenerative process.

Another way to improve metabolic control is by targeting the carotid bodies (CBs), metabolic sensors deeply involved in peripheral insulin action and glucose homeostasis [295–297]. The CBs are peripheral chemoreceptors located near the bifurcation of the common carotid artery, classically defined as oxygen, carbon dioxide, and pH sensors [298,299]. They are surrounded by a dense net of capillaries and penetrated by the sensory nerve ending of the carotid sinus nerve (CSN) a tiny branch of the glossopharyngeal nerve which does the connection from the CBs to the brainstem where their information is integrated [298,300]. In recent years, the CBs have been shown to have a key role in the control of peripheral glucose metabolism and insulin action, since it was shown that: (1) in animal models of dysmetabolism and in prediabetic patients, the CBs were overactivated, this being correlated with a state of insulin resistance and glucose intolerance [295,301,302]; (2) insulin, leptin, and GLP-1, known metabolic mediators involved in metabolic regulation, are capable of activating the CBs [295,296,303,304]; and (3) the resection or neuromodulation of the CSN prevents and reverses the pathological features associated with dysmetabolic states [295,297,301]. Considering the close association between metabolic and neurodegenerative disorders, and that the therapeutics that provide metabolic control have a huge impact on neurodegenerative processes, we anticipate that the modulation of the CBs might be a useful therapeutic strategy to improve metabolism, and therefore prevent and/or delay the progression of neurodegenerative disorders.

## 7. Conclusions

The association between dysmetabolic pathologies, like T2D or obesity, and neurodegenerative disorders is unequivocal. We have compiled the most important literature discussing the pathological mechanisms behind this relationship. Altogether it shows that the increasing incidence of both types of diseases is somehow related with worldwide aging and life habits changing, with special attention to overnutrition and low quality of nutrient intake. Insulin also has a clear central role in the relationship between metabolic and neurodegenerative disorders since it joins important peripheral and central actions for glucose homeostasis, cognitive function regulation, and food behavior control. However, it is still unclear which disease is cause or consequence. We reason that it is instead a vicious cycle. The covered literature also opens doors for possible new targets of therapeutic interventions, both by pharmacological (antidiabetic drugs) or non-pharmacologic (CBs modulation) approaches, to control these epidemics of metabolic and neurodegenerative diseases.

**Author Contributions:** A.M.C., A.C. and S.V.C. wrote the manuscript. F.O.M. and H.V.M. made a critical review. All authors have read and agreed to the published version of the manuscript.

**Funding:** AC and FOM were supported by grants and contracts from the Portuguese Foundation for Science and Technology, PD/BD/136863/2018 and CEECIND/04266/2017, respectively.

**Institutional Review Board Statement:** Not applicable.

**Informed Consent Statement:** Not applicable.

**Data Availability Statement:** Not applicable.

**Conflicts of Interest:** The authors declare no conflict of interest.

## References

1. López-Otín, C.; Blasco, M.A.; Partridge, L.; Serrano, M.; Kroemer, G. The hallmarks of aging. *Cell* **2013**, *153*, 1194–1217. [CrossRef] [PubMed]
2. Sepúlveda, J.; Murray, C. The state of global health in 2014. *Science* **2014**, *345*, 1275–1278. [CrossRef] [PubMed]
3. Aguilar, M.; Bhuket, T.; Torres, S.; Liu, B.; Wong, R.J. Prevalence of the Metabolic Syndrome in the United States, 2003–2012. *JAMA* **2015**, *313*, 1973–1974. [CrossRef]
4. Hinnouho, G.-M.; Czernichow, S.; Dugravot, A.; Nabi, H.; Brunner, E.; Kivimaki, M.; Singh-Manoux, A. Metabolically healthy obesity and the risk of cardiovascular disease and type 2 diabetes: The Whitehall II cohort study. *Eur. Heart J.* **2014**, *36*, 551–559. [CrossRef]
5. Kalyani, R.R.; Corriere, M.; Ferrucci, L. Age-related and disease-related muscle loss: The effect of diabetes, obesity, and other diseases. *Lancet Diabetes Endocrinol.* **2014**, *2*, 819–829. [CrossRef]
6. Spinelli, M.; Fusco, S.; Grassi, C. Brain Insulin Resistance and Hippocampal Plasticity: Mechanisms and Biomarkers of Cognitive Decline. *Front. Neurosci.* **2019**, *13*, 788. [CrossRef] [PubMed]
7. Profenno, L.A.; Porsteinsson, A.P.; Faraone, S.V. Meta-analysis of Alzheimer's disease risk with obesity, diabetes, and related disorders. *Biol. Psychiatry* **2010**, *67*, 505–512. [CrossRef]
8. Deng, Y.; Li, B.; Liu, Y.; Iqbal, K.; Grundke-Iqbal, I.; Gong, C.X. Dysregulation of insulin signaling, glucose transporters, O-GlcNAcylation, and phosphorylation of tau and neurofilaments in the brain: Implication for Alzheimer's disease. *Am. J. Pathol.* **2009**, *175*, 2089–2098. [CrossRef]
9. Yue, X.; Li, H.; Yan, H.; Zhang, P.; Chang, L.; Li, T. Risk of Parkinson Disease in Diabetes Mellitus: An Updated Meta-Analysis of Population-Based Cohort Studies. *Medicine* **2016**, *95*, e3549. [CrossRef]
10. Podolsky, S.; Leopold, N.A.; Sax, D.S. Increased frequency of diabetes mellitus in patients with Huntington's chorea. *Lancet* **1972**, *299*, 1356–1358. [CrossRef]
11. Hegele, R.A.; Maltman, G.M. Insulin's centenary: The birth of an idea. *Lancet Diabetes Endocrinol.* **2020**, *8*, 971–977. [CrossRef]
12. Kahn, C.R.; White, M.F. The insulin receptor and the molecular mechanism of insulin action. *J. Clin. Investig.* **1988**, *82*, 1151–1156. [CrossRef] [PubMed]
13. Tokarz, V.L.; MacDonald, P.E.; Klip, A. The cell biology of systemic insulin function. *J. Cell. Biol.* **2018**, *217*, 2273–2289. [CrossRef]
14. Lizcano, J.M.; Alessi, D.R. The insulin signalling pathway. *Curr. Biol.* **2002**, *12*, R236–R238. [CrossRef]
15. Guo, S. Insulin signaling, resistance, and the metabolic syndrome: Insights from mouse models into disease mechanisms. *J. Endocrinol.* **2014**, *220*, T1–T23. [CrossRef] [PubMed]
16. Petersen, M.C.; Shulman, G.I. Mechanisms of Insulin Action and Insulin Resistance. *Physiol. Rev.* **2018**, *98*, 2133–2223. [CrossRef]
17. Saltiel, A.R.; Kahn, C.R. Insulin signalling and the regulation of glucose and lipid metabolism. *Nature* **2001**, *414*, 799–806. [CrossRef]
18. Timper, K.; Brüning, J.C. Hypothalamic circuits regulating appetite and energy homeostasis: Pathways to obesity. *Dis. Model. Mech.* **2017**, *10*, 679–689. [CrossRef]
19. Plum, L.; Schubert, M.; Brüning, J.C. The role of insulin receptor signaling in the brain. *Trends Endocrinol. Metab.* **2005**, *16*, 59–65. [CrossRef]
20. Huang, X.; Liu, G.; Guo, J.; Su, Z. The PI3K/AKT pathway in obesity and type 2 diabetes. *Int. J. Biol. Sci.* **2018**, *14*, 1483–1496. [CrossRef]
21. Hermida, M.A.; Kumar, J.D.; Leslie, N.R. GSK3 and its interactions with the PI3K/AKT/mTOR signalling network. *Adv. Biol. Regul.* **2017**, *65*, 5–15. [CrossRef] [PubMed]
22. Koepsell, H. Glucose transporters in brain in health and disease. *Pflügers Arch. Eur. J. Physiol.* **2020**, *472*, 1299–1343. [CrossRef] [PubMed]
23. Wang, Y.; Inoue, H.; Ravnskjaer, K.; Viste, K.; Miller, N.; Liu, Y.; Hedrick, S.; Vera, L.; Montminy, M. Targeted disruption of the CREB coactivator Crtc2 increases insulin sensitivity. *Proc. Natl. Acad. Sci. USA* **2010**, *107*, 3087–3092. [CrossRef]

24. Eldin, W.S.; Emara, M.; Shoker, A. Prediabetes: A must to recognise disease state. *Int. J. Clin. Pract.* **2008**, *62*, 642–648. [CrossRef] [PubMed]
25. Saeedi, P.; Petersohn, I.; Salpea, P.; Malanda, B.; Karuranga, S.; Unwin, N.; Colagiuri, S.; Guariguata, L.; Motala, A.A.; Ogurtsova, K.; et al. Global and regional diabetes prevalence estimates for 2019 and projections for 2030 and 2045: Results from the International Diabetes Federation Diabetes Atlas. *Diabetes Res. Clin. Pract.* **2019**, *157*, 107843. [CrossRef] [PubMed]
26. IDFD Atlas. *IDF Diabetes Atlas*, 9th ed.; International Diabetes Federation: Brussels, Belgium, 2019.
27. Kahn, S.E.; Cooper, M.E.; Del Prato, S. Pathophysiology and treatment of type 2 diabetes: Perspectives on the past, present, and future. *Lancet* **2014**, *383*, 1068–1083. [CrossRef]
28. Schwartz, S.S.; Epstein, S.; Corkey, B.E.; Grant, S.F.; Gavin, J.R.; Aguilar, R.B. The Time Is Right for a New Classification System for Diabetes: Rationale and Implications of the β-Cell–Centric Classification Schema. *Diabetes Care* **2016**, *39*, 179–186. [CrossRef]
29. Tuomi, T.; Santoro, N.; Caprio, S.; Cai, M.; Weng, J.; Groop, L. The many faces of diabetes: A disease with increasing heterogeneity. *Lancet* **2013**, *383*, 1084–1094. [CrossRef]
30. Skyler, J.S.; Bakris, G.L.; Bonifacio, E.; Darsow, T.; Eckel, R.H.; Groop, L.; Groop, P.-H.; Handelsman, Y.; Insel, R.A.; Mathieu, C.; et al. Differentiation of Diabetes by Pathophysiology, Natural History, and Prognosis. *Diabetes* **2016**, *66*, 241–255. [CrossRef]
31. World Health Organization. *Classification of Diabetes Mellitus*; World Health Organization: Geneva, Switzerland, 2019.
32. Lovejoy, J.C. The influence of dietary fat on insulin resistance. *Curr. Diabetes Rep.* **2002**, *2*, 435–440. [CrossRef]
33. Sears, B.; Perry, M. The role of fatty acids in insulin resistance. *Lipids Health Dis.* **2015**, *14*, 121. [CrossRef] [PubMed]
34. Gregor, M.F.; Hotamisligil, G.S. Inflammatory Mechanisms in Obesity. *Annu. Rev. Immunol.* **2011**, *29*, 415–445. [CrossRef] [PubMed]
35. Westwater, M.L.; Fletcher, P.C.; Ziauddeen, H. Sugar addiction: The state of the science. *Eur. J. Nutr.* **2016**, *55* (Suppl. S2), 55–69. [CrossRef] [PubMed]
36. Melo, B.; Sacramento, J.F.; Ribeiro, M.J.; Prego, C.S.; Correia, M.C.; Coelho, J.C.; Cunha-Guimaraes, J.P.; Rodrigues, T.; Martins, I.B.; Guarino, M.P.; et al. Evaluating the Impact of Different Hypercaloric Diets on Weight Gain, Insulin Resistance, Glucose Intolerance, and its Comorbidities in Rats. *Nutrients* **2019**, *11*, 1197. [CrossRef]
37. Takahashi, Y.; Soejima, Y.; Fukusato, T. Animal models of nonalcoholic fatty liver disease/nonalcoholic steatohepatitis. *World J. Gastroenterol.* **2012**, *18*, 2300–2308. [CrossRef]
38. Ishimoto, T.; Lanaspa, M.A.; Rivard, C.J.; Roncal-Jimenez, C.A.; Orlicky, D.J.; Cicerchi, C.; McMahan, R.H.; Abdelmalek, M.F.; Rosen, H.R.; Jackman, M.R.; et al. High-fat and high-sucrose (western) diet induces steatohepatitis that is dependent on fructokinase. *Hepatology* **2013**, *58*, 1632–1643. [CrossRef]
39. Lionetti, L.; Mollica, M.P.; Lombardi, A.; Cavaliere, G.; Gifuni, G.; Barletta, A. From chronic overnutrition to insulin resistance: The role of fat-storing capacity and inflammation. *Nutr. Metab. Cardiovasc. Dis.* **2009**, *19*, 146–152. [CrossRef]
40. Hotamisligil, G.S. Inflammation and metabolic disorders. *Nature* **2006**, *444*, 860–867. [CrossRef]
41. He, Q.; Gao, Z.; Yin, J.; Zhang, J.; Yun, Z.; Ye, J. Regulation of HIF-1(alpha) activity in adipose tissue by obesity-associated factors: Adipogenesis, insulin, and hypoxia. *Am. J. Physiol. Endocrinol. Metab.* **2011**, *300*, E877–E885. [CrossRef]
42. Jaworski, K.; Sarkadi-Nagy, E.; Duncan, R.E.; Ahmadian, M.; Sul, H.S. Regulation of Triglyceride Metabolism. IV. Hormonal regulation of lipolysis in adipose tissue. *Am. J. Physiol. Liver Physiol.* **2007**, *293*, G1–G4.
43. Hotamisligil, G.S.; Murray, D.L.; Choy, L.N.; Spiegelman, B.M. Tumor necrosis factor alpha inhibits signaling from the insulin receptor. *Proc. Natl. Acad. Sci. USA* **1994**, *91*, 4854–4858. [CrossRef] [PubMed]
44. Zhang, H.H.; Halbleib, M.; Ahmad, F.; Manganiello, V.C.; Greenberg, A.S. Tumor necrosis factor-alpha stimulates lipolysis in differentiated human adipocytes through activation of extracellular signal-related kinase and elevation of intracellular cAMP. *Diabetes* **2002**, *51*, 2929–2935. [CrossRef] [PubMed]
45. Samuel, V.T.; Shulman, G.I. Mechanisms for insulin resistance: Common threads and missing links. *Cell* **2012**, *148*, 852–871. [CrossRef] [PubMed]
46. Freeman, C.R.; Zehra, A.; Ramirez, V.; Wiers, C.E.; Volkow, N.D.; Wang, G.J. Impact of sugar on the body, brain, and behavior. *Front. Biosci.* **2018**, *23*, 2255–2266.
47. Greenberg, D.; St Peter, J.V. Sugars and Sweet Taste: Addictive or Rewarding? *Int. J. Environ. Res. Public Health* **2021**, *18*, 9791. [CrossRef]
48. Alam, Y.H.; Kim, R.; Jang, C. Metabolism and Health Impacts of Dietary Sugars. *J. Lipid Atheroscler.* **2022**, *11*, 20–38. [CrossRef]
49. Jalal, D.I.; Smits, G.; Johnson, R.J.; Chonchol, M. Increased Fructose Associates with Elevated Blood Pressure. *J. Am. Soc. Nephrol.* **2010**, *21*, 1543–1549. [CrossRef]
50. DiNicolantonio, J.J.; O'Keefe, J.H.; Lucan, S.C. Added fructose: A principal driver of type 2 diabetes mellitus and its consequences. *Mayo Clin. Proc.* **2015**, *90*, 372–381. [CrossRef]
51. Malik, V.S.; Hu, F.B. Fructose and Cardiometabolic Health: What the Evidence From Sugar-Sweetened Beverages Tells Us. *J. Am. Coll. Cardiol.* **2015**, *66*, 1615–1624. [CrossRef]
52. Madero, M.; Arriaga, J.C.; Jalal, D.; Rivard, C.; McFann, K.; Pérez-Méndez, O.; Vázquez, A.; Ruiz, A.; Lanaspa, M.A.; Jimenez, C.R.; et al. The effect of two energy-restricted diets, a low-fructose diet versus a moderate natural fructose diet, on weight loss and metabolic syndrome parameters: A randomized controlled trial. *Metabolism* **2011**, *60*, 1551–1559. [CrossRef]
53. Aragno, M.; Mastrocola, R. Dietary Sugars and Endogenous Formation of Advanced Glycation Endproducts: Emerging Mechanisms of Disease. *Nutrients* **2017**, *9*, 385. [CrossRef] [PubMed]

54. Schwarz, J.M.; Noworolski, S.M.; Erkin-Cakmak, A.; Korn, N.J.; Wen, M.J.; Tai, V.W.; Jones, G.M.; Palii, S.P.; Velasco-Alin, M.; Pan, K.; et al. Effects of Dietary Fructose Restriction on Liver Fat, De Novo Lipogenesis, and Insulin Kinetics in Children with Obesity. *Gastroenterology* **2017**, *153*, 743–752. [CrossRef] [PubMed]
55. Lustig, R.H.; Mulligan, K.; Noworolski, S.M.; Tai, V.W.; Wen, M.J.; Erkin-Cakmak, A.; Gugliucci, A.; Schwarz, J.M. Isocaloric fructose restriction and metabolic improvement in children with obesity and metabolic syndrome. *Obesity* **2016**, *24*, 453–460. [CrossRef] [PubMed]
56. Luo, S.; Monterosso, J.R.; Sarpelleh, K.; Page, K.A. Differential effects of fructose versus glucose on brain and appetitive responses to food cues and decisions for food rewards. *Proc. Natl. Acad. Sci. USA* **2015**, *112*, 6509–6514. [CrossRef]
57. Laughlin, M.R. Normal roles for dietary fructose in carbohydrate metabolism. *Nutrients* **2014**, *6*, 3117–3129. [CrossRef]
58. Rizkalla, S.W. Health implications of fructose consumption: A review of recent data. *Nutr. Metab.* **2010**, *7*, 82. [CrossRef]
59. Blázquez, E.; Velázquez, E.; Hurtado-Carneiro, V.; Ruiz-Albusac, J.M. Insulin in the brain: Its pathophysiological implications for States related with central insulin resistance, type 2 diabetes and Alzheimer's disease. *Front. Endocrinol.* **2014**, *5*, 161. [CrossRef]
60. Benito, M. Tissue specificity on insulin action and resistance: Past to recent mechanisms. *Acta Physiol.* **2011**, *201*, 297–312. [CrossRef]
61. Daneman, R.; Prat, A. The blood-brain barrier. *Cold Spring Harb. Perspect. Biol.* **2015**, *7*, a020412. [CrossRef]
62. Banks, W.A. The source of cerebral insulin. *Eur. J. Pharmacol.* **2004**, *490*, 5–12. [CrossRef]
63. Wallum, B.J.; Taborsky, G.J.; Porte, D.; Figlewicz, D.P.; Jacobson, L.; Beard, J.C.; Ward, W.K.; Dorsa, D. Cerebrospinal Fluid Insulin Levels Increase During Intravenous Insulin Infusions in Man. *J. Clin. Endocrinol. Metab.* **1987**, *64*, 190–194. [CrossRef]
64. Bromander, S.; Anckarsäter, R.; Ahren, B.; Kristiansson, M.; Blennow, K.; Holmäng, A.; Zetterberg, H.; Anckarsäter, H.; Wass, C.E. Cerebrospinal fluid insulin during non-neurological surgery. *J. Neural Transm.* **2010**, *117*, 1167–1170. [CrossRef] [PubMed]
65. Schwartz, M.W.; Figlewicz, D.P.; Baskin, D.G.; Woods, S.C.; Porte, D. Insulin in the brain: A hormonal regulator of energy balance. *Endocr. Rev.* **1992**, *13*, 387–414.
66. Coker, G.T.; Studelska, D.; Harmon, S.; Burke, W.; O'Malley, K.L. Analysis of tyrosine hydroxylase and insulin transcripts in human neuroendocrine tissues. *Mol. Brain Res.* **1990**, *8*, 93–98. [CrossRef]
67. Pitt, J.; Wilcox, K.C.; Tortelli, V.; Diniz, L.P.; Oliveira, M.S.; Dobbins, C.; Yu, X.W.; Nandamuri, S.; Gomes, F.C.A.; DiNunno, N.; et al. Neuroprotective astrocyte-derived insulin/insulin-like growth factor 1 stimulates endocytic processing and extracellular release of neuron-bound Aβ oligomers. *Mol. Biol. Cell* **2017**, *28*, 2623–2636. [CrossRef] [PubMed]
68. Kuwabara, T.; Kagalwala, M.N.; Onuma, Y.; Ito, Y.; Warashina, M.; Terashima, K.; Sanosaka, T.; Nakashima, K.; Gage, F.H.; Asashima, M. Insulin biosynthesis in neuronal progenitors derived from adult hippocampus and the olfactory bulb. *EMBO Mol. Med.* **2011**, *3*, 742–754. [CrossRef] [PubMed]
69. Takano, K.; Koarashi, K.; Kawabe, K.; Itakura, M.; Nakajima, H.; Moriyama, M.; Nakamura, Y. Insulin expression in cultured astrocytes and the decrease by amyloid β. *Neurochem. Int.* **2018**, *119*, 171–177. [CrossRef]
70. Dakic, T.B.; Jevdjovic, T.; Peric, M.I.; Bjelobaba, I.; Markelić, M.; Milutinovic, B.S.; Lakic, I.V.; Jasnic, N.; Djordjevic, J.D.; Vujovic, P.Z. Short-term fasting promotes insulin expression in rat hypothalamus. *Eur. J. Neurosci.* **2017**, *46*, 1730–1737. [CrossRef]
71. Molnár, G.; Faragó, N.; Kocsis, K.; Rózsa, M.; Lovas, S.; Boldog, E.; Báldi, R.; Csajbók, É.; Gardi, J.; Puskás, L.G.; et al. GABAergic Neurogliaform Cells Represent Local Sources of Insulin in the Cerebral Cortex. *J. Neurosci.* **2014**, *34*, 1133–1137. [CrossRef]
72. Rhea, E.M.; Rask-Madsen, C.; Banks, W.A. Insulin transport across the blood-brain barrier can occur independently of the insulin receptor. *J. Physiol.* **2018**, *596*, 4753–4765. [CrossRef]
73. Pomytkin, I.; Costa-Nunes, J.P.; Kasatkin, V.; Veniaminova, E.; Demchenko, A.; Lyundup, A.; Lesch, K.-P.; Ponomarev, E.D.; Strekalova, T. Insulin receptor in the brain: Mechanisms of activation and the role in the CNS pathology and treatment. *CNS Neurosci. Ther.* **2018**, *24*, 763–774. [CrossRef]
74. Sciacca, L.; Cassarino, M.F.; Genua, M.; Vigneri, P.; Pennisi, M.G.; Malandrino, P.; Squatrito, S.; Pezzino, V.; Vigneri, R. Biological Effects of Insulin and Its Analogs on Cancer Cells with Different Insulin Family Receptor Expression. *J. Cell. Physiol.* **2014**, *229*, 1817–1821. [CrossRef] [PubMed]
75. Sciacca, L.; Cassarino, M.F.; Genua, M.; Pandini, G.; Le Moli, R.; Squatrito, S.; Vigneri, R. Insulin analogues differently activate insulin receptor isoforms and post-receptor signalling. *Diabetologia* **2010**, *53*, 1743–1753. [CrossRef] [PubMed]
76. Pierre-Eugene, C.; Pagesy, P.; Nguyen, T.T.; Neuillé, M.; Tschank, G.; Tennagels, N.; Hampe, C.; Issad, T. Effect of Insulin Analogues on Insulin/IGF1 Hybrid Receptors: Increased Activation by Glargine but Not by Its Metabolites M1 and M2. *PLoS ONE* **2012**, *7*, e41992. [CrossRef]
77. Havrankova, J.; Roth, J.; Brownstein, M. Insulin receptors are widely distributed in the central nervous system of the rat. *Nature* **1978**, *272*, 827–829. [CrossRef] [PubMed]
78. Banks, W.A.; Owen, J.B.; Erickson, M.A. Insulin in the brain: There and back again. *Pharmacol. Ther.* **2012**, *136*, 82–93. [CrossRef] [PubMed]
79. Ashrafi, G.; Wu, Z.; Farrell, R.; Ryan, T.A. GLUT4 Mobilization Supports Energetic Demands of Active Synapses. *Neuron* **2017**, *93*, 606–615.e3. [CrossRef]
80. Uemura, E.; Greenlee, H.W. Insulin regulates neuronal glucose uptake by promoting translocation of glucose transporter GLUT3. *Exp. Neurol.* **2006**, *198*, 48–53. [CrossRef]
81. Heidenreich, K.A.; Gilmore, P.R.; Garvey, W.T. Glucose transport in primary cultured neurons. *J. Neurosci. Res.* **1989**, *22*, 397–407. [CrossRef]

82. Apelt, J.; Mehlhorn, G.; Schliebs, R. Insulin-sensitive GLUT4 glucose transporters are colocalized with GLUT3-expressing cells and demonstrate a chemically distinct neuron-specific localization in rat brain. *J. Neurosci. Res.* **1999**, *57*, 693–705. [CrossRef]
83. Duelli, R.; Kuschinsky, W. Brain Glucose Transporters: Relationship to Local Energy Demand. *Physiology* **2001**, *16*, 71–76. [CrossRef] [PubMed]
84. Komori, T.; Morikawa, Y.; Tamura, S.; Doi, A.; Nanjo, K.; Senba, E. Subcellular localization of glucose transporter 4 in the hypothalamic arcuate nucleus of ob/ob mice under basal conditions. *Brain Res.* **2005**, *1049*, 34–42. [CrossRef] [PubMed]
85. Pearson-Leary, J.; McNay, E.C. Novel Roles for the Insulin-Regulated Glucose Transporter-4 in Hippocampally Dependent Memory. *J. Neurosci.* **2016**, *36*, 11851–11864. [CrossRef]
86. McEwen, B.S.; Reagan, L.P. Glucose transporter expression in the central nervous system: Relationship to synaptic function. *Eur. J. Pharmacol.* **2004**, *490*, 13–24. [CrossRef] [PubMed]
87. Goodner, C.J.; Hom, F.G.; Berrie, M.A. Investigation of the Effect of Insulin upon Regional Brain Glucose Metabolism in the Rat in Vivo. *Endocrinology* **1980**, *107*, 1827–1832. [CrossRef] [PubMed]
88. Hom, F.G.; Goodner, C.J.; Berrie, M.A. A [$^3$H]2-deoxyglucose method for comparing rates of glucose metabolism and insulin responses among rat tissues in vivo. Validation of the model and the absence of an insulin effect on brain. *Diabetes* **1984**, *33*, 141–152. [CrossRef] [PubMed]
89. Bingham, E.M.; Hopkins, D.; Smith, D.; Pernet, A.; Hallett, W.; Reed, L.; Marsden, P.K.; Amiel, S.A. The role of insulin in human brain glucose metabolism: An 18fluoro-deoxyglucose positron emission tomography study. *Diabetes* **2002**, *51*, 3384–3390. [CrossRef]
90. Lesniak, M.A.; Hill, J.M.; Kiess, W.; Rojeski, M.; Pert, C.B.; Roth, J. Receptors for Insulin-like Growth Factors I and II: Autoradiographic Localization in Rat Brain and Comparison to Receptors for Insulin. *Endocrinology* **1988**, *123*, 2089–2099. [CrossRef]
91. Khanh, D.V.; Choi, Y.H.; Moh, S.H.; Kinyua, A.W.; Kim, K.W. Leptin and insulin signaling in dopaminergic neurons: Relationship between energy balance and reward system. *Front. Psychol.* **2014**, *5*, 846. [CrossRef]
92. Könner, A.C.; Hess, S.; Tovar, S.; Mesaros, A.; Sánchez-Lasheras, C.; Evers, N.; Verhagen, L.A.; Brönneke, H.S.; Kleinridders, A.; Hampel, B.; et al. Role for insulin signaling in catecholaminergic neurons in control of energy homeostasis. *Cell Metab.* **2011**, *13*, 720–728. [CrossRef]
93. Heni, M.; Kullmann, S.; Ketterer, C.; Guthoff, M.; Linder, K.; Wagner, R.; Stingl, K.T.; Veit, R.; Staiger, H.; Häring, H.U.; et al. Nasal insulin changes peripheral insulin sensitivity simultaneously with altered activity in homeostatic and reward-related human brain regions. *Diabetologia* **2012**, *55*, 1773–1782. [CrossRef] [PubMed]
94. Heni, M.; Wagner, R.; Kullmann, S.; Veit, R.; Mat Husin, H.; Linder, K.; Benkendorff, C.; Peter, A.; Stefan, N.; Häring, H.U.; et al. Central insulin administration improves whole-body insulin sensitivity via hypothalamus and parasympathetic outputs in men. *Diabetes* **2014**, *63*, 4083–4088. [CrossRef] [PubMed]
95. Gauda, E.B.; Conde, S.; Bassi, M.; Zoccal, D.B.; Colombari, D.S.A.; Colombari, E.; Despotovic, N. Leptin: Master Regulator of Biological Functions that Affects Breathing. *Compr. Physiol.* **2020**, *10*, 1047–1083. [PubMed]
96. Kleinridders, A.; Könner, A.C.; Bruning, J.C. CNS-targets in control of energy and glucose homeostasis. *Curr. Opin. Pharmacol.* **2009**, *9*, 794–804. [CrossRef]
97. Könner, A.C.; Klöckener, T.; Brüning, J.C. Control of energy homeostasis by insulin and leptin: Targeting the arcuate nucleus and beyond. *Physiol. Behav.* **2009**, *97*, 632–638. [CrossRef]
98. Ferrario, C.R.; Reagan, L.P. Insulin-mediated synaptic plasticity in the CNS: Anatomical, functional and temporal contexts. *Neuropharmacology* **2018**, *136*, 182–191. [CrossRef]
99. De Felice, F.G.; Benedict, C. A Key Role of Insulin Receptors in Memory. *Diabetes* **2015**, *64*, 3653–3655. [CrossRef]
100. Dhikav, V.; Anand, K.S. Hippocampus in health and disease: An overview. *Ann. Indian Acad. Neurol.* **2012**, *15*, 239–246. [CrossRef]
101. Tyng, C.M.; Amin, H.U.; Saad, M.N.M.; Malik, A.S. The Influences of Emotion on Learning and Memory. *Front. Psychol.* **2017**, *8*, 1454. [CrossRef]
102. Mizuseki, K.; Royer, S.; Diba, K.; Buzsáki, G. Activity dynamics and behavioral correlates of CA3 and CA1 hippocampal pyramidal neurons. *Hippocampus* **2012**, *22*, 1659–1680. [CrossRef]
103. Alkadhi, K.A. Cellular and Molecular Differences between Area CA1 and the Dentate Gyrus of the Hippocampus. *Mol. Neurobiol.* **2019**, *56*, 6566–6580. [CrossRef] [PubMed]
104. Cherubini, E.; Miles, R. The CA3 region of the hippocampus: How is it? What is it for? How does it do it? *Front. Cell Neurosci.* **2015**, *9*, 19. [CrossRef] [PubMed]
105. Hunsaker, M.R.; Lee, B.; Kesner, R.P. Evaluating the temporal context of episodic memory: The role of CA3 and CA1. *Behav. Brain Res.* **2008**, *188*, 310–315. [CrossRef] [PubMed]
106. Hoge, J.; Kesner, R.P. Role of CA3 and CA1 subregions of the dorsal hippocampus on temporal processing of objects. *Neurobiol. Learn. Mem.* **2007**, *88*, 225–231. [CrossRef] [PubMed]
107. Nakahata, Y.; Yasuda, R. Plasticity of Spine Structure: Local Signaling, Translation and Cytoskeletal Reorganization. *Front. Synaptic Neurosci.* **2018**, *10*, 29. [CrossRef] [PubMed]
108. Porte, D.; Baskin, D.G., Jr.; Schwartz, M.W. Insulin signaling in the central nervous system: A critical role in metabolic homeostasis and disease from *C. elegans* to humans. *Diabetes* **2005**, *54*, 1264–1276. [CrossRef]
109. Lee, C.-C.; Huang, C.-C.; Hsu, K.-S. Insulin promotes dendritic spine and synapse formation by the PI3K/Akt/mTOR and Rac1 signaling pathways. *Neuropharmacology* **2011**, *61*, 867–879. [CrossRef]

110. Van der Heide, L.P.; Kamal, A.; Artola, A.; Gispen, W.H.; Ramakers, G.M. Insulin modulates hippocampal activity-dependent synaptic plasticity in a N-methyl-d-aspartate receptor and phosphatidyl-inositol-3-kinase-dependent manner. *J. Neurochem.* **2005**, *94*, 1158–1166. [CrossRef]
111. Choi, J.; Ko, J.; Racz, B.; Burette, A.; Lee, J.R.; Kim, S.; Na, M.; Lee, H.W.; Kim, K.; Weinberg, R.J.; et al. Regulation of dendritic spine morphogenesis by insulin receptor substrate 53, a downstream effector of Rac1 and Cdc42 small GTPases. *J. Neurosci.* **2005**, *25*, 869–879. [CrossRef]
112. Christie, J.; Wenthold, R.J.; Monaghan, D.T. Insulin Causes a Transient Tyrosine Phosphorylation of NR2A and NR2B NMDA Receptor Subunits in Rat Hippocampus. *J. Neurochem.* **2001**, *72*, 1523–1528. [CrossRef]
113. Liu, L.; Brown, J.C.; Webster, W.W.; Morrisett, R.A.; Monaghan, D.T. Insulin potentiates N-methyl-d-aspartate receptor activity in Xenopus oocytes and rat hippocampus. *Neurosci. Lett.* **1995**, *192*, 5–8. [CrossRef]
114. Martín, E.D.; Sánchez-Perez, A.; Trejo, J.L.; Martin-Aldana, J.A.; Jaimez, M.C.; Pons, S.; Umanzor, C.A.; Menes, L.; White, M.F.; Burks, D.J. IRS-2 Deficiency Impairs NMDA Receptor-Dependent Long-term Potentiation. *Cereb. Cortex* **2011**, *22*, 1717–1727. [CrossRef] [PubMed]
115. Ge, Y.; Dong, Z.; Bagot, R.C.; Howland, J.G.; Phillips, A.G.; Wong, T.P.; Wang, Y.T. Hippocampal long-term depression is required for the consolidation of spatial memory. *Proc. Natl. Acad. Sci. USA* **2010**, *107*, 16697–16702. [CrossRef] [PubMed]
116. Euston, D.R.; Gruber, A.; McNaughton, B.L. The Role of Medial Prefrontal Cortex in Memory and Decision Making. *Neuron* **2012**, *76*, 1057–1070. [CrossRef]
117. Chao, O.Y.; Silva, M.A.D.S.; Yang, Y.-M.; Huston, J.P. The medial prefrontal cortex-hippocampus circuit that integrates information of object, place and time to construct episodic memory in rodents: Behavioral, anatomical and neurochemical properties. *Neurosci. Biobehav. Rev.* **2020**, *113*, 373–407. [CrossRef]
118. Niblock, M.M.; Brunso-Bechtold, J.K.; Riddle, D.R. Insulin-like growth factor I stimulates dendritic growth in primary somatosensory cortex. *J. Neurosci.* **2000**, *20*, 4165–4176. [CrossRef]
119. Kullmann, S.; Kleinridders, A.; Small, D.M.; Fritsche, A.; Häring, H.-U.; Preissl, H.; Heni, M. Central nervous pathways of insulin action in the control of metabolism and food intake. *Lancet Diabetes Endocrinol.* **2020**, *8*, 524–534. [CrossRef]
120. Taouis, M.; Torres-Aleman, I. Editorial: Insulin and the Brain. *Front. Endocrinol.* **2019**, *10*, 299. [CrossRef]
121. Heni, M.; Schöpfer, P.; Peter, A.; Sartorius, T.; Fritsche, A.; Synofzik, M.; Häring, H.-U.; Maetzler, W.; Hennige, A.M. Evidence for altered transport of insulin across the blood–brain barrier in insulin-resistant humans. *Geol. Rundsch.* **2013**, *51*, 679–681. [CrossRef]
122. Spinelli, M.; Fusco, S.; Grassi, C. Brain insulin resistance impairs hippocampal plasticity. *Vitam. Horm.* **2020**, *114*, 281–306.
123. García-Cáceres, C.; Lechuga-Sancho, A.; Argente, J.; Frago, L.M.; Chowen, J.A. Death of Hypothalamic Astrocytes in Poorly Controlled Diabetic Rats is Associated with Nuclear Translocation of Apoptosis Inducing Factor. *J. Neuroendocr.* **2008**, *20*, 1348–1360. [CrossRef] [PubMed]
124. García-Cáceres, C.; Quarta, C.; Varela, L.; Gao, Y.; Gruber, T.; Legutko, B.; Jastroch, M.; Johansson, P.; Ninkovic, J.; Yi, C.-X.; et al. Astrocytic Insulin Signaling Couples Brain Glucose Uptake with Nutrient Availability. *Cell* **2016**, *166*, 867–880. [CrossRef] [PubMed]
125. Kodl, C.T.; Seaquist, E.R. Cognitive Dysfunction and Diabetes Mellitus. *Endocr. Rev.* **2008**, *29*, 494–511. [CrossRef] [PubMed]
126. Fadel, J.R.; Reagan, L.P. Stop signs in hippocampal insulin signaling: The role of insulin resistance in structural, functional and behavioral deficits. *Curr. Opin. Behav. Sci.* **2015**, *9*, 47–54. [CrossRef] [PubMed]
127. Arnold, S.E.; Lucki, I.; Brookshire, B.R.; Carlson, G.C.; Browne, C.A.; Kazi, H.; Bang, S.; Choi, B.-R.; Chen, Y.; McMullen, M.F.; et al. High fat diet produces brain insulin resistance, synaptodendritic abnormalities and altered behavior in mice. *Neurobiol. Dis.* **2014**, *67*, 79–87. [CrossRef]
128. Kamal, A.; Ramakers, G.M.; Gispen, W.H.; Biessels, G.J.; Al Ansari, A. Hyperinsulinemia in rats causes impairment of spatial memory and learning with defects in hippocampal synaptic plasticity by involvement of postsynaptic mechanisms. *Exp. Brain Res.* **2013**, *226*, 45–51. [CrossRef]
129. Chen, Y.; Zhao, Y.; Dai, C.L.; Liang, Z.; Run, X.; Iqbal, K.; Liu, F.; Gong, C.X. Intranasal insulin restores insulin signaling, increases synaptic proteins, and reduces Aβ level and microglia activation in the brains of 3xTg-AD mice. *Exp. Neurol.* **2014**, *261*, 610–619. [CrossRef]
130. Yang, Y.W.; Hsieh, T.F.; Li, C.I.; Liu, C.S.; Lin, W.Y.; Chiang, J.H.; Li, T.C.; Lin, C.C. Increased risk of Parkinson disease with diabetes mellitus in a population-based study. *Medicine* **2017**, *96*, e5921. [CrossRef]
131. Pagano, G.; Polychronis, S.; Wilson, H.; Giordano, B.; Ferrara, N.; Niccolini, F.; Politis, M. Diabetes mellitus and Parkinson disease. *Neurology* **2018**, *90*, e1654–e1662. [CrossRef]
132. Hardy, J.A.; Higgins, G.A. Alzheimer's disease: The amyloid cascade hypothesis. *Science* **1992**, *256*, 184–185. [CrossRef]
133. Ricciarelli, R.; Fedele, E. The Amyloid Cascade Hypothesis in Alzheimer's Disease: It's Time to Change Our Mind. *Curr. Neuropharmacol.* **2017**, *15*, 926–935. [CrossRef] [PubMed]
134. Vekrellis, K.; Xilouri, M.; Emmanouilidou, E.; Rideout, H.J.; Stefanis, L. Pathological roles of α-synuclein in neurological disorders. *Lancet Neurol.* **2011**, *10*, 1015–1025. [CrossRef]
135. Puschmann, A.; Bhidayasiri, R.; Weiner, W.J. Synucleinopathies from bench to bedside. *Park. Relat. Disord.* **2012**, *18* (Suppl. S1), S24–S27. [CrossRef]
136. Goedert, M.; Jakes, R.; Spillantini, M.G. The Synucleinopathies: Twenty Years On. *J. Parkinson's Dis.* **2017**, *7*, S51–S69. [CrossRef]

137. Spillantini, M.G.; Schmidt, M.L.; Lee, V.M.; Trojanowski, J.Q.; Jakes, R.; Goedert, M. Alpha-synuclein in Lewy bodies. *Nature* **1997**, *388*, 839–840. [CrossRef]
138. Spillantini, M.G.; Crowther, R.A.; Jakes, R.; Hasegawa, M.; Goedert, M. α-Synuclein in filamentous inclusions of Lewy bodies from Parkinson's disease and dementia with Lewy bodies. *Proc. Natl. Acad. Sci. USA* **1998**, *95*, 6469–6473. [CrossRef]
139. Spillantini, M.G.; Crowther, R.A.; Jakes, R.; Cairns, N.J.; Lantos, P.L.; Goedert, M. Filamentous α-synuclein inclusions link multiple system atrophy with Parkinson's disease and dementia with Lewy bodies. *Neurosci. Lett.* **1998**, *251*, 205–208. [CrossRef]
140. Pasinetti, G.M.; Eberstein, J.A. Metabolic syndrome and the role of dietary lifestyles in Alzheimer's disease. *J. Neurochem.* **2008**, *106*, 1503–1514. [CrossRef]
141. Eskelinen, M.H.; Ngandu, T.; Helkala, E.; Tuomilehto, J.; Nissinen, A.; Soininen, H.; Kivipelto, M. Fat intake at midlife and cognitive impairment later in life: A population-based CAIDE study. *Int. J. Geriatr. Psychiatry* **2008**, *23*, 741–747. [CrossRef]
142. De la Monte, S.M.; Wands, J.R. Alzheimer's disease is type 3 diabetes-evidence reviewed. *J. Diabetes Sci. Technol.* **2008**, *2*, 1101–1113. [CrossRef]
143. De Felice, F.G.; Lourenco, M.V. Brain metabolic stress and neuroinflammation at the basis of cognitive impairment in Alzheimer's disease. *Front. Aging Neurosci.* **2015**, *7*, 94. [CrossRef]
144. Whitmer, R.A.; Gunderson, E.P.; Barrett-Connor, E.; Quesenberry, C.P., Jr.; Yaffe, K. Obesity in middle age and future risk of dementia: A 27 year longitudinal population based study. *BMJ* **2005**, *330*, 1360. [CrossRef] [PubMed]
145. Morris, M.C.; Evans, D.A.; Bienias, J.L.; Tangney, C.C.; Wilson, R.S. Dietary fat intake and 6-year cognitive change in an older biracial community population. *Neurology* **2004**, *62*, 1573–1579. [CrossRef] [PubMed]
146. Nyaradi, A.; Foster, J.K.; Hickling, S.; Li, J.; Ambrosini, G.; Jacques, A.; Oddy, W.H. Prospective associations between dietary patterns and cognitive performance during adolescence. *J. Child Psychol. Psychiatry* **2014**, *55*, 1017–1024. [CrossRef] [PubMed]
147. Øverby, N.C.; Lüdemann, E.; Høigaard, R. Self-repor.rted learning difficulties and dietary intake in Norwegian adolescents. *Scand. J. Public Health* **2013**, *41*, 754–760. [CrossRef] [PubMed]
148. Li, Y.; Dai, Q.; Jackson, J.C.; Zhang, J. Overweight is associated with decreased cognitive functioning among school-age children and adolescents. *Obesity* **2008**, *16*, 1809–1815. [CrossRef]
149. Holloway, C.J.; E Cochlin, L.; Emmanuel, Y.; Murray, A.; Codreanu, I.; Edwards, L.M.; Szmigielski, C.; Tyler, D.J.; Knight, N.S.; Saxby, B.K.; et al. A high-fat diet impairs cardiac high-energy phosphate metabolism and cognitive function in healthy human subjects. *Am. J. Clin. Nutr.* **2011**, *93*, 748–755. [CrossRef]
150. Edwards, L.M.; Murray, A.J.; Holloway, C.J.; Carter, E.E.; Kemp, G.J.; Codreanu, I.; Brooker, H.; Tyler, D.J.; Robbins, P.A.; Clarke, K. Short-term consumption of a high-fat diet impairs whole-body efficiency and cognitive function in sedentary men. *FASEB J.* **2010**, *25*, 1088–1096. [CrossRef]
151. Luchsinger, J.; Tang, M.-X.; Shea, S.; Mayeux, R. Caloric Intake and the Risk of Alzheimer Disease. *Arch. Neurol.* **2002**, *59*, 1258–1263. [CrossRef]
152. Brands, A.M.; Biessels, G.J.; de Haan, E.H.; Kappelle, L.J.; Kessels, R.P. The effects of type 1 diabetes on cognitive performance: A meta-analysis. *Diabetes Care* **2005**, *28*, 726–735. [CrossRef]
153. Biessels, G.J.; Kappelle, L.J. Increased risk of Alzheimer's disease in Type II diabetes: Insulin resistance of the brain or insulin-induced amyloid pathology? *Biochem. Soc. Trans.* **2005**, *33 Pt 5*, 1041–1044. [CrossRef] [PubMed]
154. Ott, A.; Stolk, R.P.; van Harskamp, F.; Pols, H.A.; Hofman, A.; Breteler, M.M. Diabetes mellitus and the risk of dementia: The Rotterdam Study. *Neurology* **1999**, *53*, 1937–1942. [CrossRef] [PubMed]
155. Janson, J.; Laedtke, T.; Parisi, J.E.; O'Brien, P.; Petersen, R.C.; Butler, P.C. Increased risk of type 2 diabetes in Alzheimer disease. *Diabetes* **2004**, *53*, 474–481. [CrossRef] [PubMed]
156. Zilliox, L.A.; Chadrasekaran, K.; Kwan, J.Y.; Russell, J.W. Diabetes and Cognitive Impairment. *Curr. Diabetes Rep.* **2016**, *16*, 87. [CrossRef]
157. Li, C.Y.; Kuo, C.L.; Chang, Y.H.; Lu, C.L.; Martini, S.; Hou, W.H. Association between trajectory of severe hypoglycemia and dementia in patients with type 2 diabetes: A population-based study. *J. Epidemiol.* **2021**, JE20200518. [CrossRef]
158. Ramos-Rodriguez, J.J.; Spires-Jones, T.; Pooler, A.M.; Lechuga-Sancho, A.; Bacskai, B.J.; Garcia-Alloza, M. Progressive Neuronal Pathology and Synaptic Loss Induced by Prediabetes and Type 2 Diabetes in a Mouse Model of Alzheimer's Disease. *Mol. Neurobiol.* **2016**, *54*, 3428–3438. [CrossRef]
159. Haan, M.N. Therapy Insight: Type 2 diabetes mellitus and the risk of late-onset Alzheimer's disease. *Nat. Clin. Pract. Cardiovasc. Med.* **2006**, *2*, 159–166. [CrossRef]
160. Watson, G.; Craft, S. Modulation of memory by insulin and glucose: Neuropsychological observations in Alzheimer's disease. *Eur. J. Pharmacol.* **2004**, *490*, 97–113. [CrossRef]
161. Talbot, K.; Wang, H.Y.; Kazi, H.; Han, L.Y.; Bakshi, K.P.; Stucky, A.; Fuino, R.L.; Kawaguchi, K.R.; Samoyedny, A.J.; Wilson, R.S.; et al. Demonstrated brain insulin resistance in Alzheimer's disease patients is associated with IGF-1 resistance, IRS-1 dysregulation, and cognitive decline. *J. Clin. Investig.* **2012**, *122*, 1316–1338. [CrossRef]
162. Abbott, M.A.; Wells, D.G.; Fallon, J.R. The insulin receptor tyrosine kinase substrate p58/53 and the insulin receptor are components of CNS synapses. *J. Neurosci.* **1999**, *19*, 7300–7308. [CrossRef]
163. Llorens-Martín, M.; Jurado, J.; Hernández, F.; Avila, J. GSK-3β, a pivotal kinase in Alzheimer disease. *Front. Mol. Neurosci.* **2014**, *7*, 46. [PubMed]

164. Qu, Z.-S.; Li, L.; Sun, X.-J.; Zhao, Y.-W.; Zhang, J.; Geng, Z.; Fu, J.-L.; Ren, Q.-G. Glycogen Synthase Kinase-3 Regulates Production of Amyloid-βPeptides and Tau Phosphorylation in Diabetic Rat Brain. *Sci. World J.* **2014**, *2014*, 878123. [CrossRef] [PubMed]
165. Hooper, C.; Killick, R.; Lovestone, S. The GSK3 hypothesis of Alzheimer's disease. *J. Neurochem.* **2008**, *104*, 1433–1439. [CrossRef] [PubMed]
166. Chen, Y.; Deng, Y.; Zhang, B.; Gong, C.-X. Deregulation of brain insulin signaling in Alzheimer's disease. *Neurosci. Bull.* **2014**, *30*, 282–294. [CrossRef]
167. Liu, Z.; Patil, I.Y.; Jiang, T.; Sancheti, H.; Walsh, J.P.; Stiles, B.L.; Yin, F.; Cadenas, E. High-Fat Diet Induces Hepatic Insulin Resistance and Impairment of Synaptic Plasticity. *PLoS ONE* **2015**, *10*, e0128274. [CrossRef]
168. Hu, G.; Jousilahti, P.; Bidel, S.; Antikainen, R.; Tuomilehto, J. Type 2 Diabetes and the Risk of Parkinson's Disease. *Diabetes Care* **2007**, *30*, 842–847. [CrossRef]
169. Santiago, J.A.; Potashkin, J.A. Shared dysregulated pathways lead to Parkinson's disease and diabetes. *Trends Mol. Med.* **2013**, *19*, 176–186. [CrossRef]
170. Lu, M.; Hu, G. Targeting metabolic inflammation in Parkinson's disease: Implications for prospective therapeutic strategies. *Clin. Exp. Pharmacol. Physiol.* **2011**, *39*, 577–585. [CrossRef]
171. Abbott, R.D.; Ross, G.W.; White, L.R.; Nelson, J.S.; Masaki, K.H.; Tanner, C.M.; Curb, J.D.; Blanchette, P.L.; Popper, J.S.; Petrovitch, H. Midlife adiposity and the future risk of Parkinson's disease. *Neurology* **2002**, *59*, 1051–1057. [CrossRef]
172. Athauda, D.; Foltynie, T. Insulin resistance and Parkinson's disease: A new target for disease modification? *Prog. Neurobiol.* **2016**, *145*, 98–120. [CrossRef]
173. Gentier, I.; D'Hondt, E.; Shultz, S.; Deforche, B.; Augustijn, M.; Hoorne, S.; Verlaecke, K.; De Bourdeaudhuij, I.; Lenoir, M. Fine and gross motor skills differ between healthy-weight and obese children. *Res. Dev. Disabil.* **2013**, *34*, 4043–4051. [CrossRef] [PubMed]
174. Krombholz, H. Motor and Cognitive Performance of Overweight Preschool Children. *Percept. Mot. Skills* **2013**, *116*, 40–57. [CrossRef] [PubMed]
175. Mond, J.M.; Stich, H.; Hay, P.; Kraemer, A.; Baune, B.T. Associations between obesity and developmental functioning in pre-school children: A population-based study. *Int. J. Obes.* **2007**, *31*, 1068–1073. [CrossRef]
176. Roberts, D.; Veneri, D.; Decker, R.; Gannotti, M. Weight Status and Gross Motor Skill in Kindergarten Children. *Pediatr. Phys. Ther.* **2012**, *24*, 353–360. [CrossRef] [PubMed]
177. Poulsen, A.A.; Desha, L.; Ziviani, J.; Griffiths, L.; Heaslop, A.; Khan, A.; Leong, G. Fundamental movement skills and self-concept of children who are overweight. *Pediatr. Obes.* **2011**, *6*, e464–e471. [CrossRef] [PubMed]
178. Jones, R.A.; Okely, A.; Caputi, P.; Cliff, D. Perceived and actual competence among overweight and non-overweight children. *J. Sci. Med. Sport* **2010**, *13*, 589–596. [CrossRef] [PubMed]
179. Slining, M.; Adair, L.S.; Goldman, B.D.; Borja, J.B.; Bentley, M. Infant Overweight Is Associated with Delayed Motor Development. *J. Pediatr.* **2010**, *157*, 20–25.e1. [CrossRef]
180. Bittencourt, A.; Brum, P.O.; Ribeiro, C.T.; Gasparotto, J.; Bortolin, R.C.; de Vargas, A.R.; Heimfarth, L.; de Almeida, R.F.; Moreira, J.C.F.; de Oliveira, J.; et al. High fat diet-induced obesity causes a reduction in brain tyrosine hydroxylase levels and non-motor features in rats through metabolic dysfunction, neuroinflammation and oxidative stress. *Nutr. Neurosci.* **2020**, 1831261. [CrossRef]
181. Choi, J.Y.; Jang, E.H.; Park, C.S.; Kang, J.H. Enhanced susceptibility to 1-methyl-4-phenyl-1,2,3,6-tetrahydropyridine neurotoxicity in high-fat diet-induced obesity. *Free Radic. Biol. Med.* **2005**, *38*, 806–816. [CrossRef]
182. Bousquet, M.; St-Amour, I.; Vandal, M.; Julien, P.; Cicchetti, F.; Calon, F. High-fat diet exacerbates MPTP-induced dopaminergic degeneration in mice. *Neurobiol. Dis.* **2012**, *45*, 529–538. [CrossRef]
183. Sharma, S.; Taliyan, R. High fat diet feeding induced insulin resistance exacerbates 6-OHDA mediated neurotoxicity and behavioral abnormalities in rats. *Behav. Brain Res.* **2018**, *351*, 17–23. [CrossRef] [PubMed]
184. Morris, J.K.; Bomhoff, G.L.; Stanford, J.A.; Geiger, P.C. Neurodegeneration in an animal model of Parkinson's disease is exacerbated by a high-fat diet. *Am. J. Physiol. Regul. Integr. Comp. Physiol.* **2010**, *299*, R1082–R1090. [CrossRef] [PubMed]
185. Ma, D.; Shuler, J.M.; Raider, K.D.; Rogers, R.S.; Wheatley, J.L.; Geiger, P.C.; Stanford, J.A. Effects of discontinuing a high-fat diet on mitochondrial proteins and 6-hydroxydopamine-induced dopamine depletion in rats. *Brain Res.* **2015**, *1613*, 49–58. [CrossRef] [PubMed]
186. Rotermund, C.; Truckenmüller, F.M.; Schell, H.; Kahle, P.J. Diet-induced obesity accelerates the onset of terminal phenotypes in α-synuclein transgenic mice. *J. Neurochem.* **2014**, *131*, 848–858. [CrossRef]
187. Ekstrand, M.I.; Galter, D. The MitoPark Mouse—An animal model of Parkinson's disease with impaired respiratory chain function in dopamine neurons. *Park. Relat. Disord.* **2009**, *15*, S185–S188. [CrossRef]
188. Morris, J.; Bomhoff, G.; Gorres, B.; Davis, V.; Kim, J.; Lee, P.-P.; Brooks, W.; Gerhardt, G.; Geiger, P.; Stanford, J. Insulin resistance impairs nigrostriatal dopamine function. *Exp. Neurol.* **2011**, *231*, 171–180. [CrossRef]
189. Jang, Y.; Lee, M.J.; Han, J.; Kim, S.J.; Ryu, I.; Ju, X.; Ryu, M.J.; Chung, W.; Oh, E.; Kweon, G.R.; et al. A High-fat Diet Induces a Loss of Midbrain Dopaminergic Neuronal Function That Underlies Motor Abnormalities. *Exp. Neurobiol.* **2017**, *26*, 104–112. [CrossRef]
190. Kao, Y.-C.; Wei, W.-Y.; Tsai, K.-J.; Wang, L.-C. High Fat Diet Suppresses Peroxisome Proliferator-Activated Receptors and Reduces Dopaminergic Neurons in the Substantia Nigra. *Int. J. Mol. Sci.* **2019**, *21*, 207. [CrossRef]

191. Rotermund, C.; Machetanz, G.; Fitzgerald, J.C. The Therapeutic Potential of Metformin in Neurodegenerative Diseases. *Front. Endocrinol.* **2018**, *9*, 400. [CrossRef]
192. Hong, C.T.; Chen, K.Y.; Wang, W.; Chiu, J.Y.; Wu, D.; Chao, T.Y.; Hu, C.J.; Chau, K.D.; Bamodu, O.A. Insulin Resistance Promotes Parkinson's Disease through Aberrant Expression of α-Synuclein, Mitochondrial Dysfunction, and Deregulation of the Polo-Like Kinase 2 Signaling. *Cells* **2020**, *9*, 740. [CrossRef]
193. Wu, H.-F.; Kao, L.-T.; Shih, J.-H.; Kao, H.-H.; Chou, Y.-C.; Li, I.-H.; Kao, S. Pioglitazone use and Parkinson's disease: A retrospective cohort study in Taiwan. *BMJ Open* **2018**, *8*, e023302. [CrossRef] [PubMed]
194. Velazquez, R.; Tran, A.; Ishimwe, E.; Denner, L.; Dave, N.; Oddo, S.; Dineley, K.T. Central insulin dysregulation and energy dyshomeostasis in two mouse models of Alzheimer's disease. *Neurobiol. Aging* **2017**, *58*, 1–13. [CrossRef] [PubMed]
195. Sah, S.K.; Lee, C.; Jang, J.-H.; Park, G.H. Effect of high-fat diet on cognitive impairment in triple-transgenic mice model of Alzheimer's disease. *Biochem. Biophys. Res. Commun.* **2017**, *493*, 731–736. [CrossRef] [PubMed]
196. Thériault, P.; ElAli, A.; Rivest, S. High fat diet exacerbates Alzheimer's disease-related pathology in APPswe/PS1 mice. *Oncotarget* **2016**, *7*, 67808–67827. [CrossRef] [PubMed]
197. Valladolid-Acebes, I.; Fole, A.; Martín, M.; Morales, L.; Victoria Cano, M.; Ruiz-Gayo, M.; Del Olmo, N. Spatial memory impairment and changes in hippocampal morphology are triggered by high-fat diets in adolescent mice. Is there a role of leptin? *Neurobiol. Learn. Mem.* **2013**, *106*, 18–25. [CrossRef] [PubMed]
198. Ledreux, A.; Wang, X.; Schultzberg, M.; Granholm, A.-C.; Freeman, L.R. Detrimental effects of a high fat/high cholesterol diet on memory and hippocampal markers in aged rats. *Behav. Brain Res.* **2016**, *312*, 294–304. [CrossRef]
199. Busquets, O.; Ettcheto, M.; Pallàs, M.; Beas-Zarate, C.; Verdaguer, E.; Auladell, C.; Folch, J.; Camins, A. Long-term exposition to a high fat diet favors the appearance of β-amyloid depositions in the brain of C57BL/6J mice. A potential model of sporadic Alzheimer's disease. *Mech. Ageing Dev.* **2017**, *162*, 38–45. [CrossRef]
200. Tran, D.M.; Westbrook, R.F. A high-fat high-sugar diet-induced impairment in place-recognition memory is reversible and training-dependent. *Appetite* **2017**, *110*, 61–71. [CrossRef]
201. Spencer, S.J.; D'Angelo, H.; Soch, A.; Watkins, L.R.; Maier, S.F.; Barrientos, R.M. High-fat diet and aging interact to produce neuroinflammation and impair hippocampal- and amygdalar-dependent memory. *Neurobiol. Aging* **2017**, *58*, 88–101. [CrossRef]
202. Kothari, V.; Luo, Y.; Tornabene, T.; O'Neill, A.M.; Greene, M.; Geetha, T.; Babu, J.R. High fat diet induces brain insulin resistance and cognitive impairment in mice. *Biochim. Biophys. Acta Mol. Basis Dis.* **2017**, *1863*, 499–508. [CrossRef]
203. Fu, Z.; Wu, J.; Nesil, T.; Li, M.D.; Aylor, K.W.; Liu, Z. Long-term high-fat diet induces hippocampal microvascular insulin resistance and cognitive dysfunction. *Am. J. Physiol. Metab.* **2017**, *312*, E89–E97. [CrossRef] [PubMed]
204. Fazzari, G.; Zizza, M.; Di Vito, A.; Alò, R.; Mele, M.; Bruno, R.; Barni, T.; Facciolo, R.M.; Canonaco, M. Reduced learning and memory performances in high-fat treated hamsters related to brain neurotensin receptor1 expression variations. *Behav. Brain Res.* **2018**, *347*, 227–233. [CrossRef]
205. Abbott, K.N.; Arnott, C.K.; Westbrook, R.F.; Tran, D.M. The effect of high fat, high sugar, and combined high fat-high sugar diets on spatial learning and memory in rodents: A meta-analysis. *Neurosci. Biobehav. Rev.* **2019**, *107*, 399–421. [CrossRef] [PubMed]
206. Seshadri, S.; Wolf, P.A.; Beiser, A.; Au, R.; McNulty, K.; White, R.; D'Agostino, R.B. Lifetime risk of dementia and Alzheimer's disease. The impact of mortality on risk estimates in the Framingham Study. *Neurology* **1997**, *49*, 1498–1504. [CrossRef]
207. Plassman, B.L.; Langa, K.M.; McCammon, R.J.; Fisher, G.G.; Potter, G.G.; Burke, J.R.; Steffens, D.C.; Foster, N.L.; Giordani, B.; Unverzagt, F.W.; et al. Incidence of dementia and cognitive impairment, not dementia in the United States. *Ann. Neurol.* **2011**, *70*, 418–426. [CrossRef] [PubMed]
208. Irvine, K.; Laws, K.R.; Gale, T.M.; Kondel, T.K. Greater cognitive deterioration in women than men with Alzheimer's disease: A meta analysis. *J. Clin. Exp. Neuropsychol.* **2012**, *34*, 989–998. [CrossRef] [PubMed]
209. Hebert, L.E.; Weuve, J.; Scherr, P.A.; Evans, D.A. Alzheimer disease in the United States (2010–2050) estimated using the 2010 census. *Neurology* **2013**, *80*, 1778–1783. [CrossRef] [PubMed]
210. Ferretti, M.T.; Iulita, M.F.; Cavedo, E.; Chiesa, P.A.; Schumacher Dimech, A.; Santuccione Chadha, A.; Baracchi, F.; Girouard, H.; Misoch, S.; Giacobini, E.; et al. Sex differences in Alzheimer disease—The gateway to precision medicine. *Nat. Rev. Neurol.* **2018**, *14*, 457–469. [CrossRef]
211. Brookmeyer, R.; Gray, S.; Kawas, C. Projections of Alzheimer's disease in the United States and the public health impact of delaying disease onset. *Am. J. Public Health* **1998**, *88*, 1337–1342. [CrossRef]
212. Andersen, K.; Launer, L.J.; Dewey, M.E.; Letenneur, L.; Ott, A.; Copeland, J.R.M.; Dartigues, J.-F.; Kragh-Sorensen, P.; Baldereschi, M.; Brayne, C.; et al. Gender differences in the incidence of AD and vascular dementia: The EURODEM Studies. *Neurology* **1999**, *53*, 1992. [CrossRef]
213. Beam, C.R.; Kaneshiro, C.; Jang, J.Y.; Reynolds, C.A.; Pedersen, N.L.; Gatz, M. Differences Between Women and Men in Incidence Rates of Dementia and Alzheimer's Disease. *J. Alzheimer's Dis.* **2018**, *64*, 1077–1083. [CrossRef] [PubMed]
214. Ullah, M.F.; Ahmad, A.; Bhat, S.H.; Abu-Duhier, F.M.; Barreto, G.E.; Ashraf, G.M. Impact of sex differences and gender specificity on behavioral characteristics and pathophysiology of neurodegenerative disorders. *Neurosci. Biobehav. Rev.* **2019**, *102*, 95–105. [CrossRef]
215. Gillies, G.E.; Pienaar, I.S.; Vohra, S.; Qamhawi, Z. Sex differences in Parkinson's disease. *Front. Neuroendocrinol.* **2014**, *35*, 370–384. [CrossRef] [PubMed]

216. Solla, P.; Cannas, A.; Ibba, F.C.; Loi, F.; Corona, M.; Orofino, G.; Marrosu, M.G.; Marrosu, F. Gender differences in motor and non-motor symptoms among Sardinian patients with Parkinson's disease. *J. Neurol. Sci.* **2012**, *323*, 33–39. [CrossRef] [PubMed]
217. Elbaz, A.; Bower, J.H.; Maraganore, D.M.; McDonnell, S.; Peterson, B.J.; Ahlskog, J.; Schaid, D.J.; A Rocca, W. Risk tables for parkinsonism and Parkinson's disease. *J. Clin. Epidemiol.* **2002**, *55*, 25–31. [CrossRef]
218. Baldereschi, M.; Di Carlo, A.; Rocca, W.A.; Vanni, P.; Maggi, S.; Perissinotto, E.; Grigoletto, F.; Amaducci, L.; Inzitari, D. Parkinson's disease and parkinsonism in a longitudinal study: Two-fold higher incidence in men. *Neurology* **2000**, *55*, 1358–1363. [CrossRef] [PubMed]
219. Gaignard, P.; Liere, P.; Thérond, P.; Schumacher, M.; Slama, A.; Guennoun, R. Role of Sex Hormones on Brain Mitochondrial Function, with Special Reference to Aging and Neurodegenerative Diseases. *Front. Aging Neurosci.* **2017**, *9*, 406. [CrossRef]
220. Gaignard, P.; Fréchou, M.; Liere, P.; Thérond, P.; Schumacher, M.; Slama, A.; Guennoun, R. Sex differences in brain mitochondrial metabolism: Influence of endogenous steroids and stroke. *J. Neuroendocr.* **2018**, *30*, e12497. [CrossRef]
221. Chen, J.-Q.; Cammarata, P.R.; Baines, C.P.; Yager, J.D. Regulation of mitochondrial respiratory chain biogenesis by estrogens/estrogen receptors and physiological, pathological and pharmacological implications. *Biochim. Biophys. Acta* **2009**, *1793*, 1540–1570. [CrossRef]
222. Chen, J.-Q.; Terry, R.; Brown, T.R.; Russo, J. Regulation of energy metabolism pathways by estrogens and estrogenic chemicals and potential implications in obesity associated with increased exposure to endocrine disruptors. *Biochim. Biophys. Acta* **2009**, *1793*, 1128–1143. [CrossRef]
223. Kelly, D.M.; Jones, T.H. Testosterone: A metabolic hormone in health and disease. *J. Endocrinol.* **2013**, *217*, R25–R45. [CrossRef] [PubMed]
224. Zárate, S.; Stevnsner, T.; Gredilla, R. Role of Estrogen and Other Sex Hormones in Brain Aging. Neuroprotection and DNA Repair. *Front. Aging Neurosci.* **2017**, *9*, 430. [CrossRef] [PubMed]
225. Siddiqui, A.N.; Siddiqui, N.; Khan, R.A.; Kalam, A.; Jabir, N.R.; Kamal, M.A.; Firoz, C.K.; Tabrez, S. Neuroprotective Role of Steroidal Sex Hormones: An Overview. *CNS Neurosci. Ther.* **2016**, *22*, 342–350. [CrossRef] [PubMed]
226. Spence, R.D.; Voskuhl, R.R. Neuroprotective effects of estrogens and androgens in CNS inflammation and neurodegeneration. *Front. Neuroendocrinol.* **2012**, *33*, 105–115. [CrossRef] [PubMed]
227. Raghava, N.; Das, B.C.; Ray, S.K. Neuroprotective effects of estrogen in CNS injuries: Insights from animal models. *Neurosci. Neuroecon.* **2017**, *6*, 15–29. [CrossRef] [PubMed]
228. Schumacher, M.; Weill-Engerer, S.; Liere, P.; Robert, F.; Franklin, R.; Garcia-Segura, L.; Lambert, J.; Mayo, W.; Melcangi, C.R.; Parducz, A.; et al. Steroid hormones and neurosteroids in normal and pathological aging of the nervous system. *Prog. Neurobiol.* **2003**, *71*, 3–29. [CrossRef]
229. Armstrong, M.J.; Okun, M.S. Diagnosis and Treatment of Parkinson Disease: A Review. *JAMA* **2020**, *323*, 548–560. [CrossRef]
230. Cummings, J.L.; Tong, G.; Ballard, C. Treatment Combinations for Alzheimer's Disease: Current and Future Pharmacotherapy Options. *J. Alzheimer's Dis.* **2019**, *67*, 779–794. [CrossRef]
231. Wahlqvist, M.L.; Lee, M.-S.; Hsu, C.-C.; Chuang, S.-Y.; Lee, J.-T.; Tsai, H.-N. Metformin-inclusive sulfonylurea therapy reduces the risk of Parkinson's disease occurring with Type 2 diabetes in a Taiwanese population cohort. *Park. Relat. Disord.* **2012**, *18*, 753–758. [CrossRef]
232. Miranda, H.V.; El-Agnaf, O.M.A.; Outeiro, T.F. Glycation in Parkinson's disease and Alzheimer's disease. *Mov. Disord.* **2016**, *31*, 782–790. [CrossRef]
233. Patil, S.; Jain, P.D.; Ghumatkar, P.J.; Tambe, R.; Sathaye, S. Neuroprotective effect of metformin in MPTP-induced Parkinson's disease in mice. *Neuroscience* **2014**, *277*, 747–754. [CrossRef] [PubMed]
234. Kickstein, E.; Krauss, S.; Thornhill, P.; Rutschow, D.; Zeller, R.; Sharkey, J.; Williamson, R.; Fuchs, M.; Koehler, A.; Glossmann, H.; et al. Biguanide metformin acts on tau phosphorylation via mTOR/protein phosphatase 2A (PP2A) signaling. *Proc. Natl. Acad. Sci. USA* **2010**, *107*, 21830–21835. [CrossRef] [PubMed]
235. Kiho, T.; Kato, M.; Usui, S.; Hirano, K. Effect of buformin and metformin on formation of advanced glycation end products by methylglyoxal. *Clin. Chim. Acta* **2005**, *358*, 139–145. [CrossRef] [PubMed]
236. Beisswenger, P.; Ruggiero-Lopez, D. Metformin inhibition of glycation processes. *Diabetes Metab.* **2003**, *29*, 6S95–6S103. [CrossRef]
237. Kender, Z.; Fleming, T.; Kopf, S.; Torzsa, P.; Grolmusz, V.; Herzig, S.; Schleicher, E.; Rácz, K.; Reismann, P.; Nawroth, P. Effect of Metformin on Methylglyoxal Metabolism in Patients with Type 2 Diabetes. *Exp. Clin. Endocrinol. Diabetes* **2014**, *122*, 316–319. [CrossRef]
238. Kinsky, O.R.; Hargraves, T.L.; Anumol, T.; Jacobsen, N.E.; Dai, J.; Snyder, S.A.; Monks, T.J.; Lau, S.S. Metformin Scavenges Methylglyoxal to Form a Novel Imidazolinone Metabolite in Humans. *Chem. Res. Toxicol.* **2016**, *29*, 227–234. [CrossRef]
239. Beisswenger, P.J.; Howell, S.K.; Touchette, A.D.; Lal, S.; Szwergold, B.S. Metformin reduces systemic methylglyoxal levels in type 2 diabetes. *Diabetes* **1999**, *48*, 198–202. [CrossRef]
240. Gupta, A.; Bisht, B.; Dey, C.S. Peripheral insulin-sensitizer drug metformin ameliorates neuronal insulin resistance and Alzheimer's-like changes. *Neuropharmacology* **2011**, *60*, 910–920. [CrossRef]
241. Ou, Z.; Kong, X.; Sun, X.; He, X.; Zhang, L.; Gong, Z.; Huang, J.; Xu, B.; Long, D.; Li, J.; et al. Metformin treatment prevents amyloid plaque deposition and memory impairment in APP/PS1 mice. *Brain. Behav. Immun.* **2018**, *69*, 351–363. [CrossRef]

242. Chiang, M.-C.; Cheng, Y.-C.; Chen, S.-J.; Yen, C.-H.; Huang, R.-N. Metformin activation of AMPK-dependent pathways is neuroprotective in human neural stem cells against Amyloid-beta-induced mitochondrial dysfunction. *Exp. Cell Res.* **2016**, *347*, 322–331. [CrossRef]
243. Perez-Revuelta, B.I.; Hettich, M.M.; Ciociaro, A.; Rotermund, C.; Kahle, P.J.; Krauss, S.; Di Monte, D.A. Metformin lowers Ser-129 phosphorylated α-synuclein levels via mTOR-dependent protein phosphatase 2A activation. *Cell Death Dis.* **2014**, *5*, e1209. [CrossRef] [PubMed]
244. Katila, N.; Bhurtel, S.; Shadfar, S.; Srivastav, S.; Neupane, S.; Ojha, U.; Jeong, G.-S.; Choi, D.-Y. Metformin lowers α-synuclein phosphorylation and upregulates neurotrophic factor in the MPTP mouse model of Parkinson's disease. *Neuropharmacology* **2017**, *125*, 396–407. [CrossRef]
245. Dulovic, M.; Jovanovic, M.; Xilouri, M.; Stefanis, L.; Harhaji-Trajkovic, L.; Stevovic, T.K.; Paunovic, V.; Ardah, M.T.; El-Agnaf, O.M.; Kostic, V.; et al. The protective role of AMP-activated protein kinase in alpha-synuclein neurotoxicity in vitro. *Neurobiol. Dis.* **2014**, *63*, 1–11. [CrossRef] [PubMed]
246. Lu, M.; Su, C.; Qiao, C.; Bian, Y.; Ding, J.; Hu, G. Metformin Prevents Dopaminergic Neuron Death in MPTP/P-Induced Mouse Model of Parkinson's Disease via Autophagy and Mitochondrial ROS Clearance. *Int. J. Neuro-Psychopharmacol.* **2016**, *19*, pyw047. [CrossRef] [PubMed]
247. Ryu, Y.K.; Park, H.Y.; Go, J.; Choi, D.H.; Kim, Y.H.; Hwang, J.H.; Noh, J.R.; Lee, T.G.; Lee, C.H.; Kim, K.S. Metformin Inhibits the Development of L-DOPA-Induced Dyskinesia in a Murine Model of Parkinson's Disease. *Mol. Neurobiol.* **2018**, *55*, 5715–5726. [CrossRef] [PubMed]
248. Ng, T.P.; Feng, L.; Yap, K.B.; Lee, T.S.; Tan, C.H.; Winblad, B. Long-Term Metformin Usage and Cognitive Function among Older Adults with Diabetes. *J. Alzheimer's Dis.* **2014**, *41*, 61–68. [CrossRef]
249. Imfeld, P.; Bodmer, M.; Jick, S.S.; Meier, C.R. Metformin, other antidiabetic drugs, and risk of Alzheimer's disease: A population-based case-control study. *J. Am. Geriatr. Soc.* **2012**, *60*, 916–921. [CrossRef]
250. Moore, E.M.; Mander, A.G.; Ames, D.; Kotowicz, M.A.; Carne, R.P.; Brodaty, H.; Woodward, M.; Boundy, K.; Ellis, K.A.; Bush, A.I.; et al. Increased risk of cognitive impairment in patients with diabetes is associated with metformin. *Diabetes Care* **2013**, *36*, 2981–2987. [CrossRef]
251. Kuan, Y.C.; Huang, K.W.; Lin, C.L.; Hu, C.J.; Kao, C.H. Effects of metformin exposure on neurodegenerative diseases in elderly patients with type 2 diabetes mellitus. *Prog. Neuro-Psychopharmacol. Biol. Psychiatry* **2017**, *79 Pt B*, 77–83. [CrossRef]
252. Ping, F.; Jiang, N.; Li, Y. Association between metformin and neurodegenerative diseases of observational studies: Systematic review and meta-analysis. *BMJ Open Diabetes Res. Care* **2020**, *8*, e001370. [CrossRef]
253. Qin, X.; Zhang, X.; Li, P.; Wang, M.; Yan, L.; Bao, Z.; Liu, Q. Association Between Diabetes Medications and the Risk of Parkinson's Disease: A Systematic Review and Meta-Analysis. *Front. Neurol.* **2021**, *12*, 678649. [CrossRef] [PubMed]
254. Chen, J.; Li, S.; Sun, W.; Li, J. Anti-diabetes drug pioglitazone ameliorates synaptic defects in AD transgenic mice by inhibiting cyclin-dependent kinase5 activity. *PLoS ONE* **2015**, *10*, e0123864. [CrossRef] [PubMed]
255. Assaf, N.; El-Shamarka, M.E.; Salem, N.A.; Khadrawy, Y.A.; El Sayed, N.S. Neuroprotective effect of PPAR α and γ agonists in a mouse model of amyloidogenesis through modulation of the Wnt/β catenin pathway via targeting α- and β-secretases. *Prog. Neuro-Psychopharmacol. Biol. Psychiatry* **2020**, *97*, 109793. [CrossRef] [PubMed]
256. Searcy, J.L.; Phelps, J.T.; Pancani, T.; Kadish, I.; Popovic, J.; Anderson, K.L.; Beckett, T.L.; Murphy, M.P.; Chen, K.-C.; Blalock, E.M.; et al. Long-Term Pioglitazone Treatment Improves Learning and Attenuates Pathological Markers in a Mouse Model of Alzheimer's Disease. *J. Alzheimer's Dis.* **2012**, *30*, 943–961. [CrossRef] [PubMed]
257. Escribano, L.; Simón, A.M.; Gimeno, E.; Cuadrado-Tejedor, M.; López de Maturana, R.; García-Osta, A.; Ricobaraza, A.; Pérez-Mediavilla, A.; Del Río, J.; Frechilla, D. Rosiglitazone rescues memory impairment in Alzheimer's transgenic mice: Mechanisms involving a reduced amyloid and tau pathology. *Neuropsychopharmacology* **2010**, *35*, 1593–1604. [CrossRef]
258. Chen, H.-H.; Chang, P.-C.; Wey, S.-P.; Chen, P.-M.; Chen, C.; Chan, M.-H. Therapeutic effects of honokiol on motor impairment in hemiparkinsonian mice are associated with reversing neurodegeneration and targeting PPARγ regulation. *Biomed. Pharmacother.* **2018**, *108*, 254–262. [CrossRef]
259. Machado, M.M.F.; Bassani, T.B.; Cóppola-Segovia, V.; Moura, E.L.R.; Zanata, S.M.; Andreatini, R.; Vital, M. PPAR-γ agonist pioglitazone reduces microglial proliferation and NF-κB activation in the substantia nigra in the 6-hydroxydopamine model of Parkinson's disease. *Pharmacol. Rep.* **2019**, *71*, 556–564. [CrossRef]
260. Hassanzadeh, K.; Rahimmi, A.; Moloudi, M.R.; Maccarone, R.; Corbo, M.; Izadpanah, E.; Feligioni, M. Effect of lobeglitazone on motor function in rat model of Parkinson's disease with diabetes co-morbidity. *Brain Res. Bull.* **2021**, *173*, 184–192. [CrossRef]
261. Das, N.R.; Vaidya, B.; Khare, P.; Bishnoi, M.; Sharma, S.S. Combination of Peroxisome Proliferator-activated Receptor γ (PPARγ) Agonist and PPAR Gamma Co-Activator 1α (PGC-1α) Activator Ameliorates Cognitive Deficits, Oxidative Stress, and Inflammation in Rodent Model of Parkinson's Disease. *Curr. Neurovasc. Res.* **2021**, *18*, 497–507. [CrossRef]
262. Schintu, N.; Frau, L.; Ibba, M.; Caboni, P.; Garau, A.; Carboni, E.; Carta, A.R. PPAR-gamma-mediated neuroprotection in a chronic mouse model of Parkinson's disease. *Eur. J. Neurosci.* **2009**, *29*, 954–963. [CrossRef]
263. Breidert, T.; Callebert, J.; Heneka, M.T.; Landreth, G.; Launay, J.M.; Hirsch, E.C. Protective action of the peroxisome proliferator-activated receptor-γ agonist pioglitazone in a mouse model of Parkinson's disease. *J. Neurochem.* **2002**, *82*, 615–624. [CrossRef] [PubMed]

264. Ghosh, A.; Tyson, T.; George, S.; Hildebrandt, E.N.; Steiner, J.A.; Madaj, Z.; Schulz, E.; Machiela, E.; McDonald, W.G.; Escobar Galvis, M.L.; et al. Mitochondrial pyruvate carrier regulates autophagy, inflammation, and neurodegeneration in experimental models of Parkinson's disease. *Sci. Transl. Med.* **2016**, *8*, 368ra174. [CrossRef] [PubMed]
265. Sato, T.; Hanyu, H.; Hirao, K.; Kanetaka, H.; Sakurai, H.; Iwamoto, T. Efficacy of PPAR-γ agonist pioglitazone in mild Alzheimer disease. *Neurobiol. Aging* **2011**, *32*, 1626–1633. [CrossRef] [PubMed]
266. Watson, G.S.; Cholerton, B.A.; Reger, M.A.; Baker, L.D.; Plymate, S.R.; Asthana, S.; Fishel, M.A.; Kulstad, J.J.; Green, P.S.; Cook, D.G.; et al. Preserved cognition in patients with early Alzheimer disease and amnestic mild cognitive impairment during treatment with rosiglitazone: A preliminary study. *Am. J. Geriatr. Psychiatry* **2005**, *13*, 950–958. [CrossRef] [PubMed]
267. Cao, B.; Rosenblat, J.D.; Brietzke, E.; Park, C.; Lee, Y.; Musial, N.; Pan, Z.; Mansur, R.B.; McIntyre, R.S. Comparative efficacy and acceptability of antidiabetic agents for Alzheimer's disease and mild cognitive impairment: A systematic review and network meta-analysis. *Diabetes Obes. Metab.* **2018**, *20*, 2467–2471. [CrossRef] [PubMed]
268. Osborne, C.; West, E.; Nolan, W.; McHale-Owen, H.; Williams, A.; Bate, C. Glimepiride protects neurons against amyloid-β-induced synapse damage. *Neuropharmacology* **2016**, *101*, 225–236. [CrossRef]
269. Hsu, C.C.; Wahlqvist, M.L.; Lee, M.S.; Tsai, H.N. Incidence of dementia is increased in type 2 diabetes and reduced by the use of sulfonylureas and metformin. *J. Alzheimer's Dis.* **2011**, *24*, 485–493. [CrossRef] [PubMed]
270. Tat, V.; Forest, C.P. The role of SGLT2 inhibitors in managing type 2 diabetes. *J. Am. Acad. Physician Assist.* **2018**, *31*, 35–40. [CrossRef]
271. Lin, B.; Koibuchi, N.; Hasegawa, Y.; Sueta, D.; Toyama, K.; Uekawa, K.; Ma, M.; Nakagawa, T.; Kusaka, H.; Kim-Mitsuyama, S. Glycemic control with empagliflozin, a novel selective SGLT2 inhibitor, ameliorates cardiovascular injury and cognitive dysfunction in obese and type 2 diabetic mice. *Cardiovasc. Diabetol.* **2014**, *13*, 148. [CrossRef]
272. Naznin, F.; Sakoda, H.; Okada, T.; Tsubouchi, H.; Waise, T.Z.; Arakawa, K.; Nakazato, M. Canagliflozin, a sodium glucose cotransporter 2 inhibitor, attenuates obesity-induced inflammation in the nodose ganglion, hypothalamus, and skeletal muscle of mice. *Eur. J. Pharmacol.* **2017**, *794*, 37–44. [CrossRef]
273. Sa-Nguanmoo, P.; Tanajak, P.; Kerdphoo, S.; Jaiwongkam, T.; Pratchayasakul, W.; Chattipakorn, N.; Chattipakorn, S.C. SGLT2-inhibitor and DPP-4 inhibitor improve brain function via attenuating mitochondrial dysfunction, insulin resistance, inflammation, and apoptosis in HFD-induced obese rats. *Toxicol. Appl. Pharmacol.* **2017**, *333*, 43–50. [CrossRef] [PubMed]
274. Zhou, M.; Chen, S.; Peng, P.; Gu, Z.; Yu, J.; Zhao, G.; Deng, Y. Dulaglutide ameliorates STZ induced AD-like impairment of learning and memory ability by modulating hyperphosphorylation of tau and NFs through GSK3β. *Biochem. Biophys. Res. Commun.* **2019**, *511*, 154–160. [CrossRef] [PubMed]
275. Batista, A.F.; Forny-Germano, L.; Clarke, J.R.; E Silva, N.M.L.; Brito-Moreira, J.; Boehnke, S.; Winterborn, A.; Coe, B.; Lablans, A.; Vital, J.F.; et al. The diabetes drug liraglutide reverses cognitive impairment in mice and attenuates insulin receptor and synaptic pathology in a non-human primate model of Alzheimer's disease. *J. Pathol.* **2018**, *245*, 85–100. [CrossRef] [PubMed]
276. Duarte, A.I.; Candeias, E.; Alves, I.N.; Mena, D.; Silva, D.F.; Machado, N.J.; Campos, E.J.; Santos, M.S.; Oliveira, C.R.; Moreira, P.I. Liraglutide Protects Against Brain Amyloid-β1–42 Accumulation in Female Mice with Early Alzheimer's Disease-Like Pathology by Partially Rescuing Oxidative/Nitrosative Stress and Inflammation. *Int. J. Mol. Sci.* **2020**, *21*, 1746. [CrossRef] [PubMed]
277. McClean, P.L.; Parthsarathy, V.; Faivre, E.; Hölscher, C. The Diabetes Drug Liraglutide Prevents Degenerative Processes in a Mouse Model of Alzheimer's Disease. *J. Neurosci.* **2011**, *31*, 6587–6594. [CrossRef]
278. Labandeira, C.M.; Fraga-Bau, A.; Arias Ron, D.; Muñoz, A.; Alonso-Losada, G.; Koukoulis, A.; Romero-Lopez, J.; Rodriguez-Perez, A.I. Diabetes, insulin and new therapeutic strategies for Parkinson's disease: Focus on glucagon-like peptide-1 receptor agonists. *Front. Neuroendocrinol.* **2021**, *62*, 100914. [CrossRef]
279. Labandeira, C.; Fraga-Bau, A.; Ron, D.A.; Alvarez-Rodriguez, E.; Vicente-Alba, P.; Lago-Garma, J.; Rodriguez-Perez, A. Parkinson's disease and diabetes mellitus: Common mechanisms and treatment repurposing. *Neural Regen. Res.* **2022**, *17*, 1652. [CrossRef]
280. Aviles-Olmos, I.; Dickson, J.; Kefalopoulou, Z.; Djamshidian, A.; Ell, P.; Soderlund, T.; Whitton, P.; Wyse, R.; Isaacs, T.; Lees, A.; et al. Exenatide and the treatment of patients with Parkinson's disease. *J. Clin. Investig.* **2013**, *123*, 2730–2736. [CrossRef]
281. Aviles-Olmos, I.; Dickson, J.; Kefalopoulou, Z.; Djamshidian, A.; Kahan, J.; Ell, P.; Whitton, P.; Wyse, R.; Isaacs, T.; Lees, A.; et al. Motor and Cognitive Advantages Persist 12 Months after Exenatide Exposure in Parkinson's Disease. *J. Park. Dis.* **2014**, *4*, 337–344. [CrossRef]
282. Athauda, D.; Maclagan, K.; Skene, S.S.; Bajwa-Joseph, M.; Letchford, D.; Chowdhury, K.; Hibbert, S.; Budnik, N.; Zampedri, L.; Dickson, J.; et al. Exenatide once weekly versus placebo in Parkinson's disease: A randomised, double-blind, placebo-controlled trial. *Lancet* **2017**, *390*, 1664–1675. [CrossRef]
283. Wang, S.-Y.; Wu, S.-L.; Chen, T.-C.; Chuang, C.-S. Antidiabetic Agents for Treatment of Parkinson's Disease: A Meta-Analysis. *Int. J. Environ. Res. Public Health* **2020**, *17*, 4805. [CrossRef] [PubMed]
284. Wu, P.; Dong, Y.; Chen, J.; Guan, T.; Cao, B.; Zhang, Y.; Qi, Y.; Guan, Z.; Wang, Y. Liraglutide Regulates Mitochondrial Quality Control System through PGC-1α in a Mouse Model of Parkinson's Disease. *Neurotox. Res.* **2022**, *40*, 286–297. [CrossRef] [PubMed]
285. Cao, B.; Zhang, Y.; Chen, J.; Wu, P.; Dong, Y.; Wang, Y. Neuroprotective effects of liraglutide against inflammation through the AMPK/NF-κB pathway in a mouse model of Parkinson's disease. *Metab. Brain Dis.* **2022**, *37*, 451–462. [CrossRef] [PubMed]
286. Badawi, G.A.; Abd El Fattah, M.A.; Zaki, H.F.; El Sayed, M.I. Sitagliptin and liraglutide reversed nigrostriatal degeneration of rodent brain in rotenone-induced Parkinson's disease. *Inflammopharmacology* **2017**, *25*, 369–382. [CrossRef] [PubMed]

287. Zhang, L.; Li, L.; Hölscher, C. Neuroprotective effects of the novel GLP-1 long acting analogue semaglutide in the MPTP Parkinson's disease mouse model. *Neuropeptides* **2018**, *71*, 70–80. [CrossRef] [PubMed]
288. Zhang, L.; Li, L.; Hölscher, C. Semaglutide is Neuroprotective and Reduces α-Synuclein Levels in the Chronic MPTP Mouse Model of Parkinson's Disease. *J. Parkinson's Dis.* **2019**, *9*, 157–171. [CrossRef]
289. Kosaraju, J.; Holsinger, R.M.D.; Guo, L.; Tam, K.Y. Linagliptin, a Dipeptidyl Peptidase-4 Inhibitor, Mitigates Cognitive Deficits and Pathology in the 3xTg-AD Mouse Model of Alzheimer's Disease. *Mol. Neurobiol.* **2017**, *54*, 6074–6084. [CrossRef]
290. Kosaraju, J.; Murthy, V.; Khatwal, R.B.; Dubala, A.; Chinni, S.; Muthureddy Nataraj, S.K.; Basavan, D. Vildagliptin: An antidiabetes agent ameliorates cognitive deficits and pathology observed in streptozotocin-induced Alzheimer's disease. *J. Pharm. Pharmacol.* **2013**, *65*, 1773–1784. [CrossRef]
291. Chen, S.; Zhou, M.; Sun, J.; Guo, A.; Fernando, R.L.; Chen, Y.; Peng, P.; Zhao, G.; Deng, Y. DPP-4 inhibitor improves learning and memory deficits and AD-like neurodegeneration by modulating the GLP-1 signaling. *Neuropharmacology* **2019**, *157*, 107668. [CrossRef]
292. Li, J.; Zhang, S.; Li, C.; Li, M.; Ma, L. Sitagliptin rescues memory deficits in Parkinsonian rats via upregulating BDNF to prevent neuron and dendritic spine loss. *Neurol. Res.* **2018**, *40*, 736–743. [CrossRef]
293. Brauer, R.; Wei, L.; Ma, T.; Athauda, D.; Girges, C.; Vijiaratnam, N.; Auld, G.; Whittlesea, C.; Wong, I.; Foltynie, T. Diabetes medications and risk of Parkinson's disease: A cohort study of patients with diabetes. *Brain* **2020**, *143*, 3067–3076. [CrossRef]
294. Zhou, B.; Zissimopoulos, J.; Nadeem, H.; Crane, M.A.; Goldman, D.; Romley, J.A. Association between exenatide use and incidence of Alzheimer's disease. *Alzheimer's Dement. Transl. Res. Clin. Interv.* **2021**, *7*, e12895. [CrossRef] [PubMed]
295. Ribeiro, M.J.; Sacramento, J.F.; Gonzalez, C.; Guarino, M.P.; Monteiro, E.C.; Conde, S.V. Carotid Body Denervation Prevents the Development of Insulin Resistance and Hypertension Induced by Hypercaloric Diets. *Diabetes* **2013**, *62*, 2905–2916. [CrossRef] [PubMed]
296. Ribeiro, M.J.; Sacramento, J.F.; Gallego-Martin, T.; Olea, E.; Melo, B.F.; Guarino, M.P.; Yubero, S.; Obeso, A.; Conde, S.V. High fat diet blunts the effects of leptin on ventilation and on carotid body activity. *J. Physiol.* **2018**, *596*, 3187–3199. [CrossRef] [PubMed]
297. Sacramento, J.F.; Ribeiro, M.J.; Rodrigues, T.; Olea, E.; Melo, B.F.; Guarino, M.P.; Fonseca-Pinto, R.; Ferreira, C.R.; Coelho, J.; Obeso, A.; et al. Functional abolition of carotid body activity restores insulin action and glucose homeostasis in rats: Key roles for visceral adipose tissue and the liver. *Diabetologia* **2016**, *60*, 158–168. [CrossRef] [PubMed]
298. González, C.; López-López, J.; Obeso, A.; Pérez-García, M.T.; Rocher, A. Cellular mechanisms of oxygen chemoreception in the carotid body. *Respir. Physiol.* **1995**, *102*, 137–147. [CrossRef]
299. Nurse, C.A. Synaptic and paracrine mechanisms at carotid body arterial chemoreceptors. *J. Physiol.* **2014**, *592*, 3419–3426. [CrossRef]
300. Zera, T.; Moraes, D.J.A.; Da Silva, M.P.; Fisher, J.P.; Paton, J.F.R. The Logic of Carotid Body Connectivity to the Brain. *Physiology* **2019**, *34*, 264–282. [CrossRef]
301. Sacramento, J.F.; Chew, D.J.; Melo, B.; Donegá, M.; Dopson, W.; Guarino, M.P.; Robinson, A.; Prieto-Lloret, J.; Patel, S.; Holinski, B.J.; et al. Bioelectronic modulation of carotid sinus nerve activity in the rat: A potential therapeutic approach for type 2 diabetes. *Diabetologia* **2018**, *61*, 700–710. [CrossRef]
302. Cunha-Guimaraes, J.P.; Guarino, M.P.; Timóteo, A.T.; Caires, I.; Sacramento, J.F.; Ribeiro, M.J.; Selas, M.; Santiago, J.C.P.; Carmo, M.; Conde, S.V. Carotid body chemosensitivity: Early biomarker of dysmetabolism in humans. *Eur. J. Endocrinol.* **2020**, *182*, 549–557. [CrossRef]
303. Pauza, A.G.; Thakkar, P.; Tasic, T.; Felippe, I.; Bishop, P.; Greenwood, M.P.; Rysevaite-Kyguoliene, K.; Ast, J.; Broichhagen, J.; Hodson, D.J.; et al. GLP1R Attenuates Sympathetic Response to High Glucose via Carotid Body Inhibition. *Circ. Res.* **2022**, *130*, 694–707. [CrossRef] [PubMed]
304. Cracchiolo, M.; Sacramento, J.F.; Mazzoni, A.; Panarese, A.; Carpaneto, J.; Conde, S.V.; Micera, S. Decoding Neural Metabolic Markers from the Carotid Sinus Nerve in a Type 2 Diabetes Model. *IEEE Trans. Neural Syst. Rehabil. Eng.* **2019**, *27*, 2034–2043. [CrossRef] [PubMed]

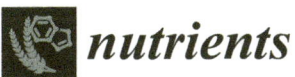

Review

# D-Pinitol—Active Natural Product from Carob with Notable Insulin Regulation

**Abdullatif Azab**

Carobway Ltd., Nes Ziona 7406520, Israel; abedazab@carobway.com; Tel.: +972-50-5650025

**Abstract:** Carob is one of the major food trees for peoples of the Mediterranean basin, but it has also been traditionally used for medicinal purposes. Carob contains many nutrients and active natural products, and D-Pinitol is clearly one of the most important of these. D-Pinitol has been reported in dozens of scientific publications and its very diverse medicinal properties are still being studied. Presently, more than thirty medicinal activities of D-Pinitol have been reported. Among these, many publications have reported the strong activities of D-Pinitol as a natural antidiabetic and insulin regulator, but also as an active anti-Alzheimer, anticancer, antioxidant, and anti-inflammatory, and is also immune- and hepato-protective. In this review, we will present a brief introduction of the nutritional and medicinal importance of Carob, both traditionally and as found by modern research. In the introduction, we will present Carob's major active natural products. The structures of inositols will be presented with a brief literature summary of their medicinal activities, with special attention to those inositols in Carob, as well as D-Pinitol's chemical structure and its medicinal and other properties. D-Pinitol antidiabetic and insulin regulation activities will be extensively presented, including its proposed mechanism of action. Finally, a discussion followed by the conclusions and future vision will summarize this article.

**Keywords:** carob; inositols; D-Pinitol; medicinal activities; antidiabetic; insulin regulator; mechanism of action

**Citation:** Azab, A. D-Pinitol—Active Natural Product from Carob with Notable Insulin Regulation. *Nutrients* 2022, 14, 1453. https://doi.org/10.3390/nu14071453

Academic Editors: Silvia V. Conde and Fatima O. Martins

Received: 3 March 2022
Accepted: 29 March 2022
Published: 30 March 2022

**Publisher's Note:** MDPI stays neutral with regard to jurisdictional claims in published maps and institutional affiliations.

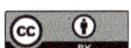

**Copyright:** © 2022 by the author. Licensee MDPI, Basel, Switzerland. This article is an open access article distributed under the terms and conditions of the Creative Commons Attribution (CC BY) license (https://creativecommons.org/licenses/by/4.0/).

## 1. Introduction

### 1.1. Carob: The Faithful Companion of Humanity

Carob (*Ceratonia siliqua* L.) is one of the most important nutritional crops for peoples of the Middle East, North Africa, and Southern Europe [1]. Carob fruits (named pods or kibbles), contain a wide range of macro- and micronutrients, as well as many other natural products. A summary of Carob fruit composition is presented in Table 1.

**Table 1.** General composition of Carob fruits [2].

| Component | Proportion (%) |
|---|---|
| Moisture | 6.3–7.6 |
| Protein | 1.7–5.9 |
| Ash | 2.3–3.2 |
| Fat | 0.2–4.4 |
| Total dietary fiber | 11.7–47 |
| Starch | 0.1 |
| Total carbohydrates | 42–86 |
| Fructose | 2–7.4 |
| Glucose | 3–7.3 |
| Sucrose | 15–34 |
| D-Pinitol | 5.5 |

However, since antiquity, humans have used different parts of the Carob tree for many and interesting purposes [3]. Among these, analgesic and anti-inflammatory activities are the most important [4,5]. Most of the traditional medicine uses have utilized different forms of fruits, including unripe pods, but these utilizations included extracts, decoctions and infusions of leaves and bark [6].

Modern research followed traditional knowledge and dozens of studies were published to date about dozens of medicinal activities of Carob's various products, including its extracts and single natural products. Consequently, many review articles that summarize the research articles can also be found [7–10]. However, one of the best review articles about Carob's composition has been published by K. Rtibi et al., where they focus on Carob-derived treatments of the gastrointestinal tract [11]. In Figure 1, major and new (red names) phenolic compounds are shown [12–14].

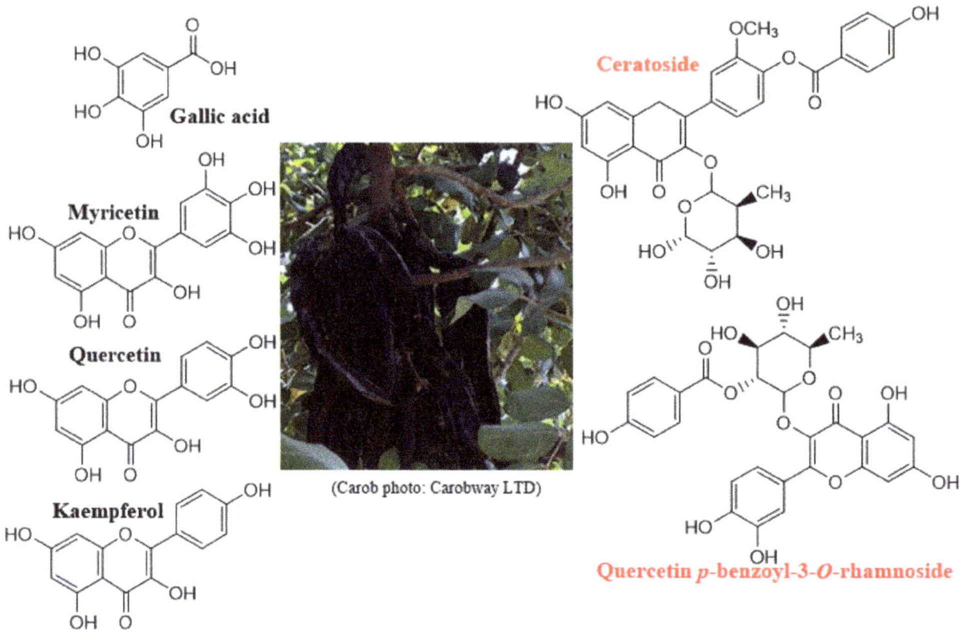

**Figure 1.** Major and new phenolic compounds found in Carob pods and leaves [12–14].

To conclude this section, it is important to indicate that in recent years there has emerged a rapidly growing interest in Carob seeds, their composition (protein rich), nutritional potential and medicinal activities [2,15,16].

### 1.2. Insulin Resistance in Type 2 Diabetes

Type 2 diabetes (T2D) is defined by the World Health Organization (WHO) as a "metabolic disorder of multiple etiology characterized by chronic hyperglycemia with disturbance of carbohydrate, fat, and protein metabolism resulting from defects in insulin secretion, insulin action, or both" [17]. The International Diabetes Federation reported that in 2018, there were 463 million people around the world affected by this disease, and the organization estimates that by 2045, there will be 700 million people affected by it [18]. It has also been reported that in 2017, the global healthcare expenditure associated with diabetes and its complications was USD 850 billion. The prevalence rate is estimated as 13.5% in low-income countries, compared with 10.4% in high-income nations. It is interesting to mention the fact that this trend is also found within different ethnicities in the same country. In the USA, the ethnic distribution of T2D follows the "rule" higher-income-lower-diabetes: Non-Hispanic Whites (highest income) 7.6%, Asians 9%, Hispanics 12.8%, and African Americans (lowest income) 13.2%, in 2017 [19]. In Israel, the author's home country, there are 12% of diabetics among Arabs (lower income) and 6.2% among Jews (higher income) [20].

Therefore, in the abovementioned definition of T2D, insulin plays a critical role, and "insulin resistance" is the major cause of this disease. This health disorder is defined as: "a defect in insulin-mediated control of glucose metabolism in tissues—prominently in muscle, fat and liver" [17], but insulin has various functions in the human body, and they are presented in Table 2 [21].

Table 2. Functions of insulin in human body [21].

| Effect Type | Role of Insulin |
|---|---|
| Metabolic | Stimulation of glucose transport and metabolism |
| | Stimulation of glycogen synthesis |
| | Stimulation of lipogenesis |
| | Inhibition of lipolysis |
| | Stimulation of ion flux |
| Growth-promoting | Stimulation of DNA synthesis |
| | Stimulation of cell growth and differentiation |
| Metabolic & Growth-promoting | Stimulation of amino acid influx |
| | Stimulation of protein synthesis |
| | Inhibition of protein degradation |
| | Stimulation of RNA synthesis |

The mechanism of action of insulin in healthy conditions can be found in many publications [22], and a simplified illustration of it is shown in Figure 2.

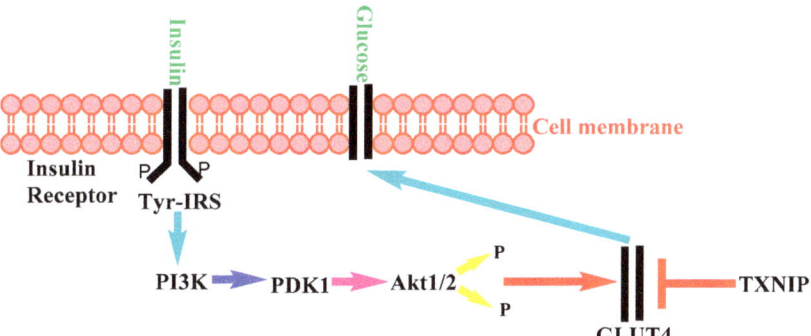

Figure 2. Insulin mechanism of action in healthy conditions.

Insulin enters the cell through an insulin receptor. As a result, tyrosine (Tyr) phosphorylation occurs on the insulin receptor substrate (IRS) protein. The resulting adduct activates phosphoinositide 3-kinase (PI3K), resulting in activation of phosphoinositide-dependent kinase-1,2 (PDK1/2). Protein kinase (AKT) gets phosphorylated by PDK1/2 and promotes glucose transporter 4 (GLUT4) translocation to plasma membrane and facilitates glucose into cell. Thioredoxin interacting protein (TXNIP) inhibits is blocked.

Numerous research articles have been published about this key factor of T2D, and dozens of review articles that summarize these research publications. However, it is important to understand the possible mechanisms of insulin resistance that were also presented in most of these scientific publications. One of the most comprehensive and illustrated review articles was published by M.C. Petersen and G.I. Shulman [23]. Insulin resistance is discussed as major and sub-major types, where each section is illustrated with many figures and graphs.

The review article of H. Yaribeygi et al. follows the previous reference, though it is far less comprehensive [24]. However, one of its clearest advantages is the table that summarizes the molecular mechanisms that are involved in insulin resistance (page 6 in Ref. [24]), and it is partially cited here as shown in Table 3.

Table 3. Molecular mechanisms of insulin resistance [24].

| Molecular Mechanism | Roles in Insulin Resistance |
|---|---|
| Upregulation of PTP1B [25] | Reverses insulin-induced phosphorylation in tyrosine residues of IRS-1 and so impairs insulin signal transduction |
| Inflammatory mediators and adipokines | Activation of IKKβ/NF-κB and JNK pathways, serine phosphorylation of IRS-1 in the site of 307, declines GLUT-4 expression, reduces IRS-1 expression via ERK1/2, induce IRS degradation through SOCS1- and SOCS3-dependent mechanisms |
| Free radical overload | Activates several serine–threonine kinase pathways, i.e., IKKβ/NF-κB and JNK, IRS degradation, suppresses GLUT-4 expression and localization in cell membrane, decreases insulin-induced IRS-1 and PIP-kinase relocation between cytoplasm and microsomes, decreases PKB phosphorylation, serine phosphorylation at site of serine 307 of IRS-1, activates inflammatory responses |
| Defects in serine phosphorylation of IRS-1 | Decrease in insulin receptor phosphorylation, phosphorylation in serine 307 which blocks signaling |
| Obesity and adipocytes importance | Decrease in insulin receptor phosphorylation, phosphorylation in serine 307 which blocks signaling |
| Accelerated insulin degradation | Autoimmune antibodies against insulin or abnormal insulin structure due to mutation |
| Mitochondrial dysfunction | Induces oxidative stress, impairs insulin signaling |
| Reduced the capacity of receptors to binding to insulin | Decrease in number of insulin receptors, reduction in functional receptors due to mutation, autoimmune antibodies against insulin receptors |
| Mutations of GLUT-4 | Point mutation changes normal modification of GLUT-4, inhibits glucose entering into dependent cells and impairs subsequent signaling pathways |
| ER stress | Disrupts proper protein folding leading to accumulation of misfolded proteins |

PTP1B [25], protein tyrosine phosphatase 1B; IRS-1, insulin receptor substrates-1; IKKβ/NF-κB, central regulator of NF-κB; GLUT-4, type 4 glucose transporter; ERK, extracellular signal-regulated kinase SOCS1/3, suppressor of cytokine signaling; JNK, c-Jun N-terminal kinase; ER, endoplasmic reticulum.

The review article of D.E. James has special importance for two major reasons [26]. First, it includes excellent figures that explain the putative factors that contribute to insulin resistance (Figure 4, page 12 in Ref. [26]). Second, it discusses the situation of fasting in insulin resistance conditions. This situation has great relevance for hundreds of millions of people around the world. Another review article with special importance about insulin resistance has been recently published by W.A. Banks and E.M. Rhea [27]. This article is important for three major reasons. First, it links insulin resistance with the brain–blood barrier (BBB); second, it discusses the relation of insulin signaling and oxidative stress manifestation in T2D and Alzheimer's disease; and third, it contains excellent illustrations, especially the figure that shows the interactions between insulin and oxidative stress.

*1.3. Treatment of Insulin Resistance with Natural Products*

As mentioned in the previous section, T2D is a severe global health issue and a major cause of financial burden. Consequently, many methods have been developed to target this disorder. However, before presenting treatments that are based on natural products, we will briefly present some selected synthetic pharmaceuticals.

C.L. Reading et al. have reported the anti-inflammatory activity and improvement of the insulin-sensitivity activity of synthetic sterol (Figure 3) in insulin-resistant obese-impaired glucose tolerance [28].

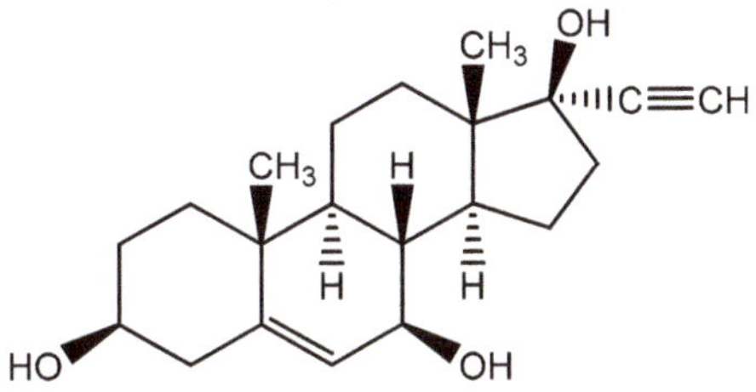

17$\alpha$-ethynylandrost-5-ene-3$\beta$,7$\beta$,17$\beta$-triol

**Figure 3.** Synthetic sterol with insulin-sensitivity improvement activity [29].

A significantly different approach has been reported by S. Xue et al. who report a treatment for hepatogenous diabetes using Oleanolic acid, which triggered the expression of short-peptide genetic synthesis [30]. The synergistic activity of Oleanolic acid and the peptide (researchers have named it shGLP-1), proved to be more efficient than the activity of each component separately. To conclude this part, we indicate the review article of R. Vieira et al. which is very informative and comprehensive [31].

Many natural products have been tested and published for their insulin regulation activity. F.S. Saadeldeen et al. list in their excellent review article 98 naturally occurring compounds that regulate glucose metabolism and treat insulin resistance [32]. This article provides the structure of each compound, its botanical source, and its activity.

Following traditional Chinese medicine therapeutic methods, J. Li et al. list pure natural products and herbal formulations used to treat insulin resistance [33]. Formulations are listed with their Chinese names, and detailed information about methods and purposes of use.

In addition to D-Pinitol, which will be discussed in Section 3, numerous natural products have been published in research articles for having insulin regulation activity. We limit our presentation here to two of these compounds that have been mentioned in very recent publications. First, R. Alaaeldin et al. reported the amelioration of insulin resistance of Carpachromene (Figure 4), a natural product that can be found in Banyan (*Ficus binghalensis* L.) [34].

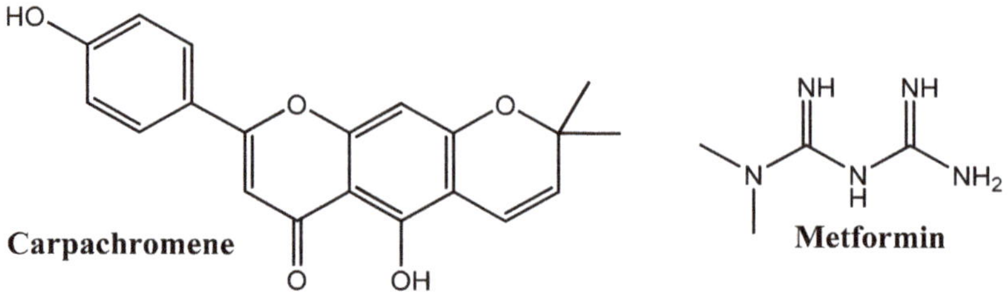

**Figure 4.** Carpachromene and Metformin.

They found (in vitro model) that Carpachromene has significant insulin resistance amelioration compared with Metformin, a synthetic drug widely used for treating this disorder.

The second report was published by A. Deenadayalan et al. who tested the effect of Stevioside (Figure 5) on insulin resistance, in both in vivo (rats) and in silico models [35].

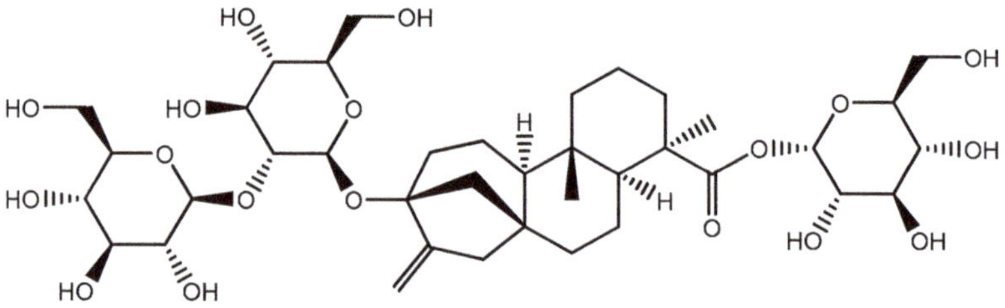

**Figure 5.** Stevioside (*Stevia rebaudiana* Bertoni).

Their findings indicate that this compound has similar activity to metformin.

Finally, it is important to mention very recent research published by H. Sanz-Lamora et al. that found that treatment with pure polyphenol supplementation (D18060501) worsened insulin resistance in diet-induced obese mice [36].

## 2. Inositols—A Brief Presentation

Inositols are naturally occurring *Cyclitols* or *Polyols*, and they can be found in mammalian and plant kingdoms [37]. In terms of more specific chemical structure, these natural products are stereoisomers of hexahydroxy cyclohexane. In Figure 6, the structures of naturally occurring inositols are shown.

The biological properties of inositols have been extensively studied and published. Most of these activities have been summarized by O.C. Watkins et al. [38]. These properties include insulin regulation, antidiabetic, antioxidant, antibacterial, female fertility enhancer, metabolic syndrome treatment, antidepressant, gastroprotective, hepatoprotective, hypolipidemic and antiaging. However, in this review and in most published literature about the properties of these compounds, it is clear that most studies have focused on two activities: insulin regulation and treatment of female fertility disorders. In Table 4 we cite some of these notable publications, in chronological order.

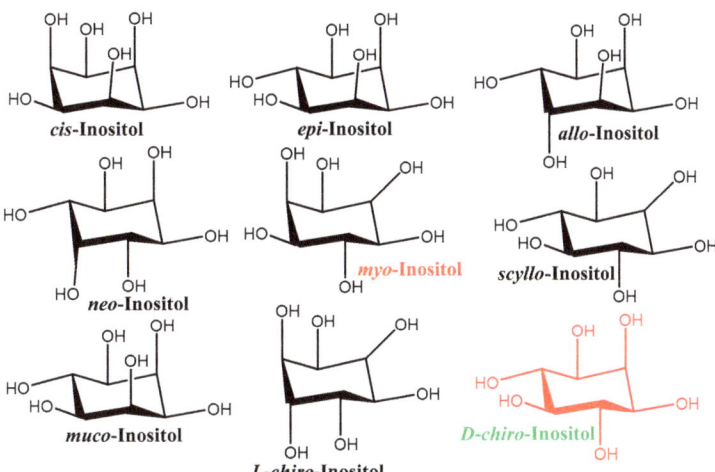

**Figure 6.** Structures of naturally occurring inositols.

**Table 4.** Selected publications of insulin regulation and women fertility disorders treatment of inositols.

| Property Short Description | Type of Publication | Ref., Year |
|---|---|---|
| Insulin regulation in human diabetics | research | [39], 1990 |
| Treatment respiratory disorders in infants | research | [40], 1992 |
| Insulin regulation in human diabetics | research | [41], 1993 |
| Treatments of psychiatric disorders | review | [42], 1997 |
| Treatment of polycystic ovary syndrome (PCOS) | research | [43], 1999 |
| Treatment of Alzheimer disease, in vitro | research | [44], 2000 |
| Insulin regulation in human diabetics | research | [45], 2005 |
| Treatment of endothelial dysfunction, antioxidant, animal model | research | [46], 2006 |
| Biological roles | review | [47], 2007 |
| Derivatives and their functions | review | [48], 2008 |
| Treatment of PCOS | review | [49], 2014 |
| Insulin regulation in obese male children | research | [50], 2016 |
| Treatment of PCOS | review | [51], 2016 |
| Treatment of PCOS | research | [52], 2017 |
| Bioavailability for treatment of PCOS | review | [53], 2017 |
| Treatment of PCOS in subfertile women | review | [54], 2018 |
| Effects on glucose homeostasis | review | [55], 2019 |
| General presentation of medicinal activities | review | [56], 2019 |
| Treatment of PCOS | review | [57], 2020 |
| Treatment of PCOS, with other technologies | review | [58], 2021 |
| Treatment of preterm birth | review | [59], 2021 |
| Treatment of psychological symptoms in PCOS | review | [60], 2021 |
| Insulin regulation in pregnancy | review | [38], 2022 |

From Carob, six inositols and their derivatives (methyl ethers) were isolated and characterized [61]. Their structures are shown in Figure 7.

*myo*-Inositol is the most abundant compound of this family in all life forms, followed by D-Pinitol and its precursor, D-*chiro*-Inositol, in the plant kingdom. D-Bornesitol and D-Sequoyitol are relatively rare, and their properties are almost unknown. D-Ononitol has been very limitedly studied [62,63].

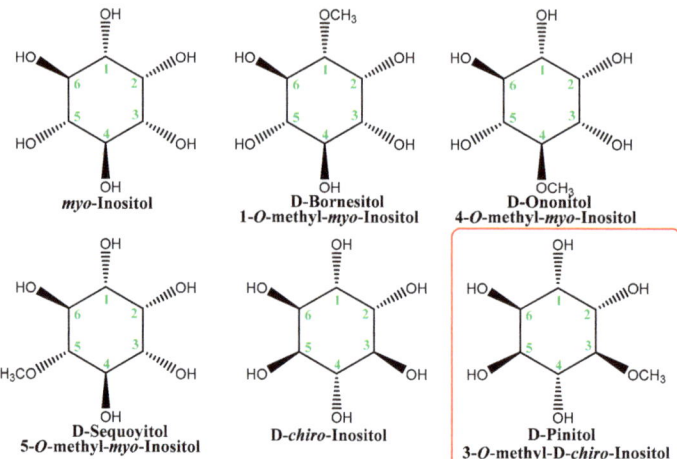

**Figure 7.** Inositols and their methyl ethers isolated from Carob.

## 3. D-Pinitol: Occurrence, Isolation, and Properties

D-Pinitol can be found in more than 20 plant sources, and its highest content is in Carob pods, at 5.5% [2,64]. To date, more than 40 publications have reported the quantification and/or isolation of this important natural product. One of the most notable works has been published by O. Negishi et al. [65]. They determined the content of methylated inositols in 43 edible plants by the HPAE-PAD analytical method. J. Qiu et al. reported the determination of D-Pinitol in rat plasma [66]. This study is highly important since it provides understanding of the pharmacokinetics and bioavailability of D-Pinitol in vivo.

The medicinal and other properties of D-Pinitol have been extensively studied and published. In Table 5, we list most of these reports, excluding publications that report no or low results.

**Table 5.** Published properties of D-Pinitol.

| Activity/Property | Testing Method | Ref. |
| --- | --- | --- |
| Anti-Alzheimer | In vivo, mice | [67] |
| Anti-Alzheimer | In vitro, hippocampal cultures | [68] |
| Anti-Alzheimer | In vivo, *C. elegans*, mice | [69] |
| Antiaging | In vivo, *D. Melanogaster* | [70] |
| Antibacterial | *M. smegmatis* | [71] |
| Anticancer | In vitro, human cancer cells | [72–77] |
| Anticancer | In vivo, rats | [78–83] |
| Anti-colitis | In vivo, rats | [84] |
| Antidepressant | In vivo, mice | [85] |
| Antidiabetic | In vivo, mice/rats | [86–92] |
| Antidiabetic | In vivo, humans | [93–98] |
| Antidiabetic | Theoretical evaluation | [99] |
| Antidiarrheal | In vivo, mice | [100] |
| Antifibrotic | In vivo, mice | [101] |
| Antihyperlipidemic | In vivo, rats | [64,102] |
| Anti-inflammatory | In vivo, mice/rats | [103–106] |
| Anti-inflammatory | In vitro, Human cells | [72,107,108] |
| Anti-inflammatory | In vitro, BV2 microglial cells | [109] |

Table 5. *Cont.*

| Activity/Property | Testing Method | Ref. |
|---|---|---|
| Antinociceptive | In vivo, mice | [100] |
| Anti-obesity | In vivo, humans | [110] |
| Anti-obesity | In vivo, rats | [111] |
| Anti-osteoclastic | In vitro, UAMS32 cells | [112] |
| Antioxidant | In vivo, rats | [78,81,82,88,113] |
| Anti-psoriatic | In vivo, mice | [114] |
| Antiviral | Theoretical evaluation | [115] |
| Asthma treatment | In vivo, mice | [116] |
| Bone protection | In vitro, Bone marrow cell lines, rats | [117] |
| Bone protection | In vivo, rats | [118] |
| Cardioprotective | In vivo, humans | [93] |
| Cardioprotective | In vivo, mice/rats | [119,120] |
| Cytotoxic | In vitro, human cancer cell lines | [121] |
| Diuretic | In vivo, mice | [122] |
| Geno-protective | In vitro, monkey liver cell lines | [123] |
| Hepatoprotective | In vivo, humans | [124] |
| Hepatoprotective | In vivo, mice/rats | [125–131] |
| Hydration biomarker | In vivo, humans | [132,133] |
| Hypotensive | In vivo, mice | [134] |
| Immuno-protective | Theoretical evaluation | [99] |
| Immuno-protective | In vivo, mice | [116,135,136] |
| Immunosuppressive | In vivo, mice | [137] |
| Insulin regulation | In vivo, mice/rats | [111,131,138–141] |
| Insulin regulation | In vivo, humans | [96,142] |
| Insulin regulation | In vitro, 3T3-L1, HUVEC cells | [143,144] |
| Memory enhancement | In vivo, rats | [90] |
| Nanoparticles loaded | In vitro, against *M. smegmatis* | [29] |
| Nephroprotective | In vivo, mice/rats | [105,145] |
| Neuroprotective | In vivo, mice/rats | [85,122,146–148] |
| Sleep enhancer | In vivo, *D. melanogaster*, in vitro PC12 cells | [149] |
| Synergism w/ curcumin | In vitro, PC12 cells, against $As^{+3}$ toxicity | [150] |
| Wound healing | In vivo, rats, in vitro, HaCaT cells | [151] |

## 4. D-Pinitol as Insulin Regulator

In Section 3, we cited eight important published studies about the activity of D-Pinitol as insulin regulator (Table 5). In fact, the number of publications about this topic is much higher, and many review articles have published about it and other medicinal properties of D-Pinitol. These review articles and the research publications that they cite, conclude that D-Pinitol has two mechanisms of action as an insulin regulator [152]: insulin sensitizing and insulin mimetic.

K. Srivastava et al. present the insulin-sensitizing effect of D-Pinitol in their review article about this natural product [153], and a simplified illustration of this effect is shown in Figure 8.

Interestingly, in a table that lists the botanical sources of D-Pinitol in Ref. [153] (page 3), the authors do not mention the three plants with the highest content of this natural product: Carob, Bougainvillea and Soybean [64].

T. Antonowski et al. present the insulin-like (insulin-mimetic) activity of D-Pinitol [154]. This publication, and others, demonstrates the simplified mechanism shown in Figure 9.

This minireview article is notably useful for understanding the structures of cyclitols and their role in ameliorating metabolic syndrome and diabetes.

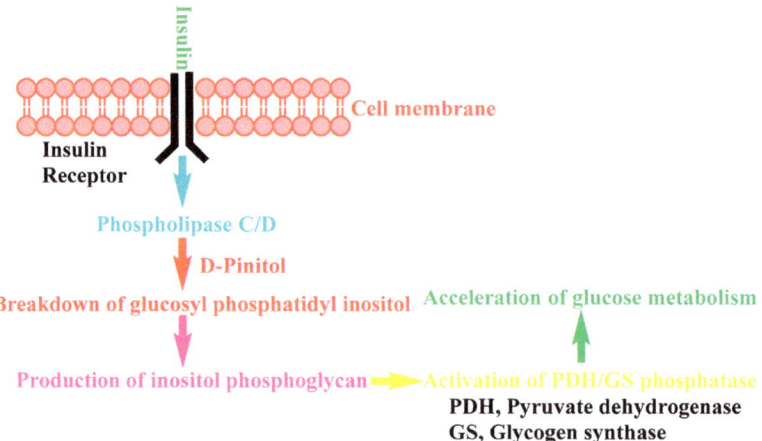

**Figure 8.** Insulin-sensitizing mechanism of D-Pinitol.

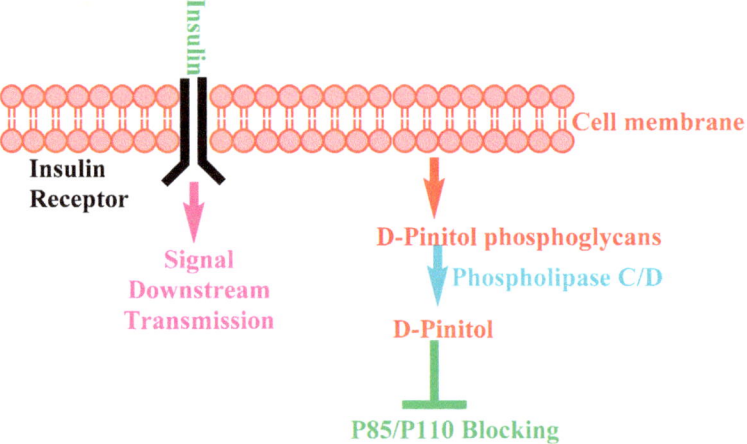

**Figure 9.** Insulin-mimetic mechanism of D-Pinitol.

## 5. Discussion

D-Pinitol is a naturally occurring inositol that can be found in many plant species. Carob has the highest content of D-Pinitol, which has a wide range of medicinal and other properties (Section 3). One of these, and probably the most important, is insulin regulation, which has two major mechanisms: insulin-sensitizing and insulin-mimetic [152].

Many natural products have one or both properties of insulin regulation, including plant extracts and other mixed compounds. For example, S.A. Kalekar et al. have reported on the in vitro insulin-sensitizing activity of hydroethanolic extracts of three plants: *Phyllanthus emblica* L., *Tinospora cordifolia* (Thunb.) Miers and *Curcuma longa* L. [155]. In a more recent study, V. Stadlbauer et al. tested more than 600 plant extracts and found three of them to have clear in vivo insulin-mimetic activity: *Xysmalobium undulatum* L., *Sapindus mukorossi* L., *Chelidonium majus* L. [156]. It is important to mention that in this study Carob is not included.

Despite the abovementioned, D-Pinitol, and D-Pinitol-containing products of Carob, have several advantages over other insulin-regulating plant products, due to the following reasons:

(A) D-Pinitol content of Carob (pods) is the highest of all plants [64].
(B) D-Pinitol-containing products of Carob such as molasses, have important health benefits [157].
(C) Compared with most other natural products that have insulin-regulation activity, such as polyphenols, D-Pinitol is more stable in biological gastric conditions [48]. This property increases its bioavailability in the human body.
(D) In addition to that which is mentioned in C, D-Pinitol is generally stable, but even if it undergoes methoxy group hydrolysis, the resulting compound is *chiro*-Inositol, which is an active insulin-regulator as well [158]. See Figure 6.
(E) Even though there is a limited number of studies that indicate it, it is evident that D-Pinitol's activities are significantly increased when it synergistically acts with other natural products [25,92,150,159].
(F) D-Pinitol has wide range of medicinal activities (Table 5), so it is a multi-functional natural product. This property increases its potential as a drug.

## 6. Conclusions and Future Horizons

Most of the medicinal properties of D-Pinitol have been studied and published. Some of these have been extensively investigated, while others were limitedly or even not published. It is very important to conduct further studies of all activities of D-Pinitol, but activities such as insulin regulation, anti-Alzheimer, antiaging and possible anti-Parkinson activities must draw more attention.

The synergistic effect of D-Pinitol with other natural products of Carob and other plants is in its beginnings, so this topic must also be thoroughly studied.

Our group is currently investigating some known and unpublished activities of D-Pinitol, and we are examining possible clinical and other applications that will hopefully lead to healthy foods, food-additives, and other healthy products.

**Funding:** This research received no external funding.

**Conflicts of Interest:** The author declares no conflict of interest.

## References

1. Azab, A. Carob (*Ceratonia siliqua*): Super Food and Medicine. Literature Update. *Eur. Chem. Bull.* **2020**, *9*, 306–312. [CrossRef]
2. Brassesco, M.E.; Brandao, T.; Silva, C.; Pintado, M. Carob bean (*Ceratonia siliqua* L.): A new perspective for functional food. *Trends Food Sci. Technol.* **2021**, *114*, 310–322. [CrossRef]
3. Azab, A. Carob (*Ceratonia siliqua*): Health, medicine and chemistry. *Eur. Chem. Bull.* **2017**, *6*, 456–469. [CrossRef]
4. Ben Ayache, S.; Behija Saafi, E.; Emhemmed, F.; Flamini, G.; Achour, L.; Muller, C.D. Biological activities of aqueous extracts from Carob plant (*Ceratonia siliqua* L.) by antioxidant, analgesic and proapoptotic properties evaluation. *Molecules* **2020**, *25*, 3120. [CrossRef]
5. Khalifa, A.B. *Herbs: Nature's Pharmacy*, 1st ed.; Arab Cultural Center: Casablanca, Morocco, 2004; pp. 286–288.
6. Saad, B.; Said, O. *Greco-Arab and Islamic Herbal Medicine*; John Wiley & Sons, Inc.: Hoboken, NJ, USA, 2011; p. 308. [CrossRef]
7. Nasar-Abbas, S.M.; E-Huma, Z.; Vu, T.H.; Khan, M.K.; Esbenshade, H.; Jayasena, V. Carob kibble: A bioactive-rich food ingredient. *Compr. Rev. Food Sci. Food Saf.* **2016**, *15*, 63–72. [CrossRef]
8. Stavrou, I.J.; Christou, A.; Kapnissi-Christodoulou, C.P. Polyphenols in carobs: A review on their composition, antioxidant capacity and cytotoxic effects, and health impact. *Food Chem.* **2018**, *269*, 355–374. [CrossRef]
9. Lakkab, I.; El Hajaji, H.; Lachkar, N.; El Bali, B.; Lachkar, M.; Ciobica, A. Phytochemistry, bioactivity: Suggestion of *Ceratonia siliqua* L. as neurodegenerative disease therapy. *J. Complement. Integr. Med.* **2018**, *15*, 20180013. [CrossRef]
10. Zhu, B.J.; Zayed, M.Z.; Zhu, H.-X.; Zhao, J.; Li, S.-P. Functional polysaccharides of carob fruit: A review. *Chin. Med.* **2019**, *14*, 40. [CrossRef]
11. Rtibi, K.; Selmi, S.; Grami, D.; Amri, M.; Eto, B.; El-Benna, J.; Sebai, H.; Marzouki, L. Chemical constituents and pharmacological actions of carob pods and leaves (*Ceratonia siliqua* L.) on the gastrointestinal tract: A review. *Biomed. Pharmacother.* **2017**, *93*, 522–528. [CrossRef]
12. Papagiannopoulos, M.; Wollseifen, H.R.; Mellenthin, A.; Haber, B.; Galensa, R. Identification and quantification of polyphenols in carob fruits (*Ceratonia siliqua* L.) and derived products by HPLC-UV-ESI/MS. *J. Agric. Food Chem.* **2004**, *52*, 3784–3791. [CrossRef]

13. Gohar, A.; Gedara, S.R.; Baraka, H.N. New acylated flavonol glycoside from *Ceratonia siliqua* L. seeds. *J. Med. Plants Res.* **2009**, *3*, 424–428. [CrossRef]
14. Cavdarova, M.; Makris, D.P. Extraction Kinetics of Phenolics from Carob (*Ceratonia siliqua* L.) Kibbles Using Environmentally Benign Solvents. *Waste Biomass Valori.* **2014**, *5*, 773–779. [CrossRef]
15. Benković, M.; Bosiljkov, T.; Semić, A.; Ježek, D.; Srečec, S. Influence of Carob Flour and Carob Bean Gum on Rheological Properties of Cocoa and Carob Pastry Fillings. *Foods* **2019**, *8*, 66. [CrossRef]
16. Santonocito, D.; Granata, G.; Geraci, C.; Panico, A.; Siciliano, E.A.; Raciti, G.; Puglia, C. Carob Seeds: Food Waste or Source of Bioactive Compounds? *Pharmaceutics* **2020**, *12*, 1090. [CrossRef]
17. Reed, J.; Bain, S.; Kanamarlapudi, V. A Review of Current Trends with Type 2 Diabetes Epidemiology, Aetiology, Pathogenesis, Treatments and Future Perspectives. *Diabetes Metab. Syndr. Obes.* **2021**, *14*, 3567–3602. [CrossRef]
18. Ganasegeran, K.; Hor, C.P.; Jamil, M.F.; Loh, H.C.; Noor, J.M.; Hamid, N.A.; Suppiah, P.D.; Abdul Manaf, M.R.; Ch'ng, A.S.; Looi, I. A Systematic Review of the Economic Burden of Type 2 Diabetes in Malaysia. *Int. J. Environ. Res. Public Health* **2020**, *17*, 5723. [CrossRef]
19. Rodríguez, J.E.; Campbell, K.M. Racial and Ethnic Disparities in Prevalence and Care of Patients with Type 2 Diabetes. *Clin. Diabetes* **2017**, *35*, 66–70. [CrossRef]
20. Peleg, O. The Relationship between Type 2 Diabetes, Differentiation of Self, and Emotional Distress: Jews and Arabs in Israel. *Nutrients* **2022**, *14*, 39. [CrossRef]
21. Kahn, C.R. The molecular mechanism of insulin action. *Annu. Rev. Med.* **1985**, *36*, 429–451. [CrossRef]
22. Ingle, P.V.; Yin, S.B.; Ying, B.J.; Leong, B.K.; Xin, T.Z.; Hwa, L.T.; Mun, L.T. Current Trends in Pharmacological Treatment of Type II Diabetes Mellitus. *Int. J. Pharm. Res. Rev.* **2018**, *7*, 1–15.
23. Petersen, M.C.; Shulman, G.I. Mechanisms of Insulin Action and Insulin Resistance. *Physiol. Rev.* **2018**, *98*, 2133–2223. [CrossRef]
24. Yaribeygi, H.; Farrokhi, F.R.; Butler, A.E.; Sahebkar, A. Insulin resistance: Review of the underlying molecular mechanisms. *J. Cell Physiol.* **2019**, *234*, 8152–8161. [CrossRef]
25. Ahmad, F.; Misra, L.; Gupta, V.K.; Darokar, M.P.; Prakash, O.; Khan, F.; Shukla, R. Synergistic effect of (+)-pinitol from *Saraca asoca* with β-lactam antibiotics and studies on the in silico possible mechanism. *J. Kor. Diabetes Assoc.* **2005**, *29*, 344–351, Reprinted in *J. Assian Nat. Prod. Res.* **2015**, *18*, 72–183. [CrossRef]
26. James, D.E.; Stöckli, J.; Birnbaum, M.J. The aetiology and molecular landscape of insulin resistance. *Nat. Rev. Mol. Cell Biol.* **2021**, *22*, 751–771. [CrossRef]
27. Banks, W.A.; Rhea, E.M. The Blood-Brain Barrier, Oxidative Stress, and Insulin Resistance. *Antioxidants* **2021**, *10*, 1695. [CrossRef]
28. Reading, C.L.; Stickney, D.R.; Flores-Riveros, J.; Destiche, D.A.; Ahlem, C.N.; Cefalu, W.T.; Frincke, J.M. A synthetic anti-inflammatory sterol improves insulin sensitivity in insulin-resistant obese impaired glucose tolerance subjects. *Obesity* **2013**, *21*, E343–E349. [CrossRef]
29. Ravindran, R.; Mitra, K.; Arumugam, S.K.; Doble, M. Preparation of Curdlan sulphate–Chitosan nanoparticles as a drug carrier to target *Mycobacterium smegmatis* infected macrophages. *Carbohydr. Polym.* **2021**, *258*, 117686. [CrossRef]
30. Xue, S.; Yin, J.; Shao, J.; Yu, Y.; Yang, L.; Wang, Y.; Xie, M.; Fussenegger, M.; Ye, H. A Synthetic-Biology-Inspired Therapeutic Strategy for Targeting and Treating Hepatogenous Diabetes. *Mol. Ther.* **2017**, *25*, 443–455. [CrossRef]
31. Vieira, R.; Souto, S.B.; Sánchez-López, E.; Machado, A.L.; Severino, P.; Jose, S.; Santini, A.; Fortuna, A.; García, M.L.; Silva, A.M.; et al. Sugar-Lowering Drugs for Type 2 Diabetes Mellitus and Metabolic Syndrome-Review of Classical and New Compounds: Part-I. *Pharmaceuticals* **2019**, *12*, 152. [CrossRef]
32. Saadeldeen, F.S.; Niu, Y.; Wang, H.; Zhou, L.; Meng, L.; Chen, S.; Sun-Waterhouse, D.; Waterhouse, G.I.; Liu, Z.; Kang, W. Natural Products: Regulating Glucose Metabolism and Improving Insulin Resistance. *Food Sci. Hum. Wellness* **2020**, *9*, 214–228. [CrossRef]
33. Li, J.; Bai, L.; Wei, F.; Zhao, J.; Wang, D.; Xiao, Y.; Yan, W.; Wei, J. Therapeutic Mechanisms of Herbal Medicines against Insulin Resistance: A Review. *Front. Pharmacol.* **2019**, *10*, 661. [CrossRef] [PubMed]
34. Alaaeldin, R.; Abdel-Rahman, I.A.; Hassan, H.A.; Youssef, N.; Allam, A.E.; Abdelwahab, S.F.; Zhao, Q.L.; Fathy, M. Carpachromene Ameliorates Insulin Resistance in HepG2 Cells via Modulating IR/IRS1/PI3k/Akt/GSK3/FoxO1 Pathway. *Molecules* **2021**, *26*, 7629. [CrossRef] [PubMed]
35. Deenadayalan, A.; Subramanian, V.; Paramasivan, V.; Veeraraghavan, V.P.; Rengasamy, G.; Sadagopan, J.C.; Rajagopal, P.; Jayaraman, S. Stevioside Attenuates Insulin Resistance in Skeletal Muscle by Facilitating IR/IRS-1/Akt/GLUT 4 Signaling Pathways: An In Vivo and In Silico Approach. *Molecules* **2021**, *26*, 7689. [CrossRef] [PubMed]
36. Sanz-Lamora, H.; Marrero, P.F.; Haro, D.; Relat, J. A Mixture of Pure, Isolated Polyphenols Worsens the Insulin Resistance and Induces Kidney and Liver Fibrosis Markers in Diet-Induced Obese Mice. *Antioxidants* **2022**, *11*, 120. [CrossRef] [PubMed]
37. Hoffmann-Ostenhof, O.; Pittner, F. The biosynthesis of *myo*-inositol and its isomers. *Can. J. Chem.* **1982**, *60*, 1863–1871. [CrossRef]
38. Watkins, O.C.; Yong, H.E.; Sharma, N.; Chan, S.-Y. A review of the role of inositols in conditions of insulin dysregulation and in uncomplicated and pathological pregnancy. *Crit. Rev. Food Sci. Nutr.* **2022**, *62*, 1626–1673. [CrossRef]
39. Kennington, A.S.; Hill, C.R.; Craig, J.; Bogardus, C.; Raz, I.; Ortmeyer, H.K.; Hansen, B.C.; Romero, G.; Larner, J. Low urinary chiro-inositol excretion in non-insulin-dependent diabetes mellitus. *N. Engl. J. Med.* **1990**, *323*, 373–378. [CrossRef]
40. Hallman, M.; Bry, K.; Hoppu, K.; Lappi, M.; Pohjavuori, M. Inositol supplementation in premature infants with respiratory distress syndrome. *N. Engl. J. Med.* **1992**, *326*, 1233–1239. [CrossRef]

41. Asplin, I.; Galasko, G.; Larner, J. Chiro-inositol deficiency and insulin resistance: A comparison of the chiro-inositol- and the myo-inositol-containing insulin mediators isolated from urine, hemodialysate, and muscle of control and type II diabetic subjects. *Proc. Natl. Acad. Sci. USA* **1993**, *90*, 5924–5928. [CrossRef]
42. Levine, J. Controlled trials of inositol in psychiatry. *Eur. Neuropsychopharmacol.* **1997**, *7*, 147–155. [CrossRef]
43. Nestler, J.E.; Jakubowicz, D.J.; Reamer, P.; Gunn, R.D.; Allan, G. Ovulatory and metabolic effects of D-chiro-inositol in the polycystic ovary syndrome. *N. Engl. J. Med.* **1999**, *340*, 1314–1320. [CrossRef]
44. McLaurin, J.; Golomb, R.; Jurewicz, A.; Antel, J.P.; Fraser, P.E. Inositol stereoisomers stabilize an oligomeric aggregate of Alzheimer amyloid beta peptide and inhibit Aβ-induced toxicity. *J. Biol. Chem.* **2000**, *275*, 18495–18502. [CrossRef]
45. Jung, T.S.; Hahm, J.R.; Kim, J.J.; Jung, J.H.; Kang, M.Y.; Moon, S.W.; Lee, K.W.; Kim, H.C.; Lee, J.D.; Kim, J.H.; et al. Determination of urinary Myo-/chiro-inositol ratios from Korean diabetes patients. *Yonsei Med. J.* **2005**, *46*, 532–538. [CrossRef]
46. Nascimento, N.R.; Lessa, L.M.; Kerntopf, M.R.; Sousa, C.M.; Alves, R.S.; Queiroz, M.G.; Price, J.; Heimark, D.B.; Larner, J.; Du, X.; et al. Inositols prevent and reverse endothelial dysfunction in diabetic rat and rabbit vasculature metabolically and by scavenging superoxide. *Proc. Natl. Acad. Sci. USA* **2006**, *103*, 218–223. [CrossRef]
47. Michell, R.H. Evolution of the diverse biological roles of inositols. *Biochem. Soc. Symp.* **2007**, *74*, 223–246. [CrossRef]
48. Michell, R.H. Inositol derivatives: Evolution and functions. *Nat. Rev. Mol. Cell Biol.* **2008**, *9*, 151–161. [CrossRef]
49. Bizzarri, M.; Carlomagno, G. Inositol: History of an effective therapy for Polycystic Ovary Syndrome. *Eur. Rev. Med. Pharmacol. Sci.* **2014**, *18*, 1896–1903. [PubMed]
50. Mancini, M.; Andreassi, A.; Salvioni, M.; Pelliccione, F.; Mantellassi, G.; Banderali, G. Myoinositol and D-Chiro Inositol in Improving Insulin Resistance in Obese Male Children: Preliminary Data. *Int. J. Endocrinol.* **2016**, 8720342. [CrossRef]
51. Kalra, B.; Kalra, S.; Sharma, J.B. The inositols and polycystic ovary syndrome. *Indian J. Endocrinol. Metab.* **2016**, *20*, 720–724. [CrossRef]
52. Hanna, R.; Wehbe, T.; Abou Jaoude, E. Metabolic Effects of D-Chiro-Inositol and Myo-Inositol in Polycystic Ovary Syndrome. *Int. J. Clin. Endocrinol. Metab.* **2017**, *3*, 029–033. [CrossRef]
53. Orrù, B.; Circo, R.; Logoteta, P.; Petousis, S.; Carlomagno, G. Finding the best therapeutic approach for PCOS: The importance of inositol(s) bioavailability. *Eur. Rev. Med. Pharmacol. Sci.* **2017**, *21*, 83–88. [PubMed]
54. Showell, M.G.; Mackenzie-Proctor, R.; Jordan, V.; Hodgson, R.; Farquhar, C. Inositol for subfertile women with polycystic ovary syndrome. *Cochrane Database Syst. Rev.* **2018**, *12*, CD012378. [CrossRef]
55. Miñambres, I.; Cuixart, G.; Gonçalves, A.; Corcoy, R. Effects of inositol on glucose homeostasis: Systematic review and meta-analysis of randomized controlled trials. *Clin. Nutr.* **2019**, *38*, 1146–1152. [CrossRef]
56. Chhetri, D.R. *Myo*-Inositol and Its Derivatives: Their Emerging Role in the Treatment of Human Diseases. *Front Pharmacol.* **2019**, *10*, 1172. [CrossRef]
57. Roseff, S.; Montenegro, M. Inositol Treatment for PCOS Should Be Science-Based and Not Arbitrary. *Int. J. Endocrinol.* **2020**, *2020*, 6461254. [CrossRef]
58. Merviel, P.; James, P.; Bouée, S.; Le Guillou, M.; Rince, C.; Nachtergaele, C.; Kerla, V. Impact of myo-inositol treatment in women with polycystic ovary syndrome in assisted reproductive technologies. *Reprod. Health* **2021**, *18*, 13. [CrossRef] [PubMed]
59. Sharma, N.; Watkins, O.C.; Chu, A.H.; Cutfield, W.; Godfrey, K.M.; Yong, H.E.; Chan, S.Y. *Myo*-inositol: A potential prophylaxis against premature onset of labour and preterm birth. *Nutr. Res. Rev.* **2021**, *34*, 1–9. [CrossRef] [PubMed]
60. Cantelmi, T.; Lambiase, E.; Unfer, V.R.; Gambioli, R.; Unfer, V. Inositol treatment for psychological symptoms in Polycystic Ovary Syndrome women. *Eur. Rev. Med. Pharmacol Sci.* **2021**, *25*, 2383–2389. [CrossRef] [PubMed]
61. Goulas, V.; Stylos, E.; Chatziathanasiadou, M.V.; Mavromoustakos, T.; Tzakos, A.G. Functional Components of Carob Fruit: Linking the Chemical and Biological Space. *Int. J. Mol. Sci.* **2016**, *17*, 1875. [CrossRef] [PubMed]
62. Skøt, L.; Egsgaard, H. Identification of ononitol and O-methyl-scyllo-inositol in pea root nodules. *Planta* **1984**, *161*, 32–36. [CrossRef]
63. Sheveleva, E.; Chmara, W.; Bohnert, H.J.; Jensen, R.G. Increased Salt and Drought Tolerance by D-Ononitol Production in Transgenic *Nicotiana tabacum* L. *Plant Physiol.* **1997**, *115*, 1211–1219. [CrossRef]
64. Kim, J.I.; Kim, J.C.; Joo, H.J.; Jung, S.H.; Kim, J.J. Determination of total chiro-inositol content in selected natural materials and evaluation of the antihyperglycemic effect of pinitol isolated from soybean and carob. *Food Sci. Biotechnol.* **2005**, *14*, 441–445.
65. Negishi, O.; Mun'im, A.; Negishi, Y. Content of methylated inositols in familiar edible plants. *J. Agric. Food Chem.* **2015**, *63*, 2683–2688. [CrossRef]
66. Qiu, J.; Yan, X.; Liao, Y.; Yu, D.; Wen, C.; Xiang, Z. An UPLC-MS/MS method for quantification of D-pinitol in rat plasma and its application to a pharmacokinetic and bioavailability study. *J. Chromatogr. B Analyt. Technol. Biomed. Life Sci.* **2021**, *1163*, 122498. [CrossRef]
67. Fenili, D.; Weng, Y.Q.; Aubert, I.; Nitz, M.; McLaurin, J. Sodium/myo-Inositol transporters: Substrate transport requirements and regional brain expression in the TgCRND8 mouse model of amyloid pathology. *PLoS ONE* **2011**, *6*, e24032. [CrossRef]
68. Pitt, J.; Thorner, M.; Brautigan, D.; Larner, J.; Klein, W.L. Protection against the synaptic targeting and toxicity of Alzheimer's-associated Aβ oligomers by insulin mimetic chiro-inositols. *FASEB J.* **2013**, *27*, 199–207. [CrossRef]
69. Griñán-Ferré, C.; Bellver-Sanchis, A.; Olivares-Martín, M.; Bañuelos-Hortigüela, O.; Pallàs, M. Synergistic Neuroprotective Effects of a Natural Product Mixture against AD Hallmarks and Cognitive Decline in *Caenorhabditis elegans* and an SAMP8 Mice Model. *Nutrients* **2021**, *13*, 2411. [CrossRef]

70. Hada, B.; Yoo, M.R.; Seong, K.M.; Jin, Y.W.; Myeong, H.K.; Min, K.J. D-chiro-inositol and pinitol extend the life span of Drosophila melanogaster. *J. Gerontol. A Biol. Sci. Med. Sci.* **2013**, *68*, 226–234. [CrossRef]
71. Ravindran, R.; Chakrapani, G.; Mitra, K.; Doble, M. Inhibitory activity of traditional plants against Mycobacterium smegmatis and their action on Filamenting temperature sensitive mutant Z (FtsZ)-A cell division protein. *PLoS ONE* **2020**, *15*, e0232482. [CrossRef]
72. Sethi, G.; Ahn, K.S.; Sung, B.; Aggarwal, B.B. Pinitol targets nuclear factor-kappaB activation pathway leading to inhibition of gene products associated with proliferation, apoptosis, invasion, and angiogenesis. *Mol. Cancer Ther.* **2008**, *7*, 1604–1614. [CrossRef]
73. Lin, T.H.; Tan, T.W.; Tsai, T.H.; Chen, C.C.; Hsieh, T.F.; Lee, S.S.; Liu, H.H.; Chen, W.C.; Tang, C.H. D-pinitol inhibits prostate cancer metastasis through inhibition of αVβ3 integrin by modulating FAK, c-Src and NF-κB pathways. *Int. J. Mol. Sci.* **2013**, *14*, 9790–9802. [CrossRef] [PubMed]
74. Rengarajan, T.; Nandakumar, N.; Rajendran, P.; Haribabu, L.; Nishigaki, I.; Balasubramanian, M.P. D-pinitol promotes apoptosis in MCF-7 cells via induction of p53 and Bax and inhibition of Bcl-2 and NF-κB. *Asian Pac. J. Cancer Prev.* **2014**, *15*, 1757–1762. [CrossRef] [PubMed]
75. Jayasooriya, R.G.; Kang, G.-H.; Park, S.R.; Choi, Y.-H.; Kim, G.-Y. Pinitol Suppresses Tumor Necrosis Factor-α-Induced Invasion of Prostate Cancer LNCaP Cells by Inhibiting Nuclear Factor-κB-Mediated Matrix Metalloproteinase-9 Expression. *Trop. J. Pharm. Res.* **2015**, *14*, 1357–1364. [CrossRef]
76. Shin, H.-C.; Bang, T.-H.; Kang, H.-M.; Park, B.-S.; Kim, I.-R. Anticancer effects of D-pinitol in human oral squamous carcinoma cells. *Int. J. Oral Biol.* **2020**, *45*, 152–161. [CrossRef]
77. Yao, X.; Shi, K.; Yang, Y.; Gu, X.; Tan, W.; Wang, Q.; Gao, X.; Veeraraghavan, V.P.; Mohan, S.K.; Jin, S. D-Pinitol treatment induced the apoptosis in human leukemia MOLT-4 cells by improved apoptotic signaling pathway. *Saudi J. Biol. Sci.* **2020**, *27*, 2134–2138. [CrossRef]
78. Rengarajan, T.; Jagadeesan, A.J.; Balamurugan, A.; Balasubramanian, M.P. Chemotherapeutic potential of D-Pinitol against 7, 12 dimethylbenz (a) (DMBA) induced mammary carcinoma in Sprague Dawley rats. *Int. J. Pharm. BioSci.* **2011**, *2*, 232–241.
79. Rengarajan, T.; Nandakumar, N.; Balasubramanian, M.P. D-Pinitol a low-molecular cyclitol prevents 7,12-Dimethylbenz a anthracene induced experimental breast cancer through regulating anti-apoptotic protein Bcl-2, mitochondrial and carbohydrate key metabolizing enzymes. *Biomed. Prevent. Nutr.* **2012**, *2*, 25–30. [CrossRef]
80. Rengarajan, T.; Nandakumar, N.; Balasubramanian, M.P. D-Pinitol attenuates 7, 12 dimethylbenz a anthracene induced hazards through modulating protein bound carbohydrates, adenosine triphosphatases and lysosomal enzymes during experimental mammary carcinogenesis. *J. Exp. Ther. Oncol.* **2012**, *10*, 39–49.
81. Rengarajan, T.; Nandakumar, N.; Balasubramanian, M.P. D-Pinitol prevents rat breast carcinogenesis induced by 7, 12 - Dimethylbenz aanthracene through inhibition of Bcl-2 and induction of p53, caspase-3 proteins and modulation of hepatic biotransformation enzymes and antioxidants. *Biomed. Prevent. Nutr.* **2013**, *3*, 31–41. [CrossRef]
82. Venkatachalam, S.; Boobathi, L.; Balasubramanian, B.M. D-Pinitol Prevents Rat Colon Carcinogenesis Induced by Azoxymethane through Free Radical Formation Induced Cell Damage and Affects Enzymes and Antioxidants. *Res. J. Pharm. Technol.* **2014**, *7*, 845–849.
83. Rengarajan, T.; Nandakumar, N.; Rajendran, P.; Ganesh, M.K.; Balasubramanian, M.P.; Nishigaki, I. D-pinitol mitigates tumor growth by modulating interleukins and hormones and induces apoptosis in rat breast carcinogenesis through inhibition of NF-κB. *J. Physiol. Biochem.* **2015**, *71*, 191–204. [CrossRef]
84. Lin, Y.; Wu, Y.; Su, J.; Wang, M.; Wu, X.; Su, Z.; Yi, X.; Wei, L.; Jian Cai, J.; Sun, Z. Therapeutic role of D-pinitol on experimental colitis via activating Nrf2/ARE and PPAR-γ/NF-κB signaling pathways. *Food Funct.* **2021**, *12*, 2554–2568. [CrossRef]
85. Alonso-Castro, A.J.; Alba-Betancourt, C.; Rocha-González, E.; Ruiz-Arredondo, A.; Zapata-Morales, J.R.; Gasca-Martínez, D.; Pérez-Gutiérrez, S. Neuropharmacological effects of d-pinitol and its possible mechanisms of action. *J. Food Biochem.* **2019**, *43*, e13070. [CrossRef]
86. Narayanan, C.R.; Joshi, D.D.; Muhumdar, A.M.; Dhekne, V.V. Pinitol—A new anti-diabetic compound from the leaves of *Bougainvillea spectabilis*. *Curr. Sci.* **1987**, *56*, 139–141.
87. Sivakumar, S.; Subramanian, S.P. D-pinitol attenuates the impaired activities of hepatic key enzymes in carbohydrate metabolism of streptozotocin-induced diabetic rats. *Gen. Physiol. Biophys.* **2009**, *28*, 233–241. [CrossRef]
88. Sivakumar, S.; Subramanian, S.P. Pancreatic tissue protective nature of D-Pinitol studied in streptozotocin-mediated oxidative stress in experimental diabetic rats. *Eur. J. Pharmacol.* **2009**, *622*, 65–70. [CrossRef]
89. Dang, N.T.; Mukai, R.; Yoshida, K.; Ashida, H. D-pinitol and myo-inositol stimulate translocation of glucose transporter 4 in skeletal muscle of C57BL/6 mice. *Biosci. Biotechnol. Biochem.* **2010**, *74*, 1062–1067. [CrossRef]
90. Lee, B.H.; Lee, C.C.; Wu, S.C. Ice plant (*Mesembryanthemum crystallinum*) improves hyperglycaemia and memory impairments in a Wistar rat model of streptozotocin-induced diabetes. *J. Sci Food Agric.* **2014**, *94*, 2266–2273. [CrossRef]
91. Huang, B.; Wang, Z.; Park, J.H.; Ryu, O.H.; Choi, M.K.; Lee, J.Y.; Kang, Y.H.; Lim, S.S. Anti-diabetic effect of purple corn extract on C57BL/KsJ db/db mice. *Nutr. Res. Pract.* **2015**, *9*, 22–29. [CrossRef]
92. Srivastava, K.; Dubey, A.; Tiwari, M.; Dubey, A. To evaluate the synergistic effect of Pinitol with Glimepride in diabetic Wistar rats. *J. Crit. Rev.* **2020**, *7*, 2058–2062.

93. Kim, J.I.; Kim, J.C.; Kang, M.J.; Lee, M.S.; Kim, J.J.; Cha, I.J. Effects of pinitol isolated from soybeans on glycaemic control and cardiovascular risk factors in Korean patients with type II diabetes mellitus: A randomized controlled study. *Eur. J. Clin. Nutr.* **2005**, *59*, 456–458. [CrossRef]
94. Kang, M.J.; Kim, J.I.; Yoon, S.Y.; Kim, J.C.; Cha, I.J. Pinitol from soybeans reduces postprandial blood glucose in patients with type 2 diabetes mellitus. *J. Med. Food* **2006**, *9*, 182–186. [CrossRef]
95. Kim, M.J.; Yoo, K.H.; Kim, J.H.; Seo, Y.T.; Ha, B.W.; Kho, J.H.; Shin, Y.G.; Chung, C.H. Effect of pinitol on glucose metabolism and adipocytokines in uncontrolled type 2 diabetes. *Diabetes Res. Clin. Pract.* **2007**, *77*, S247–S251. [CrossRef]
96. Hernández-Mijares, A.; Bañuls, C.; Peris, J.E.; Monzó, N.; Jover, A.; Bellod, L.; Victor, V.M.; Rocha, M. A single acute dose of pinitol from a naturally-occurring food ingredient decreases hyperglycaemia and circulating insulin levels in healthy subjects. *Food Chem.* **2013**, *141*, 1267–1272. [CrossRef]
97. Lambert, C.; Cubedo, J.; Padró, T.; Vilahur, G.; López-Bernal, S.; Rocha, M.; Hernández-Mijares, A.; Badimon, L. Effects of a Carob-Pod-Derived Sweetener on Glucose Metabolism. *Nutrients* **2018**, *10*, 271. [CrossRef]
98. Suzuki, Y.; Sakuraba, K.; Wada, T.; Watabane, N.; Wada, S.; Kitabayashi, Y.; Sunohara, M. Single-Dose Pinitol Ingestion Suppresses Post-Prandial Glucose Levels: A Randomized, Double-Blind, Placebo-Controlled, Crossover Trial. *Nat. Prod. Commun.* **2019**, *14*, 1–5. [CrossRef]
99. Mishra, A.K.; Tewari, S.P. Theoretical evaluation of the bioactivity of plant-derived natural molecule D-Pinitol and other derived structure. *AIP Conf. Proc.* **2019**, *2142*, 150019. [CrossRef]
100. Alonso-Castro, A.J.; Zapata-Morales, J.R.; Arana-Argáez, V.; Torres-Romero, J.C.; Ramírez-Villanueva, E.; Pérez-Medina, S.E.; Ramírez-Morales, M.A.; Juárez-Méndez, M.A.; Infante-Barrios, Y.P.; Martínez-Gutiérrez, F.; et al. Pharmacological and toxicological study of a chemical-standardized ethanol extract of the branches and leaves from *Eysenhardtia polystachya* (Ortega) Sarg. (Fabaceae). *J. Ethnopharmacol.* **2018**, *224*, 314–322. [CrossRef]
101. Koh, E.S.; Kim, S.; Kim, M.; Hong, Y.A.; Shin, S.J.; Park, C.W.; Chang, Y.S.; Chung, S.; Kim, H.S. D-Pinitol alleviates cyclosporine A-induced renal tubulointerstitial fibrosis via activating Sirt1 and Nrf2 antioxidant pathways. *Int. J. Mol. Med.* **2018**, *41*, 1826–1834. [CrossRef]
102. Geethan, P.K.; Prince, P.S. Antihyperlipidemic effect of D-pinitol on streptozotocin-induced diabetic Wistar rats. *J. Biochem. Mol. Toxicol.* **2008**, *22*, 220–224. [CrossRef]
103. Singh, R.K.; Pandey, B.L.; Tripathi, M.; Pandey, V.B. Anti-inflammatory effect of (+)-pinitol. *Fitoterapia* **2001**, *72*, 168–170. [CrossRef]
104. Kim, J.C.; Shin, J.Y.; Shin, D.H.; Kim, S.H.; Park, S.H.; Park, R.D.; Park, S.C.; Kim, Y.B.; Shin, Y.C. Synergistic antiinflammatory effects of pinitol and glucosamine in rats. *Phytother. Res.* **2005**, *19*, 1048–1051. [CrossRef] [PubMed]
105. Sivakumar, S.; Palsamy, P.; Subramanian, S.P. Impact of D-pinitol on the attenuation of proinflammatory cytokines, hyperglycemia-mediated oxidative stress and protection of kidney tissue ultrastructure in streptozotocin-induced diabetic rats. *Chem. Biol. Interact.* **2010**, *188*, 237–245. [CrossRef]
106. Zheng, K.; Zhao, Z.; Lin, N.; Wu, Y.; Xu, Y.; Zhang, W. Protective Effect of Pinitol Against Inflammatory Mediators of Rheumatoid Arthritis via Inhibition of Protein Tyrosine Phosphatase Non-Receptor Type 22 (PTPN22). *Med. Sci. Monit.* **2017**, *23*, 1923–1932. [CrossRef] [PubMed]
107. Choi, M.S.; Lee, W.H.; Kwon, E.Y.; Kang, M.A.; Lee, M.K.; Park, Y.B.; Jeon, S.M. Effects of soy pinitol on the pro-inflammatory cytokines and scavenger receptors in oxidized low-density lipoprotein-treated THP-1 macrophages. *J. Med. Food.* **2007**, *10*, 594–601. [CrossRef] [PubMed]
108. Eser, F.; Altundag, E.M.; Gedik, G.; Demirtas, I.; Onal, A.; Selvi, B. Anti-inflammatory effect of D-pinitol isolated from the leaves of *Colutea cilicica* Boiss et Bal. on K562 cells. *Turk. J. Biochem.* **2017**, *42*, 445–450. [CrossRef]
109. Kong, J.; Du, Z.; Dong, L. Pinitol Prevents Lipopolysaccharide (LPS)-Induced Inflammatory Responses in BV2 Microglia Mediated by TREM2. *Neurotox. Res.* **2020**, *38*, 96–104. [CrossRef]
110. López-Domènech, S.; Bañuls, C.; de Marañón, A.M.; Abab-Jiménez, Z.; Morillas, C.; Gómez-Abril, S.Á.; Rovira-Llopis, S.; Víctor, V.M.; Hernández-Mijares, A.; Rocha, M. Pinitol alleviates systemic inflammatory cytokines in human obesity by a mechanism involving unfolded protein response and sirtuin 1. *Clin. Nutr.* **2018**, *37*, 2036–2044. [CrossRef]
111. Navarro, J.A.; Decara, J.; Medina-Vera, D.; Tovar, R.; Suarez, J.; Pavón, J.; Serrano, A.; Vida, M.; Gutierrez-Adan, A.; Sanjuan, C.; et al. D-Pinitol from *Ceratonia siliqua* Is an Orally Active Natural Inositol That Reduces Pancreas Insulin Secretion and Increases Circulating Ghrelin Levels in Wistar Rats. *Nutrients* **2020**, *12*, 2030. [CrossRef]
112. Yu, J.; Choi, S.; Park, E.S.; Shin, B.; Yu, J.; Lee, S.H.; Takami, M.; Kang, J.S.; Meong, H.; Rho, J. D-chiro-inositol negatively regulates the formation of multinucleated osteoclasts by down-regulating NFATc1. *J. Clin. Immunol.* **2012**, *32*, 1360–1371. [CrossRef]
113. Rengarajan, T.; Rajendran, P.; Nandakumar, N.; Balasubramanian, M.P.; Nishigaki, I. Free radical scavenging and antioxidant activity of D-pinitol against 7, 12 dimethylbenz(a) anthracene induced breast cancer in sprague dawley rats. *Asian Pac. J. Trop. Dis.* **2014**, *4*, 384–390. [CrossRef]
114. Ma, J.; Feng, S.; Ai, D.; Liu, Y.; Yang, X. D-Pinitol Ameliorates Imiquimod-Induced PsoriasisLike Skin Inflammation in a Mouse Model via the NF-κB Pathway. *J. Environ. Pathol. Toxicol. Oncol.* **2019**, *38*, 285–295. [CrossRef]
115. Suresh, K.G.; Manivannan, R.; Nivetha, B. In-silico docking analysis of phytochemicals from *mimosa pudica l.* Leaves as an antiviral agent against herpes simplex virus type I. *Int. J. Biomed. NanoLet.* **2021**, *1*, 1–9.
116. Lee, J.S.; Lee, C.M.; Jeong, Y.I.; Jung, I.D.; Kim, B.H.; Seong, E.Y.; Kim, J.I.; Choi, I.W.; Chung, H.Y.; Park, Y.M. D-pinitol regulates Th1/Th2 balance via suppressing Th2 immune response in ovalbumin-induced asthma. *FEBS Lett.* **2007**, *581*, 57–64. [CrossRef]

117. Liu, S.C.; Chuang, S.M.; Tang, C.H. D-pinitol inhibits RANKL-induced osteoclastogenesis. *Int. Immunopharmacol.* **2012**, *12*, 494–500. [CrossRef]
118. Sudha, M.; Vetrichelvan, T. Protective effect of D-Pinitol isolated from aerial parts of soybean plants on haematological profile against Doxorubicin-induced cyto-toxicity in mice. *Int. J. Pharm. Sci. Res.* **2021**, *12*, 2926–2932. [CrossRef]
119. Li, X.L.; Xu, M.; Yu, F.; Fu, C.L.; Yu, X.; Cheng, M.; Gao, H.Q. Effects of D-pinitol on myocardial apoptosis and fibrosis in streptozocin-induced aging-accelerated mice. *J. Food Biochem.* **2021**, *45*, e13669. [CrossRef]
120. Hu, X.; Zhu, Y.; LV, X.; Feng, Z. Elucidation of the mechanism of action of pinitol against pressure overload-induced cardiac hypertrophy and fibrosis in an animal model of aortic stenosis. *Biosci. Biotechnol. Biochem.* **2021**, *85*, 643–655. [CrossRef]
121. Cordero, C.P.; Pinzon, R.; Aristizabal, F.A. Cytotoxicity of bixin, rutin, pinitol B and ent-16-kauren-19-oic acid isolated from Colombian plants. *Rev. Col. Cienc. Quím. Farm.* **2003**, *32*, 137–140.
122. Alonso-Castro, A.J.; Alba-Betancourt, C.; Yáñez-Barrientos, E.; Luna-Rocha, C.; Páramo-Castillo, A.S.; Aragón-Martínez, O.H.; Zapata-Morales, J.R.; Cruz-Jiménez, G.; Gasca-Martínez, D.; González-Ibarra, A.A.; et al. Diuretic activity and neuropharmacological effects of an ethanol extract from *Senna septemtrionalis* (Viv.) H.S. Irwin & Barneby (Fabaceae). *J. Ethnopharmacol.* **2019**, *239*, 111923. [CrossRef]
123. Sudha, M.; Vetrichelvan, T. Genoprotective effect of D-Pinitol isolated from aerial parts of Soybean plants against Doxorubicin-induced genotoxicity evaluated by in vitro comet assay in Vero cell lines. *Int. J. Res. Pharm. Sci.* **2021**, *12*, 1379–1384. [CrossRef]
124. Lee, E.; Lim, Y.; Kwon, S.W.; Kwon, O. Pinitol consumption improves liver health status by reducing oxidative stress and fatty acid accumulation in subjects with non-alcoholic fatty liver disease: A randomized, double-blind, placebo-controlled trial. *J. Nutr. Biochem.* **2019**, *68*, 33–41. [CrossRef]
125. Ostlund, R.E.; Seemayer, R.; Gupta, S.; Kimmel, R.; Ostlund, E.L.; Sherman, W.R. A stereospecific myo-inositol/D-chiro-inositol transporter in HepG2 liver cells. Identification with D-chiro-3-3Hinositol. *J. Biol. Chem.* **1996**, *271*, 10073–10078. [CrossRef]
126. Zhou, Y.; Park, C.M.; Cho, C.W.; Song, Y.S. Protective effect of pinitol against D-galactosamine-induced hepatotoxicity in rats fed on a high-fat diet. *Biosci. Biotechnol. Biochem.* **2008**, *72*, 1657–1666. [CrossRef]
127. Sivakumar, S.; Palsamy, P.; Subramanian, S.P. Attenuation of oxidative stress and alteration of hepatic tissue ultrastructure by D-pinitol in streptozotocin-induced diabetic rats. *Free Radic. Res.* **2010**, *44*, 668–678. [CrossRef]
128. Magielse, J.; Arcoraci, T.; Breynaert, A.; van Dooren, I.; Kanyanga, C.; Fransen, E.; Van Hoof, V.; Vlietinck, A.; Apers, S.; Pieters, L.; et al. Antihepatotoxic activity of a quantified Desmodium adscendens decoction and D-pinitol against chemically-induced liver damage in rats. *J. Ethnopharmacol.* **2013**, *146*, 250–256. [CrossRef]
129. Rengarajan, T.; Rajendran, P.; Nandakumar, N.; Lokeshkumar, B.; Balasubramanian, M.P. D-Pinitol Protects Against Carbon Tetrachloride-Induced Hepatotoxicity in Rats. *J. Environ. Pathol. Toxicol. Oncol.* **2015**, *34*, 287–298. [CrossRef]
130. Yan, L.; Luo, H.; Li, X.; Li, Y. d-Pinitol protects against endoplasmic reticulum stress and apoptosis in hepatic ischemia-reperfusion injury via modulation of AFT4-CHOP/GRP78 and caspase-3 signaling pathways. *Int. J. Immunopathol. Pharmacol.* **2021**, *35*, 20587384211032098. [CrossRef]
131. Da Silva, J.A.; Da Silva, A.C.; Figueiredo, L.S.; Araujo, T.R.; Freitas, I.N.; Carneiro, E.M.; Ribeiro, E.S.; Ribeiro, R.A. D-Pinitol Increases Insulin Secretion and Regulates Hepatic Lipid Metabolism in Msg-Obese Mice. *An. Acad. Bras. Cienc.* **2020**, *92*, e20201382. [CrossRef]
132. Muñoz, C.X.; Johnson, E.C.; Kunces, L.J.; McKenzie, A.L.; Wininger, M.; Butts, C.L.; Caldwell, A.; Seal, A.; McDermott, B.P.; Vingren, J.; et al. Impact of Nutrient Intake on Hydration Biomarkers Following Exercise and Rehydration Using a Clustering-Based Approach. *Nutrients* **2020**, *12*, 1276. [CrossRef]
133. Adams, W.M.; Wininger, M.; Zaplatosch, M.E.; Hevel, D.J.; Maher, J.P.; McGuirt, J.T. Influence of Nutrient Intake on 24 Hour Urinary Hydration Biomarkers Using a Clustering-Based Approach. *Nutrients* **2020**, *12*, 2933. [CrossRef] [PubMed]
134. Moreira, L.N.; Silva, J.F.; Silva, G.C.; Lemos, V.S.; Cortes, S.F. Activation of eNOS by D-pinitol Induces an Endothelium-Dependent Vasodilatation in Mouse Mesenteric Artery. *Front. Pharmacol.* **2018**, *9*, 528. [CrossRef] [PubMed]
135. Lee, J.S.; Jung, I.D.; Jeong, Y.I.; Lee, C.M.; Shin, Y.K.; Lee, S.Y.; Suh, D.S.; Yoon, M.S.; Lee, K.S.; Choi, Y.H.; et al. D-pinitol inhibits Th1 polarization via the suppression of dendritic cells. *Int. Immunopharmacol.* **2007**, *7*, 791–804. [CrossRef] [PubMed]
136. Bae, C.J.; Lee, J.W.; Shim, S.B.; Jee, S.W.; Lee, S.H.; Woo, J.M.; Lee, C.K.; Hwang, D.Y. GATA binding protein 3 overexpression and suppression significantly contribute to the regulation of allergic skin inflammation. *Int. J. Mol. Med.* **2011**, *28*, 171–179. [CrossRef] [PubMed]
137. Chauhan, P.S.; Gupta, K.K.; Bani, S. The immunosuppressive effects of *Agyrolobium roseum* and pinitol in experimental animals. *Int. Immunopharmacol.* **2011**, *11*, 286–291. [CrossRef] [PubMed]
138. Brautigan, D.L.; Brown, M.; Grindrod, S.; Chinigo, G.; Kruszewski, A.; Lukasik, S.M.; Bushweller, J.H.; Horal, M.; Keller, S.; Tamura, S.; et al. Allosteric activation of protein phosphatase 2C by D-chiro-inositol-galactosamine, a putative mediator mimetic of insulin action. *Biochemistry* **2005**, *44*, 11067–11173. [CrossRef] [PubMed]
139. Kim, U.H.; Yoon, J.H.; Li, H.; Kang, J.H.; Ji, H.S.; Park, K.H.; Shin, D.H.; Park, H.Y.; Jeong, T.S. Pterocarpan-enriched soy leaf extract ameliorates insulin sensitivity and pancreatic β-cell proliferation in type 2 diabetic mice. *Molecules* **2014**, *19*, 18493–18510. [CrossRef]
140. Gao, Y.; Zhang, M.; Wu, T.; Xu, M.; Cai, H.; Zhang, Z. Effects of D-Pinitol on Insulin Resistance through the PI3K/Akt Signaling Pathway in Type 2 Diabetes Mellitus Rats. *J. Agric. Food Chem.* **2015**, *63*, 6019–6026. [CrossRef]

141. Medina-Vera, D.; Navarro, J.A.; Tovar, R.; Rosell-Valle, C.; Gutiérrez-Adan, A.; Ledesma, J.C.; Sanjuan, C.; Pavón, F.J.; Baixeras, E.; Rodríguez de Fonseca, F.; et al. Activation of PI3K/Akt Signaling Pathway in Rat Hypothalamus Induced by an Acute Oral Administration of D-Pinitol. *Nutrients* **2021**, *13*, 2268. [CrossRef]
142. Kim, H.J.; Park, K.S.; Lee, S.K.; Min, K.W.; Han, K.A.; Kim, Y.K.; Ku, B.J. Effects of pinitol on glycemic control, insulin resistance and adipocytokine levels in patients with type 2 diabetes mellitus. *Ann. Nutr. Metab.* **2012**, *60*, 1–5. [CrossRef]
143. Do, G.M.; Choi, M.S.; Kim, H.J.; Woo, M.N.; Lee, M.K.; Jeon, S.M. Soy pinitol acts partly as an insulin sensitizer or insulin mediator in 3T3-L1 preadipocytes. *Genes Nutr.* **2008**, *2*, 359–364. [CrossRef]
144. Siracusa, L.; Occhiuto, C.; Molonia, M.S.; Cimino, F.; Palumbo, M.; Saija, A.; Speciale, A.; Rocco, C.; Ruberto, G.; Cristani, M. A pinitol-rich *Glycyrrhiza glabra* L. leaf extract as functional supplement with potential in the prevention of endothelial dysfunction through improving insulin signalling. *Arch. Physiol. Biochem.* **2020**, 1–10. [CrossRef]
145. Vasaikar, N.; Mahajan, U.; Patil, K.R.; Suchal, K.; Patil, C.R.; Ojha, S.; Goyal, S.N. D-pinitol attenuates cisplatin-induced nephrotoxicity in rats: Impact on pro-inflammatory cytokines. *Chem. Biol. Interact.* **2018**, *290*, 6–11. [CrossRef]
146. Farias, V.X.; Macêdo, F.H.; Oquendo, M.B.; Tomé, A.R.; Báo, S.N.; Cintra, D.O.; Santos, C.F.; Albuquerque, A.A.; Heimark, D.B.; Larner, J.; et al. Chronic treatment with D-chiro-inositol prevents autonomic and somatic neuropathy in STZ-induced diabetic mice. *Diabetes Obes. Metab.* **2011**, *13*, 243–250. [CrossRef]
147. Dong, W.; Zhao, S.; Wen, S.; Dong, C.; Chen, Q.; Gong, T.; Chen, W.; Liu, W.; Mu, L.; Shan, H.; et al. A preclinical randomized controlled study of ischemia treated with Ginkgo biloba extracts: Are complex components beneficial for treating acute stroke? *Curr. Res. Transl. Med.* **2020**, *68*, 197–203. [CrossRef]
148. An, Y.; Li, J.; Liu, Y.; Fan, M.; Tian, W. Protective effect of D-pinitol on the experimental spinal cord injury in rats. *Metab. Brain Dis.* **2020**, *35*, 473–482. [CrossRef]
149. Sakata, K.; Kawasaki, H.; Suzuki, T.; Ito, K.; Negishi, O.; Tsuno, T.; Tsuno, H.; Yamazaki, Y.; Ishida, N. Inositols affect the mating circadian rhythm of Drosophila melanogaster. *Front. Pharmacol.* **2005**, *6*, 111. [CrossRef]
150. Rahaman, M.S.; Yamasaki, S.; Binte Hossain, K.F.; Hosokawa, T.; Saito, T.; Kurasaki, M. Effects of curcumin, D-pinitol alone or in combination in cytotoxicity induced by arsenic in PC12 Cells. *Food Chem. Toxicol.* **2020**, *144*, 111577. [CrossRef]
151. Juneja, K.; Mishra, R.; Chauhan, S.; Gupta, S.; Roy, P.; Sircar, D. Metabolite profiling and wound-healing activity of *Boerhavia diffusa* leaf extracts using in vitro and in vivo models. *J. Trad. Complement. Med.* **2020**, *10*, 52–59. [CrossRef]
152. López-Gambero, A.J.; Sanjuan, C.; Serrano-Castro, P.J.; Suárez, J.; Rodríguez de Fonseca, F. The Biomedical Uses of Inositols: A Nutraceutical Approach to Metabolic Dysfunction in Aging and Neurodegenerative Diseases. *Biomedicines* **2020**, *8*, 295. [CrossRef]
153. Srivastava, K.; Tiwari, M.; Dubey, A.; Dubey, A. D-Pinitol—A Natural Phytomolecule and its Pharmacological effect. *Int. J. Pharm. Life Sci.* **2020**, *11*, 6609–6623.
154. Antonowski, T.; Osowski, A.; Lahuta, L.; Górecki, R.; Rynkiewicz, A.; Wojtkiewicz, J. Health-Promoting Properties of Selected Cyclitols for Metabolic Syndrome and Diabetes. *Nutrients* **2019**, *11*, 2314. [CrossRef]
155. Kalekar, S.A.; Munshi, R.P.; Bhalerao, S.S.; Thatte, U.M. Insulin sensitizing effect of 3 Indian medicinal plants: An in vitro study. *Indian J. Pharmacol.* **2013**, *45*, 30–33. [CrossRef]
156. Stadlbauer, V.; Neuhauser, C.; Aumiller, T.; Stallinger, A.; Iken, M.; Weghuber, J. Identification of Insulin-Mimetic Plant Extracts: From an In Vitro High-Content Screen to Blood Glucose Reduction in Live Animals. *Molecules* **2021**, *26*, 4346. [CrossRef]
157. Papaefstathiou, E.; Agapiou, A.; Giannopoulos, S.; Kokkinofta, R. Nutritional characterization of carobs and traditional carob products. *Food Sci. Nutr.* **2018**, *6*, 2151–2161. [CrossRef]
158. Kim, I.-S.; Kim, C.-H.; Yang, W.-S. Physiologically Active Molecules and Functional Properties of Soybeans in Human Health—A Current Perspective. *Int. J. Mol. Sci.* **2021**, *22*, 4054. [CrossRef]
159. Tewari, R.; Gupta, M.; Ahmad, F.; Rout, P.K.; Misra, L.; Patwardhan, A.; Vasudeva, R. Extraction, quantification and antioxidant activities of flavonoids, polyphenols and pinitol from wild and cultivated *Saraca asoca* bark using RP-HPLC-PDA-RI method. *Ind. Crops Prod.* **2017**, *103*, 73–80. [CrossRef]

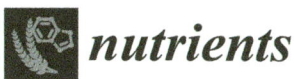

# Review
# Metabolic Effects of an Oral Glucose Tolerance Test Compared to the Mixed Meal Tolerance Tests: A Narrative Review

Marlene Lages [1,2,3], Renata Barros [2,3], Pedro Moreira [2,3,4] and Maria P. Guarino [2,5,*]

[1] ciTechCare—Center for Innovative Care and Health Technology, Polytechnic of Leiria, 2410-541 Leiria, Portugal; marlene.c.lages@ipleiria.pt
[2] Faculty of Nutrition and Food Science, University of Porto, 4150-180 Porto, Portugal; renatabarros@fcna.up.pt (R.B.); pedromoreira@fcna.up.pt (P.M.)
[3] EPIUnit—Instituto de Saude Publica, Universidade do Porto, 4200-450 Porto, Portugal
[4] Laboratorio Para a Investigação Integrativa e Translacional em Saude Populacional (ITR), Portugal Centre in Physical Activity, Health and Leisure, University of Porto, 4200-450 Porto, Portugal
[5] School of Health Sciences, Polytechnic of Leiria, 2411-901 Leiria, Portugal
* Correspondence: maria.guarino@ipleiria.pt

**Abstract:** The oral glucose tolerance test (OGTT) is recommended for assessing abnormalities in glucose homeostasis. Recognised as the gold standard test for diagnosing diabetes, the OGTT provides useful information about glucose tolerance. However, it does not replicate the process of absorption and digestion of complex foods, such as that which occurs with a mixed meal tolerance test (MMTT), an alternative that is still not well explored in the diagnosis of metabolic alterations. The MMTT could be an asset in detecting glucose homeostasis disorders, including diabetes since it has more similarities to the common dietary pattern, allowing early detection of subtle changes in metabolic homeostasis in response to combined nutrients. This alternative has the advantage of being more tolerable and pleasant to patients since it induces a more gradual increase in blood glucose, thus reducing the risk of rebound hypoglycemia and other related complications. The present article reviewed the clinical data available regarding the possibility of screening or diagnosing altered glucose homeostasis, including type 2 diabetes mellitus, with the MMTT.

**Keywords:** diabetes; diagnosis; insulin resistance; fasting plasma glucose; impaired fasting glycemia; impaired glucose tolerance

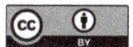

## 1. Introduction

Diabetes mellitus (DM) includes a cluster of metabolic conditions defined by hyperglycemia that can result from insufficient insulin secretion, defects in insulin action, or both [1]. The global prevalence of DM continues to increase, placing an ever-increasing burden on healthcare systems due to the disease and its complications [2]. Currently, 351.7 million people aged between 20 and 64 years have diabetes, whether it is diagnosed or undiagnosed diabetes. By 2030, it is expected that this number will increase to 417.3 million and by 2045 it will reach 486.1 million people [3]. Globally, 213.9 million of the 463 million, or half of the adults that live with diabetes, do not know that they have this disease [3]. In Portugal, in 2018, the estimated prevalence of diabetes was 13.6% in the population aged between 20 and 79 years old. According to these numbers, more than 1 million Portuguese in this age group have diabetes, of which 56% have already been diagnosed and 44% have not yet been diagnosed [4].

Early screening and detection are of crucial importance since continued undiagnosed diabetes increases the risk of having diabetes-related complications [5]. Most cases of DM-associated morbidity and mortality are caused by macrovascular and microvascular complications, some associated with late diagnosis [6]. Diagnosis and classification of diabetes are important for determining the more effective treatment, whether this is based on lifestyle changes, pharmacological therapy, or a combination of both therapeutic approaches.

A report from the World Health Organization (WHO) and the International Diabetes Federation considered the OGTT as the gold standard test used to diagnose diabetes [7]. Despite providing useful information about glucose tolerance, it does not provide information about insulin sensitivity or resistance mostly due to its main limitation, which is that it does not mimic the physiological postprandial metabolism.

The standardized mixed meal has been pointed out as a substitute for the glucose solution administered in the OGTT. In addition, the administration of 75 g of glucose may cause unpleasant symptoms, such as nausea, vomiting, diarrhoea, bloating and anxiety [8–10]. The metabolic feedback to a mixed meal is a better indication of beta-cell function under normal daily life conditions compared with the standard OGTT since the mixed meal contains proteins and fatty acids, which are components that can stimulate insulin secretion [11–13]. In the literature, some studies compare blood glucose levels and insulin sensitivity and resistance during the OGTT and a mixed meal tolerance test (MMTT) [14]. However, the meals used in these clinical studies are diverse and sometimes have a different nutritional composition, leading to heterogeneous results. To the best of our knowledge, there are no previous review articles published that directly compare the results of an OGTT to the different mixed meal tests. Thus, the present review aimed to assess and compare the metabolic effects of the OGTT and mixed meal tests in clinical studies and provide a comprehensive overview of this area of research.

## 2. Materials and Methods

The search was conducted between October and November 2021 using the Scopus database. MeSH terms were applied when possible, and different search strategies were used combining the following keywords: "oral glucose tolerance test", "mixed meal tolerance test", "meal test", "meal tolerance test", "diabetes", and "gestational diabetes".

The search strategies had no date restrictions and included articles published in English and Portuguese. The exclusion criteria were: protocols, letters, commentaries, and studies that were not carried out within the scope of this review, including studies conducted in animals models and studies where the participants, or at least a subsample of participants, did not perform both the OGTT and MMTT to allow comparison. The date last searched was 31 December 2021. Hand searching and references from the extracted articles were also consulted. After selecting the original articles to include and discuss in the present review, the information about their results was synthesized in a table format, including the study design, characteristics of the participants, index test information (sensitivity, specificity, positive predictive value (PPV), negative predictive value (NPV)), and 2-h glucose correlation for the OGTT and MMTT whenever this was available.

## 3. Standard Methods for the Diagnosis of Diabetes

The diagnosis of diabetes is based on plasma glucose criteria, which include the value of fasting plasma glucose (FPG) or the 2-h plasma glucose (2-h PG) value during a 75 g OGTT, or glycated haemoglobin A1c (HbA1c) criteria [1]. The American Diabetes Association (ADA) considers that HbA1c values above 6.5% diagnose diabetes and are considered a significant marker to develop long-term diabetes complications. The use of HbA1c as a clinical endpoint has the advantage that it can be performed without the need for a fasting period, contrary to the FPG or the OGTT. Additionally, this biomarker has greater preanalytical stability and is an indirect measure of mean blood glucose values over the past three months, which eliminates day-to-day variability as a confounding factor in the assessment of impaired glucose tolerance (IGT) or impaired fasting glucose (IFG) [15]. Nonetheless, the use of a single biomarker to detect glucose disturbances has inherent limitations, including lower sensitivity and specificity, and inaccuracy since HbA1c can be affected by ethnicity, haemoglobin variants, and other clinical conditions [16–18].

Fasting plasma glucose is a method with sensitivity but has poor reproducibility. To measure this biomarker, it is required that patients have fasted for at least 8 h before the blood sample collection, and the value can still be affected by short-term factors such as stress and exercise [19,20]. The current recommendations for diabetes diagnosis are established based on studies that measure plasma glucose in blood samples collected in the morning following an overnight fast of a minimum of 8 h. However, some patients may perform this test in the afternoon after an 8 h day fast and, since plasma glucose values are elevated in the morning, it is uncertain if FPG criteria should remain the same for this situation [21,22]. Additionally, when FPG values are used isolated for diagnosis of diabetes, people with an FPG below 126 mg/dL may be misdiagnosed because results from this test can show a discordance from the 2-h PG [23–25]. Additionally, the degree of hyperglycemia changes over time and may present as glucose tolerance abnormalities without reaching the criteria for diabetes, depending on the time from diagnosis and progression of the disease process. Thus, IFG is identified as having FPG levels from 100 mg/dL to 125 mg/dL and IGT as 2-h values in the OGTT of 140 mg/dL to 199 mg/dL [26].

The OGTT is the reference method to diagnose type 2 diabetes mellitus (T2DM) and to define the categories of glucose intolerance that result from higher-than-normal blood glucose levels in the absence of frank diabetes mellitus [26]. The cut-off points allow detecting the intermediate conditions between normal glucose tolerance and diabetes, namely, IGT and IFG [26]. This test was standardized by the administration of a glucose load that contains the equivalent of 75 g of sugar dissolved in water. To screen for diabetes, the 2-h PG after the OGTT and the FPG are more accurate when there is a discordance between the HbA1c and glucose value [26,27].

## 4. Oral Glucose Tolerance Test and Mixed Meal Tolerance Tests

The OGTT and the MMTT are generally used in clinical research related to metabolism as well as diabetes drug development. These tests provide an integrated assessment of the β-cell response to an insulin secretory stimulus that comprises activation of the incretin axis. The main incretin hormones involved in this process are glucagon-like peptide 1, secreted by the L cells, and glucose-dependent insulinotropic peptide, secreted by the K cells. The activation of these incretins includes enhancement of glucose-stimulated insulin secretion from islet β-cells in combination with reduced glucagon release from α-cells [28]. However, a mixed meal is a more physiologic stimulus to insulin secretion because β-cells are also responsive to certain amino acids and fatty acids in addition to glucose [29,30].

The OGTT may reveal both glucose and insulin secretion/action disturbances, but it is important to point out that the liquid glucose can be quickly absorbed, causing an early release of insulin. This can cause false reactive hypoglycemia associated with adverse epigastric symptoms, which do not replicate the usual glucose excursion and insulin responses in daily life conditions. From a clinical perspective, the incidence of reactive hypoglycemia is important. There are reports of hypoglycemia-induced ischemic electrocardiogram changes [31,32], which can indicate a need for caution when performing an OGTT in patients with coronary heart disease. Reactive hypoglycemia can also be challenging in dumping syndrome patients since the liquid glucose promotes rapid gastric emptying [33,34]. Considering this, the exchange of the traditional glucose drink with a standard mixed meal could be beneficial to patients and provide a similar clinical insight into glucose homeostasis.

Regarding the patient's preparation to perform the OGTT and MMTT, there are no considerable differences. The tests are both performed after an 8 h overnight fast and patients are advised not to consume alcohol, caffeine, or tobacco and to abstain from vigorous exercise since these factors can influence insulin sensitivity. Besides, around 100 g to 150 g of carbohydrates should be consumed daily for three days before the test since the dietary restriction of this macronutrient may impair glucose tolerance [26]. Glucose tolerance can also be influenced by other macro and micronutrients, for example, the percentage of energy resulting from fat and protein. However, the effect of these other macronutrients on glucose tolerance is not as immediate as in the case of carbohydrates. Therefore, it is not necessary to make changes in the amounts of fat and protein ingested in the days before the tests [35].

## 5. Mixed Meal Tolerance Test as a Method to Screen Glucose Disturbances

As previously mentioned, the MMTT provides a more physiological stimulus to insulin secretion. From a clinical perspective, performing this test could present some advantages in the screening of glucose and insulin disorders. Patients would also benefit from performing a more pleasant and palatable test with potentially fewer side effects and significantly less discomfort.

Some authors have already conducted clinical studies to compare the metabolic responses of OGTT to the MMTT and some of the main results of these studies are presented in Table 1. The correlations between the 2-glucose values for both tests were classified according to Evans (1996) [36].

**Table 1.** Characteristics and main results of the selected studies comparing the metabolic effects of the oral glucose tolerance test to the meal tolerance tests.

| Ref. | Participants | Main Results | 2-h Glucose Correlations |
|---|---|---|---|
| **Randomized cross-over studies** | | | |
| Chanprasertpinyo et al., 2017 [37] | Healthy adults without DM ($n = 104$) 30 M; 74 F | **2-h glucose levels (OGTT/ice cream * test)**: $\rho = 0.82$; $p < 0.001$; 9.61% discordant diagnostic results **Ice cream test**: 5.76% of missed DM cases | + Very strong |
| Wolever et al., 1998 [38] | Adults with normal weight, obesity, IGT, or diabetes ($n = 36$) 15 M; 21 F | **2-h glucose levels (OGTT/MMTT)**: $r = 0.97$ **1-h glucose (MMTT)/2-h glucose (OGTT)**: $r = 0.96$ **1-h glucose (OGTT)/2-h glucose (MMTT)**: $r = 0.91$ | + Very strong |
| Marena et al., 1992 [39] | Adults with NGT, IGT, mild NIDDM, or NIDDM ($n = 40$; 10 by group) 20 M; 20 F | **Glucose incremental areas (OGTT/mixed meal *)**: $r = 0.511$, $p < 0.001$ **2-h glucose values (OGTT/mixed meal)**: $r = 0.956$, $p < 0.001$ | + Very strong |
| **Non-randomized cross-over studies** | | | |
| Meier et al., 2009 [14] | Adults with NGT, IGT, or diabetes ($n = 60$) | **2-h glucose levels (OGTT/MMTT)**: $r^2 = 0.78$, $p < 0.0001$ | + Strong |
| Harano et al., 2006 [40] | Healthy adults ($n = 19$) 6 M; 13 F | **Cookie * test**: 1 (5%) IGT **OGTT**: 19 (100%) normal blood glucose | n.s. |
| **Cross-sectional studies** | | | |
| Traub et al., 2012 [41] | Healthy early postmenopausal women ($n = 12$) | **MMTT**: 1 (8%) of 2 (16%) participants identified with IGT (confirmed with the OGTT). The second participant had abnormal fasting glucose with the OGTT | n.s. |
| Freeman et al., 2010 [42] | Women with PCOS ($n = 8$) | **Blood glucose levels** **OGTT and MMTT**: 1 (12%) IGT **OGTT**: 1 (12%) IFG (not with MMTT) **MMTT**: 1 (12%) diabetes (not with OGTT) **Blood insulin levels** **OGTT and MMTT**: 4 (57%) IGT | n.s. |

Table 1. Cont.

| Ref. | Participants | Main Results | 2-h Glucose Correlations |
|---|---|---|---|
| **Retrospective study** | | | |
| Forbes et al., 2018 [43] | Adults with T1DM and stable transplant grafts (n = 13) 9 M; 4 F | 2-h glucose values (OGTT and MMTT *): r = 0.45; p = 0.07 90-min MMTT glucose ≥ 144 mg/dL: equivalent to 2-h OGTT glucose ≥ 199.8 mg/dL | + Moderate |

* Nutritional composition described in Table 2. DM, Diabetes Mellitus; M, Male; F, Female; OGTT, Oral Glucose Tolerance Test; IGT, Impaired Glucose Tolerance; NGT, Normal Glucose Tolerance; NIDDM, Non-Insulin-Dependent Diabetes Mellitus; MMTT, Mixed Meal Tolerance Test; PCOS, Polycystic Ovarian Syndrome; T1DM, Type 1 Diabetes Mellitus. n.s., not stated.

Table 2. Nutritional characteristics of the products and/or meals tested.

| Ref. | Product | Energy (kcal) | Carbohydrates (% TE, g) | Protein (% TE, g) | Fat (% TE, g) |
|---|---|---|---|---|---|
| Forbes et al., 2018 [43] | Ensure HP | 1.1 kcal/mL | 55% | 22% | 23% |
| Marais et al., 2018 [44] | Future Life Excel meal | n.d. | 75.0 g | n.d. | n.d. |
| Chanprasertpinyo et al., 2017 [37] | Ice cream | 620.9 | 73.9 g | 18.9 g | 27.7 g |
| Racusin et al., 2015 [45] | 10 strawberry-flavored candy twists (Twizzlers) | n.d. | 50.0 g (91.968%) | 3.515% | 4.527% |
| Traub et al., 2012 [41] | Muffin (Beigel's Bakery) | 410.0 | 56.0 g | 6.0 g | 18.0 g |
| Traub et al., 2012 [41] | Shake | 600.0 | 75.0 g | 30.0 g | 20.0 g |
| Freeman et al., 2010 [42] | Muffin (Costco) and orange juice (Tropicana) | 800.0 | 105.0 g | 12.0 g | 38.0 g |
| Meier et al., 2009 [14] | Continental breakfast [1] | 820.0 | 90.0 g | 26.8 g | 39.2 g |
| Harano et al., 2006 [40] | Cookie | 533.0 | 75.0 g | 7.0 g | 25.0 g |
| Wolever et al., 1998 [38] | 5 wafers (DSP) | 345.0 | 50.0 g | 12.1 g | 10.7 g |
| Roberts et al., 1997 [46] | Standardized breakfast [2] | 300.0 | 45.0 g | 10.0 g | 9.0 g |
| Marena et al., 1992 [39] | Standard mixed meal [3] | 590.0 | 69.0 g (44.0%) | 22.6 g (15.0%) | 27.0 g (41.0%) |
| Coustan et al., 1987 [47] | Standard test breakfast [4] | 600.0 | 52.0 g | 28.0 g | 31.0 g |

TE, total energy; n.d., not defined; DSP, diabetes screening product. [1] Two European bread rolls; 20 g of butter; 40 g of gouda cheese; 30 g of jam; one egg; 150 g of yogurt; 200 mL of tea. [2] Breakfast cereal with milk; toast and butter; tea (amounts not expressed). [3] 125 g of fruit juice; 75 g of ham; 89 g of white bread. [4] Two scrambled eggs; two slices of toast or one English muffin; two pats of butter or margarine; 8 oz orange juice; 8 oz whole or skim milk; one cup of coffee or tea (no sugar).

In a cross-over study conducted by Chanprasertpinyo et al. [37], the authors assessed the effectiveness of using ice cream (described in Table 2) as an alternative to the 75 g oral glucose solution to diagnose diabetes and IGT in 104 healthy participants with no previous history of diabetes. The 2-h plasma glucose values were lower after the ice cream test compared with the OGTT (97.52 ± 40.71 mg/dL and 110 ± 55.53 mg/dL, respectively), but without statistical significance (Table 1). The discordance rate between the two tests was 9.61% when using the 2-h glucose values as the diagnostic criteria for diabetes. By combining the FPG values with the 2-h plasma glucose levels, the ice cream test would have missed 5.76% of the participants with a high risk of having diabetes. Two (1.9%) participants had hypoglycemia (38 and 49 mg/dL) after completing the OGTT, even though they did not demonstrate any symptoms. The authors also assessed the preferences and side-effects of the participants using a questionnaire and, according to this, 63% preferred the ice cream test and 36% reported more unpleasant symptoms with the OGTT.

Wolever et al. [38]'s results showed that the 2-h plasma glucose coefficient of variation of the mixed meal composed of wafers (described in Table 2) and the 75 g OGTT was not significant in people with diabetes. The plasma glucose levels 2-h following the mixed meal were closely associated with the ones 2-h after the OGTT, showing a linear correlation.

Marena et al. [39] compared the effects of a standard mixed meal (described in Table 2) and an OGTT on plasma glucose values on 40 participants equally distributed as healthy participants, IGT patients, mild non-insulin-dependent patients, and non-insulin-dependent with secondary failure to oral agent treatment. The levels of plasma glucose following the OGTT were significantly higher compared with the mixed meal in all groups. After the mixed meal, there was a statically significant difference in the mean 2-h plasma glucose levels among the four groups of participants. Regarding the plasma glucose incremental areas, these were significantly higher following the OGTT compared with the mixed meal, with exception to the healthy group. A significant correlation was found between plasma glucose incremental areas following the OGTT and the mixed meal ($r = 0.511$, $p < 0.001$). A highly significant ($r = 0.956$, $p < 0.001$) correlation between glucose values during the OGTT and mixed meal was also found. The values of glucose variation following the mixed meal were identical to the ones after the OGTT for the group with healthy participants.

The study conducted by Meier et al. [14], in a group of 60 participants, including 16 (26.7%) patients with T2DM, found a strong correlation between the 2-h glucose values after the 75 g OGTT and the corresponding glucose values following the test meal (described in Table 2) ($r^2 = 0.78$, $p < 0.0001$). Additionally, peak glucose excursions following the glucose load were strongly associated with the correspondent maximum glucose values after the mixed meal administration [14]. Besides, there were statically significant correlations among the 120 min glucose values following the OGTT and the glucose values measured at all time points during the test meal (every 30 min until reaching 240 min).

Harano et al. [40] developed a cookie (described in Table 2) test to determine glucose, insulin, and lipids disturbances. The mean glucose and insulin values at 0, 1, and 2 h after the cookie test and the 75 g OGTT, performed on 19 healthy participants, were not statistically different. However, in two (11%) participants insulin response was earlier and higher in amplitude with the oral glucose solution. Similar to other studies, the 2-h glucose value with OGTT tended to be lower compared with the cookie test. According to the WHO criteria for evaluation of diabetes and IGT, 18 (94.7%) participants were classified as normal and one (5.3%) participant with IGT with the cookie test, whereas with oral glucose solution all 19 participants had normal glucose values. Reactive hypoglycemia was noted in five (26.3%) participants with the OGTT, and one (5.3%) with the cookie test. Participants reported epigastric symptoms only with the oral glucose solution.

This cookie test was also performed on a subgroup of 64 participants with lifestyle diseases and a subgroup of 26 participants that acted as the control for the lifestyle diseases subgroup. In the participants with diabetes ($n = 14$) (21.9%) from the subgroup with lifestyle diseases, glucose values were above 138.6 mg/dL following the cookie test. The insulin area under the curve (AUC) after the cookie test was used to measure insulin resistance and it showed that the participants with obesity ($n = 24$) (37.5%) and IGT ($n = 6$) (9.4%) had significantly higher values with the cookie test [40].

Traub et al. [41] compared the effectiveness of a muffin test to a 75 g OGTT in diagnosing IGT. Participants were 73 healthy adult women in the early postmenopausal stage. After an overnight 10-h fast, participants consumed a commercially available muffin (described in Table 2) and a coffee or tea with insignificant carbohydrate content. A subgroup of 12 (16%) participants performed the OGTT at a separate visit and an MMTT on a third visit. To perform the MMTT, the 12 participants were stabilized for 120 min before they ingested an oral shake with 600 kcal (described in Table 2). Compared with the MMTT and the OGTT, the muffin test worked well as a screening method to detect abnormal glucose metabolism. The mean 2-h glucose levels were significantly lower after the OGTT compared with the MMTT ($p = 0.0002$) and after the muffin test, but without being statistically significant ($p > 0.05$). Two (17%) participants of the subgroup were classified with IGT based on the muffin test but only one of these two women was identified in the OGTT. However, it should be noticed that the second participant had altered fasting glucose in the OGTT. Out of the 73 participants, eight (11%) were identified with IGT by the 2-h muffin test glucose. The screening of impaired glucose metabolism using the FPG cut-off (less than 126 mg/dL) would have a prevalence of missed cases of 63% (five in eight women). The data analysis demonstrated a significant correlation between the mean FPG and the 2-h muffin test glucose. These results were similar to the ones from a study by Freeman and colleagues [42]. They chose a meal that combined a commercially accessible muffin and orange juice (described in Table 2) to perform the MMTT in 13 women with polycystic ovarian syndrome (PCOS) since postprandial values may give a better representation of day-to-day glucose and insulin variations in these women. Only women diagnosed with PCOS without diabetes were included. In this study, the authors did not perform a statistical comparison between the results of the OGTT and the MMTT since the timing of the blood sample collection was different in the two tests (every 30 min in the MMTT and hourly in the OGTT). Only eight (62%) women performed the OGTT, thus having glucose measured with both the MMTT and the OGTT, and for one of these eight women insulin levels were not assessed during the OGTT. At the timepoints that coincided (60 and 120 min), glucose levels were lower in the MMTT in comparison with the OGTT (60 min: 111.40 ± 35.24 mg/dL and 142.57 ± 34.87 mg/dL; 120 min: 106.6 ± 30.78 mg/dL and 112.43 ± 25.79 mg/dL, respectively) and insulin levels were higher in the MMTT in comparison with the OGTT (60 min: 169.8 ± 132.9 µIU/mL and 154.62 ± 81.76 µIU7mL; 120 min: 152.05 ± 120.37 µIU/mL and 118.50 ± 97.34 µIU/mL, respectively). According to the cut-offs defined by ADA in 2008 [48], one (12%) woman showed IGT on both tests, one (12%) woman had IFG only on the OGTT, and one (12%) woman was classified as to have diabetes according to the results of the MMTT, but the values obtained in the OGTT were within the normal range. Out of the seven women that performed both tests, four (57%) had IGT on both the OGTT and MMTT [42]. No adverse effects were reported by the participants during and after the MMTT.

In a more recent study, Forbes et al. [43] studied 13 insulin-independent islet transplant patients. Twelve (92%) of the patients performed both tests, namely, the MMTT and the 75 g OGTT. In the MMTT a drink was administered, Ensure HP (Table 2), according to the participant's body weight. Although there was no statistical significance, the data analysis showed a correlation between the glucose levels after the OGTT and MMTT. The results also demonstrated an association between the 90-min glucose $\geq$ 144.0 mg/dL following the MMTT and the 120-min OGTT cut-off point for diabetes diagnosis.

## 6. Meal Tolerance Tests to Screen for Gestational Diabetes Mellitus

Some authors have also been assessing the efficacy of meal tests in screening GDM and the main results of the selected studies are presented in Table 3. Currently, to diagnose GDM there are two possible approaches [26]: the one-step 75 g OGTT derived from the International Association of the Diabetes and Pregnancy Study Groups, where glucose is measured at a fasted state, 1-h and 2-h after the glucose load; and the two-step approach with a first screen, the glucose challenge test (GCT), using a 50 g glucose solution (nonfasting) and the assessment of 1-h plasma glucose value, followed by the second step, which is performing a 3-h 100 g OGTT for women who screen positive according to the Carpenter and Coustan criteria [26,49]. The summary of the main results is presented in Table 3.

**Table 3.** Main characteristics and results of the selected studies that used the meal tests to screen gestational diabetes mellitus.

| Ref. | Participants | Main Results | 2-h Glucose Correlations |
|---|---|---|---|
| **Case-control study** | | | |
| Eslamian and Ramezani 2006 [50] | Pregnant women ($n = 141$) | **GCT:** 41 (29.3%) GDM<br>**OGTT:** 12 (8.57%) GDM<br>**Breakfast test:** 28 (20%) GDM<br>Optimal cut-off value: 130 mg/dL at 60 min (83.3% sensitivity; 85.9% specificity; 35.7% PPV; 98.2% NPV) | n.s. |
| **Randomized cross-over studies** | | | |
| Marais et al. 2018 [44] | Pregnant women with a high risk of GDM ($n = 51$) | **2-h OGTT (venous):** 5 (10%) GDM<br>**2-h OGTT (capillary):** 6 (12%) GDM<br>**2-h DBGP test (capillary):** 7 (14%) GDM; 3 (6%) missed GDM cases; 5 (10%) false-positive cases<br>**DBGP test:** 25% sensitivity; 96% specificity; 33% PPV; 95% NPV | n.s. |
| Coustan et al. 1987 [47] | Pregnant women with GDM ($n = 20$) | 16 (80%) of the 20 subjects with GDM had a 1-h breakfast test plasma glucose level $\geq$ 120 mg/dL (threshold defined by the 1-h mean glucose + 2 SD)<br>**MMTT:** 75% sensitivity; 94% specificity | n.s. |
| **Non-randomized cross-over studies** | | | |
| Racusin et al. 2015 [45] | Pregnant women screened positive for GDM ($n = 20$) | **1-h candy twists test:**<br>100% sensitivity; 50% specificity; 18% PPV; 100% NPV; 82% false-referral rate; 18% detection rate | +<br>Moderate ** |
| Roberts et al. 1997 [46] | Non-diabetic pregnant women ($n = 102$) | **OGTT (cut-off 144 mg/dL):** 7 (7%) IGT<br>**Breakfast (cut-off 144 mg/dL):** 0 (0%) IGT<br>**OGTT (cut-off 162 mg/dL):** 2 (2%) IGT<br>**OGTT (cut off 192 mg/dL):** 0 (0%) GDM | n.s. |

GDM, Gestational Diabetes Mellitus; OGTT, Oral Glucose Tolerance Test; GCT, Glucose Challenge Test; PPV, Positive Predictive Value; NPV, Negative Predictive Value; DBGP, Design Breakfast Glucose Profile; SD, standard deviation; MMTT, Mixed Meal Tolerance Test; IGT, Impaired Glucose Tolerance. n.s., not stated; ** $p < 0.05$.

Eslamian and Ramezani [50] also tested a standard breakfast containing 50 g of glucose, the equivalent of the first step to screen for GDM in the two-step approach. The 141 pregnant women enrolled in this randomized cross-over study performed both the 50-g glucose breakfast study and the standard 50-g GCT. Women with blood glucose values above 130 mg/dL after 60 min performed the 100 g 3-h OGTT to confirm the diagnosis. The breakfast test results were positive for 28 women (20%) while the GCT positively screened 41 women (29.3%). After performing the OGTT, it was confirmed that only 12 women (8.57%) had GDM. However, it was not reported how many of these pregnant women had been positively screened with the breakfast test. The concordance between the OGTT and GCT and breakfast test were 0.429 and 0.432, respectively ($p < 0.001$, Kappa test). The authors highlighted that the breakfast was tolerated by all the participants while the 50-g GCT was not tolerated by three women.

In the study by Marais et al. [44] conducted on 51 pregnant women, the 75-g OGTT with venous blood sampling diagnosed GDM in five (10%) patients, while the 75-g OGTT with capillary blood sampling diagnosed GDM in six (12%) women. The design breakfast glucose profile (DBGP) (described in Table 2) with capillary blood sampling diagnosed GDM in seven (14%) patients. The correlations between fasting capillary OGTT and DBGP ($r = 0.639$), 2-h capillary OGTT and DBGP ($r = 0.542$), fasting venous OGTT and fasting capillary DBGP ($r = 0.608$), and 2-h venous OGTT and 2-h capillary DBGP ($r = 0.598$) were statistically significant ($p < 0.001$). Comparing the diagnostic capacity of the gold standard, the DBGP test missed three (6%) women with GDM and gave five (10%) false-positive results, though three (6%) of these cases were due to higher values of fasting capillary glucose.

Coustan et al. [47] compared the plasma glucose values determined after a GCT with the value measured 1 h after a 600-kcal MMTT (Table 2) on 70 pregnant women, 20 (29%) of which were already diagnosed with GDM. In the subgroup of 50 pregnant women with presumed normal glucose, 24 (48%) performed the 100-g OGTT because one or both 50 g screening tests exceeded 130 mg/dL and four (8%) were diagnosed with GDM. For a cut-point of $\geq 120$ mg/dL, out of the 20 women in the group with known GDM, 16 (80%) women were screened positive with the MMTT. Including the 24 cases of GDM, and for a threshold of $\geq 120$ mg/dL, the sensitivity of the MMTT was 75% and the specificity was 94%.

Racusin and colleagues [45] tested strawberry candy twists (described in Table 2) as an alternative to the 50-g glucose solution (glucola) used in the GCT. The authors set the value to screen-positive for GDM as blood glucose equal to or above 130 mg/dL 1-h following the candy twists to ensure maximum detection of GDM. The two (10%) women diagnosed with GDM with the 3-h 100 g OGTT according to the National Diabetes Data Group criteria and the Carpenter and Coustan criteria [49,51] were screened as positive with the candy twists and the glucola drink. The candy twists screening would have prevented nine (45%) women from performing the 3-h OGTT. The results showed that the positive predictive value of the candy twists was higher than the glucola drink. However, only 11 (55%) of the 20 participants screened positive with the candy twists when all the participants had previously screened positive with the 50-g glucose beverage.

In the cross-over study conducted by Roberts et al. [46], 102 non-diabetic pregnant women performed both a 75-g OGTT and a standardized breakfast test (described in Table 2) on separated days within one week. Plasma glucose values were measured before and 2 h after the standardized meal. The correlation between the OGTT and breakfast test glucose values at 1-h ($r = 0.36$) and 2-h ($r = 0.15$) was weak. The authors used the WHO recommendations for diabetes diagnosis [52] from 1979 and identified seven (7%) women with IGT, established with a cut-off value of 144 mg/dL after the OGTT. However, when using the cut-off value of 162 mg/dL recommended by the Diabetic Pregnancy Study Group [53], only two (2%) women had IGT. Regarding the 2-h glucose values after the breakfast test, no women had values above 144 mg/dL. No women were diagnosed with GDM according to the 2-h OGTT glucose above 198 mg/dL.

In this same article [46], the authors also studied a group of pregnant women with IGT according to the WHO criteria [52]. Similarly, they did not find a significant correlation between the 2-h glucose values after the OGTT and the breakfast test ($r = 0.35$). Roberts and colleagues compared the 2-h glucose values after the OGTT with the highest glucose values after the breakfast test, and out of the 104 pregnant women with IGT, only 15 (14%) had values above 144 mg/dL.

## 7. Discussion

Some studies suggest that the MMTT is more similar to the physiological postprandial metabolic responses compared with the OGTT. In this review, we analyzed the results from 13 studies, five of them conducted in pregnant women, that compared the efficacy of an MMTT in screening or diagnosing DM and GDM. Half of the studies not performed in the context of GDM showed a strong or very strong correlation between the 2-h glucose values of both tests [14,37–39] and low percentages of missed or misdiagnosed cases [37,40–42], which may indicate that the MMTT could serve as an alternative to the OGTT. As for GDM, the results showed that a high number of women screened positive for GDM using the MMTT without having that condition, as proven by the low percentage of PPV and sensitivity [45,50,54]. The results are promising, and in the future, the MMTT could be a valid alternative to the OGTT. However, considering the current data and options available, it is not yet possible to make this transition. There are still some key points that should be taken into consideration, including the definition of cut-off points to screen and diagnose diabetes with the MMTT and the standardization of a mixed meal.

When comparing both tests, gastric emptying is a factor that should be considered since it is quicker after the OGTT compared with a mixed meal, which leads to a fast release of glucose to the duodenum and the portal venous circulation [55–57]. Additionally, the protein and fat content present in the mixed meals delay gastrointestinal glucose absorption, which leads to lower profiles of postprandial glucose and different insulin secretion profiles [58,59]. The types of mixed meals used in the tolerance tests are also, generally, more palatable and acceptable than the OGTT, causing fewer side effects such as stomach discomfort, headache, dizziness, hunger, and nausea [38]. The high glucose content of the solution used in the OGTT leads to a fast increase in blood glucose and, consequently, in most cases, a fast rise in insulin values, which next provokes a sudden decline in blood glucose with dizziness and syncope risk. Reactive hypoglycemia is one of the unpleasant side effects of this test and, according to the study by Harano and colleagues [40], it was more prevalent in this test than in the meal tolerance test. Preventing these symptoms and side effects can be particularly important in pregnant women, who are usually more sensitive to this type of test. These solutions could also prevent the need to repeat the OGTT in pregnant women due to the vomiting induced by the glucose solution, as occurred in the study by Roberts and colleagues [46]. According to the results of the study conducted by Forbes and colleagues [43], the MMTT could even reduce the time necessary to perform a diagnostic test. In this study, the 90-min glucose values after the MMTT were associated with the 120-min OGTT cut-off point for the diagnosis of diabetes, which could spare 30 min in test time.

The administration of a standard mixed meal as the challenge test for screening diabetes and impaired glucose tolerance may be an alternative to the glucose load, providing that the standardized meal has an expected effect on glucose levels [47]. Brodovicz et al. [10] suggested that a liquid meal test could also be another solution to explore since it may be easier to standardize and administer. In their study, postprandial metabolic responses were very similar and well-correlated after a mixed or liquid meal test with comparable nutritional and energetic value; however, the participants did not perform an OGTT to compare the metabolic responses. Although, when looking for a more physiological stimulus to diagnose impaired glucose metabolism, the liquid meal approaches an OGTT in the sense that it is not as physiological as a solid mixed meal due to the more rapid delivery of nutrients to the duodenum. It has, however, the advantage of avoiding the confounding factor of delayed gastric emptying [43,60].

The non-completion of OGTT delays the diagnosis of diabetes, which increases the risk of developing complications associated with this condition. One of the main reasons cited for non-completion of the OGTT by pregnant women is related to the fact that they cannot tolerate the test procedure [61]. The results of the study by Roberts and colleagues [46] showed that pregnant women that performed the OGTT first had a higher withdrawal rate, which can be an indicator that this procedure was less tolerable. Investigating new methods and/or alternatives for the glucose solution used in the diagnosis of diabetes, which are easier and more tolerated, has significant clinical importance but also shortcomings. Though the mixed meal tolerance tests can be recognized as a substitute test for postprandial responses, comparisons of metabolic responses to the MMTT among studies cannot be made due to the diversity of meal sizes and nutritional contents that have a different impact on gastric distension, gastric emptying, and incretin response [59,62–65]. An MMTT performed with a standard mixed meal would simplify comparisons of results across countries and studies, reduce the variability, and contribute to the validation of this methodology. The standardization of the meals used to screen for diabetes was previously emphasized by Marais et al. [54]. They performed a study on 50 pregnant women to measure the carbohydrate quantity of non-standardized breakfast meal tests used to screen GDM. Although the carbohydrate content median was 71 g, similar to the 75 g oral glucose solution, the values ranged from 55 g to 145 g. Though the standardized meal could represent a substitute for the oral glucose solution, the authors advise against using non-standardized meals since only seven of the meals (14%) fell within the 10% of 75 g carbohydrate target [54]. Besides, similarly to the OGTT, to guarantee homogeneity in the meal test is necessary to ensure that the patients ingest the food in its entirety and in an equal interval to minimize the effect of confounding factors. In the case of the study by Harano et al. [40], participants had 10 to 15 min to eat the cookie, but if they were used to a small breakfast or if they did not like the cookie, they could eat half of it within 10 min and the other half within an additional 10 to 20 min.

Regarding costs, the meal tests are, in general, more affordable than the oral glucose solution. Some authors set the cost of the oral glucose solution at $6 per unit [40], others at $5.20 [41], while others just mention that the costs range from $3.41 to a lot higher [45]. Besides, a recent literature review emphasized the need to perform more studies comparing the composition and homogeneity of different oral glucose solutions since there is only a small number of studies and most of them are not appropriately designed [66]. The composition of these solutions, including the components added to improve organoleptic characteristics such as taste and smell, may influence blood glucose and endogenous insulin secretion.

In addition to being more equivalent to people's dietary patterns, the meal tolerance tests can provide valuable information concerning the different categories of glucose intolerance and insulin resistance. Though, more research is needed to define the threshold of blood glucose values when using the MMTT as a screen or diagnosis method for diabetes or other glucose intolerances. In the study by Coustan et al. [47], when the threshold was lowered to 100 mg/dL, the sensitivity increased from 75% to 96%; however, the specificity lowered from 94% to 74%. To screen for glucose disturbances, the definition of the cut-off point is of the utmost importance to avoid the administration of unnecessary OGTT, but with this value, the healthcare professionals need to be able to detect people with middle abnormal glucose tolerance tests.

Some limitations were identified while conducting this review that may be important to consider in the design of future studies. The studies included in this review presented some heterogeneity regarding the tests performed and the screening and diagnostic criteria selected by the authors. The differences in both quantity and nutritional values of the food items administered in the diverse MMTT can influence the metabolic responses of the participants [29,30]. Besides, some of the studies included herein compared the MMTT to a 75 g [14,37–43,46] or 100 g glucose load [45,47,50], while others compared it to a GCT [47,50], and one study used capillary glucose values [44] instead of blood glucose. A few of the studies included were performed more than twenty years ago; thus, some of the methodologies may be outdated (i.e., Roberts et al. [46] assessed IGT in pregnant women using the WHO criteria from 1980, which are currently outdated). Besides, none of the articles explained the process behind the formulation or choice of the meals tested, and some of them did not provide the nutritional information of the meal.

Future research in the area can address the limitations of previous studies and contribute with more information such as the acceptability and palatability of the alternative tests to the participants.

Currently, there is still a lack of clinical studies testing this hypothesis of a mixed meal as an equivalent to the glucose solution. To validate the MMTT as an alternative to the OGTT for a specific population, there is a need to design and perform more multicenter randomized clinical trials with larger sample sizes. However, designing a trial to assess and compare the diagnostic accuracy of an MMTT with the OGTT may be challenging due to the sensitivity and specificity of the OGTT being equivalent to 100%. Thus, to demonstrate a greater accuracy and precision in diagnosis, it is still necessary to show a better degree of concordance among repeated tests in clinical studies with a much larger number of participants than those present in this article.

## 8. Conclusions

A complete nutritional challenge that incorporates all the macronutrients (carbohydrates, proteins, and fat) such as the mixed meal tolerance tests is theoretically more physiological. Therefore, this type of test is likely to provide more insightful and comprehensive information concerning metabolic and glucose homeostasis compared with a single macronutrient challenge. However, the diversity of mixed meal challenges already tested highlights the need to perform larger trials to compare the effectiveness in diagnosing glucose disturbances with a standardized mixed meal and the oral glucose solution administered in the OGTT. The clinical application of the MMTT as a validated test to diagnose glucose disturbances in patients warrants further investigation.

**Author Contributions:** M.L. and M.P.G. contributed to the drafting, editing and revision of this review. R.B. and P.M. reviewed the manuscript. All authors have approved the submitted version and agree to be personally accountable for its accuracy and integrity. All authors have read and agreed to the published version of the manuscript.

**Funding:** This research received no external funding. The APC was funded by national funds from the Fundação para a Ciência e Tecnologia (UI/05704/2020). M.L. has a PhD scholarship from the Fundação para a Ciência e Tecnologia (2021.07673.BD).

**Institutional Review Board Statement:** Not applicable.

**Informed Consent Statement:** Not applicable.

**Conflicts of Interest:** The authors declare no conflict of interest.

## References

1. American Diabetes Association. Diagnosis and Classification of Diabetes Mellitus. *Diabetes Care* **2014**, *37*, S81–S90. [CrossRef] [PubMed]
2. Zheng, Y.; Ley, S.H.; Hu, F.B. Global aetiology and epidemiology of type 2 diabetes mellitus and its complications. *Nat. Rev. Endocrinol.* **2018**, *14*, 88–98. [CrossRef] [PubMed]
3. International Diabetes Federation. *IDF Diabetes Atlas*, 9th ed.; International Diabetes Federation: Brussels, Belgium, 2019; pp. 36–43.
4. Raposo, J.F. Diabetes: Factos e Números 2016, 2017 e 2018. *Rev. Port. Diabetes* **2020**, *15*, 19–27.
5. Saeedi, P.; Petersohn, I.; Salpea, P.; Malanda, B.; Karuranga, S.; Unwin, N.; Colagiuri, S.; Guariguata, L.; Motala, A.A.; Ogurtsova, K.; et al. Global and regional diabetes prevalence estimates for 2019 and projections for 2030 and 2045: Results from the International Diabetes Federation Diabetes Atlas, 9th edition. *Diabetes Res. Clin. Pract.* **2019**, *157*, 107843. [CrossRef]
6. Beckman, J.A.; Creager, M.A.; Libby, P. Diabetes and atherosclerosis epidemiology, pathophysiology, and management. *J. Am. Med. Assoc.* **2002**, *287*, 2570–2581. [CrossRef]
7. World Health Organization; International Diabetes Federation. *Definition and Diagnosis of Diabetes Mellitus and Intermediate Hyperglycemia: Report of a WHO/IDF Consultation*; World Health Organization: Geneva, Switzerland, 2006. Available online: http://apps.who.int/iris/bitstream/handle/10665/43588/9241594934_eng.pdf?sequence=1 (accessed on 4 February 2022).
8. Daniells, S.; Grenyer, B.F.S.; Davis, W.S.; Coleman, K.J.; Burgess, J.A.P.; Moses, R.G. Gestational diabetes mellitus: Is a diagnosis associated with an increase in maternal anxiety and stress in the short and intermediate term? *Diabetes Care* **2003**, *26*, 385–389. [CrossRef]
9. Hillier, T.A.; Vesco, K.K.; Pedula, K.L.; Beil, T.L.; Whitlock, E.P.; Pettitt, D.J. Screening for gestational diabetes mellitus: A systematic review for the U.S. preventive services task force. *Ann. Intern. Med.* **2008**, *148*, 766–775. [CrossRef]
10. Brodovicz, K.G.; Girman, C.J.; Simonis-Bik, A.M.C.; Rijkelijkhuizen, J.M.; Zelis, M.; Bunck, M.C.; Mari, A.; Nijpels, G.; Eekhoff, E.M.W.; Dekker, J.M. Postprandial metabolic responses to mixed versus liquid meal tests in healthy men and men with type 2 diabetes. *Diabetes Res. Clin. Pract.* **2011**, *94*, 449–455. [CrossRef]
11. Nuttall, F.Q.; Gannon, M.C.; Wald, J.L.; Ahmed, M. Plasma glucose and insulin profiles in normal subjects ingesting diets of varying carbohydrate, fat, and protein content. *J. Am. Coll. Nutr.* **1982**, *4*, 437–450. [CrossRef]

12. Nuttall, F.Q.; Mooradian, A.D.; Gannon, M.C.; Billington, C.J.; Krezowski, P. Effect of protein ingestion on the glucose and insulin response to a standardized oral glucose load. *Diabetes Care* **1984**, *7*, 465–470. [CrossRef]
13. Denis McGarry, J. Dysregulation of fatty acid metabolism in the etiology of type 2 diabetes. *Diabetes* **2002**, *51*, 7–18. [PubMed]
14. Meier, J.J.; Baller, B.; Menge, B.A.; Gallwitz, B.; Schmidt, W.E.; Nauck, M.A. Excess glycaemic excursions after an oral glucose tolerance test compared with a mixed meal challenge and self-measured home glucose profiles: Is the OGTT a valid predictor of postprandial hyperglycaemia and vice versa? *Diabetes Obes. Metab.* **2009**, *11*, 213–222. [CrossRef] [PubMed]
15. Sequeira, I.R.; Poppitt, S.D. HbA1c as a Marker of Prediabetes: A Reliable Screening Tool or Not. *Insights Nutr. Metab.* **2017**, *1*, 11–20.
16. Barry, E.; Roberts, S.; Oke, J.; Vijayaraghavan, S.; Normansell, R.; Greenhalgh, T. Efficacy and Effectiveness of Screen and Treat Policies in Prevention of Type 2 Diabetes: Systematic Review and Meta-Analysis of Screening Tests and Interventions. *BMJ* **2017**, *356*, i6538. [CrossRef] [PubMed]
17. Dorcely, B.; Katz, K.; Jagannathan, R.; Chiang, S.S.; Oluwadare, B.; Goldberg, I.J.; Bergman, M. Novel Biomarkers for Prediabetes, Diabetes, and Associated Complications. *Diabetes Metab. Syndr. Obes. Targets Ther.* **2017**, *10*, 345–361. [CrossRef] [PubMed]
18. Hostalek, U. Global Epidemiology of Prediabetes—Present and Future Perspectives. *Clin. Diabetes Endocrinol.* **2019**, *5*, 5. [CrossRef]
19. Chung, J.K.O.; Xue, H.; Pang, E.W.H.; Tam, D.C.C. Accuracy of fasting plasma glucose and hemoglobin A1c testing for the early detection of diabetes: A pilot study. *Front. Lab. Med.* **2017**, *1*, 76–81. [CrossRef]
20. Newsholme, P.; Cruzat, V.; Arfuso, F.; Keane, K. Nutrient Regulation of Insulin Secretion and Action. *J. Endocrinol.* **2014**, *221*, R105–R120. [CrossRef]
21. Bolli, G.B.; de Feo, P.; de Cosmo, S.; Perriello, G.; Ventura, M.M.; Calcinaro, F.; Lolli, C.; Campbell, P.; Brunetti, P.; Gerich, J.E. Demonstration of a Dawn Phenomenon in Normal Human Volunteers. *Diabetes* **1984**, *33*, 1150–1153. [CrossRef]
22. Troisi, R.J.; Cowie, C.C.; Harris, M.I. Diurnal Variation in Fasting Plasma Glucose: Implications for Diagnosis of Diabetes in Patients Examined in the Afternoon. *JAMA* **2000**, *284*, 3157–3159. [CrossRef]
23. Jeon, J.Y.; Ko, S.H.; Kwon, H.S.; Kim, N.H.; Kim, J.H.; Kim, C.S.; Song, K.H.; Won, J.C.; Lim, S.; Choi, S.H.; et al. Prevalence of Diabetes and Prediabetes according to Fasting Plasma Glucose and HbA1c. *Diabetes Metab. J.* **2013**, *37*, 349–357. [CrossRef] [PubMed]
24. Lee, E.T.; Howard, B.V.; Go, O.; Savage, P.J.; Fabsitz, R.R.; Robbins, D.C.; Welty, T.K. Prevalence of Undiagnosed Diabetes in Three American Indian Populations. A Comparison of the 1997 American Diabetes Association Diagnostic Criteria and the 1985 World Health Organization Diagnostic Criteria: The Strong Heart Study. *Diabetes Care* **2000**, *23*, 181–186. [CrossRef] [PubMed]
25. Al-Bahrani, A.I.; Charles, B.; Raid, B.; Al-Yahyaee, S.A. Diagnostic Accuracy of the American Diabetes Association Criteria in the Diagnosis of Glucose Intolerance among High-Risk Omani Subjects. *Ann. Saudi Med.* **2004**, *24*, 183–185.
26. American Diabetes Association Professionals Committee Classification and Diagnosis of Diabetes: Standards of Medical Care in Diabetes—2022. *Diabetes Care* **2022**, *45*, S17–S38. [CrossRef] [PubMed]
27. Gonzalez, A.; Deng, Y.; Lane, A.N.; Benkeser, D.; Cui, X.; Staimez, L.R.; Ford, C.N.; Khan, F.N.; Markley Webster, S.C.; Leong, A.; et al. Impact of Mismatches in HbA1c vs Glucose Values on the Diagnostic Classification of Diabetes and Prediabetes. *Diabet. Med.* **2020**, *37*, 689–696. [CrossRef] [PubMed]
28. Fu, Z.; Gilbert, E.R.; Liu, D. Regulation of Insulin Synthesis and Secretion and Pancreatic Beta-Cell Dysfunction in Diabetes. *Curr. Diabetes Rev.* **2012**, *9*, 25–53. [CrossRef]
29. Nolan, C.J.; Prentki, M. The Islet β-Cell: Fuel Responsive and Vulnerable. *Trends Endocrinol. Metab.* **2008**, *19*, 285–291. [CrossRef]
30. Newsholme, P.; Krause, M. Nutritional Regulation of Insulin Secretion: Implications for Diabetes. *Clin. Biochem. Rev.* **2012**, *33*, 35.
31. Desouza, C.; Salazar, H.; Cheong, B.; Murgo, J.; Fonseca, V. Association of Hypoglycemia and Cardiac Ischemia. *Diabetes Care* **2003**, *26*, 1485–1489. [CrossRef]
32. Miura, J.; Uchigata, Y.; Sato, A.; Matsunaga, R.; Fujito, T.; Borgeld, H.-J.; Tanaka, M.; Babazono, T.; Takahashi, C.; Iwamoto, Y. An IDDM Patient Who Complained of Chest Oppression with Ischemic Changes on ECG in Insulin-Induced Hypoglycemia. *Diabetes Res. Clin. Pract.* **1998**, *39*, 31–37. [CrossRef]
33. Scarpellini, E.; Arts, J.; Karamanolis, G.; Laurenius, A.; Siquini, W.; Suzuki, H.; Ukleja, A.; van Beek, A.; Vanuytsel, T.; Bor, S.; et al. International Consensus on the Diagnosis and Management of Dumping Syndrome. *Nat. Rev. Endocrinol.* **2020**, *16*, 448–466. [CrossRef] [PubMed]
34. Frank, J.W.; Saslow, S.B.; Camilleri, M.; Thomforde, G.M.; Dinneen, S.; Rizza, R.A. Mechanism of Accelerated Gastric Emptying of Liquids and Hyperglycemia in Patients with Type II Diabetes Mellitus. *Gastroenterology* **1995**, *109*, 755–765. [CrossRef]
35. Nesti, L.; Mengozzi, A.; Tricò, D. Impact of Nutrient Type and Sequence on Glucose Tolerance: Physiological Insights and Therapeutic Implications. *Front. Endocrinol.* **2019**, *10*, 144. [CrossRef] [PubMed]
36. Evans, J.D. *Straightforward Statistics for the Behavioral Sciences*; Brooks/Cole Publishing: Pacific Groove, CA, USA, 1996.
37. Chanprasertpinyo, W.; Bhirommuang, N.; Surawattanawiset, T.; Tangsermwong, T.; Phanachet, P.; Sriphrapradang, C. Using Ice Cream for Diagnosis of Diabetes Mellitus and Impaired Glucose Tolerance: An Alternative to the Oral Glucose Tolerance Test. *Am. J. Med. Sci.* **2017**, *354*, 581–585. [CrossRef]
38. Wolever, T.M.S.; Chiasson, J.L.; Csima, A.; Hunt, J.A.; Palmason, C.; Ross, S.A.; Ryan, E.A. Variation of Postprandial Plasma Glucose, Palatability, and Symptoms Associated with a Standardized Mixed Test Meal versus 75 g Oral Glucose. *Diabetes Care* **1998**, *21*, 336–340. [CrossRef]

39. Marena, S.; Montegrosso, G.; de Michieli, F.; Pisu, E.; Pagano, G. Comparison of the Metabolic Effects of Mixed Meal and Standard Oral Glucose Tolerance Test on Glucose, Insulin and C-Peptide Response in Healthy, Impaired Glucose Tolerance, Mild and Severe Non-Insulin-Dependent Diabetic Subjects. *Acta Diabetol.* **1992**, *29*, 29–33. [CrossRef]
40. Harano, Y.; Miyawaki, T.; Nabiki, J.; Shibachi, M.; Adachi, T.; Ikeda, M.; Ueda, F.; Nakano, T. Development of Cookie Test for the Simultaneous Determination of Glucose Intolerance, Hyperinsulinemia, Insulin Resistance and Postprandial Dyslipidemia. *Endocr. J.* **2006**, *53*, 173–180. [CrossRef]
41. Traub, M.L.; Jain, A.; Maslow, B.-S.; Pal, L.; Stein, D.T.; Santoro, N.; Freeman, R. The "Muffin Test"—An Alternative to the Oral Glucose Tolerance Test for Detecting Impaired Glucose Tolerance. *Menopause* **2012**, *19*, 62–66. [CrossRef]
42. Freeman, R.; Pollack, R.; Rosenbloom, E. Assessing Impaired Glucose Tolerance and Insulin Resistance in Polycystic Ovarian Syndrome with A Muffin Test: An Alternative to the Glucose Tolerance Test. *Endocr. Pract.* **2010**, *16*, 810–817. [CrossRef]
43. Forbes, S.; Lam, A.; Koh, A.; Imes, S.; Dinyari, P.; Malcolm, A.J.; Shapiro, A.M.J.; Senior, P.A. Comparison of Metabolic Responses to the Mixed Meal Tolerance Test vs the Oral Glucose Tolerance Test after Successful Clinical Islet Transplantation. *Clin. Transplant.* **2018**, *32*, e13301. [CrossRef]
44. Marais, C.; Hall, D.R.; van Wyk, L.; Conradie, M. Randomized Cross-Over Trial Comparing the Diagnosis of Gestational Diabetes by Oral Glucose Tolerance Test and a Designed Breakfast Glucose Profile. *Int. J. Gynecol. Obstet.* **2018**, *141*, 85–90. [CrossRef] [PubMed]
45. Racusin, D.A.; Antony, K.; Showalter, L.; Sharma, S.; Haymond, M.; Aagaard, K.M. Candy Twists as an Alternative to the Glucola Beverage in Gestational Diabetes Mellitus Screening. *Am. J. Obstet. Gynecol.* **2015**, *212*, 522.e1–522.e5. [CrossRef] [PubMed]
46. Roberts, R.N.; McManus, J.; Dobbs, S.; Hadden, D.R. A Standardised Breakfast Tolerance Test in Pregnancy: Comparison with the 75 g Oral Glucose Tolerance Test in Unselected Mothers and in Those with Impaired Glucose Tolerance. *Ulster Med. J.* **1997**, *66*, 18. [PubMed]
47. Coustan, D.R.; Widness, J.A.; Carpenter, M.W.; Rotondo, L.; Pratt, D.C. The "Breakfast Tolerance Test": Screening for Gestational Diabetes with a Standardized Mixed Nutrient Meal. *Am. J. Obstet. Gynecol.* **1987**, *157*, 1113–1117. [CrossRef]
48. American Diabetes Association. Diagnosis and Classification of Diabetes Mellitus. *Diabetes Care* **2008**, *31*, S55–S60. [CrossRef]
49. Carpenter, M.W.; Coustan, D.R. Criteria for Screening Tests for Gestational Diabetes. *Am. J. Obstet. Gynecol.* **1982**, *144*, 768–773. [CrossRef]
50. Eslamian, L.; Ramezani, Z. Breakfast as a Screening Test for Gestational Diabetes. *Int. J. Gynecol. Obstet.* **2006**, *96*, 34–35. [CrossRef]
51. Group, N.D.D. Classification and Diagnosis of Diabetes Mellitus and Other Categories of Glucose Intolerance. *Diabetes* **1979**, *28*, 1039–1057.
52. World Health Organization. *WHO Expert Committee on Diabetes Mellitus: Second Report*; WHO Technical Report Series; World Health Organization: Geneva, Switzerland, 1980; Volume 646. Available online: https://apps.who.int/iris/handle/10665/41399 (accessed on 10 January 2022).
53. Lind, T.; Phillips, P.R. Diabetic Pregnancy Study Group of the European Association for the Study of Diabetes Influence of Pregnancy on the 75-g OGTT: A Prospective Multicenter Study. *Diabetes* **1991**, *40*, 8–13. [CrossRef]
54. Marais, C.; van Wyk, L.; Conradie, M.; Hall, D. Screening for Gestational Diabetes: Examining a Breakfast Meal Test. *S. Afr. J. Clin. Nutr.* **2016**, *29*, 118–121. [CrossRef]
55. Meier, J.J.; Kemmeries, G.; Holst, J.J.; Nauck, M.A. Erythromycin Antagonizes the Deceleration of Gastric emptying by Glucagon-Like Peptide 1 and Unmasks Its Insulinotropic Effect in Heathy Subjects. *Diabetes* **2005**, *54*, 2212–2218. [CrossRef] [PubMed]
56. Meier, J.J.; Gallwitz, B.; Salmen, S.; Goetze, O.; Holst, J.J.; Schmidt, W.E.; Nauck, M.A. Normalization of Glucose Concentrations and Deceleration of Gastric Emptying after Solid Meals during Intravenous Glucagon-Like Peptide 1 in Patients with Type 2 Diabetes. *J. Clin. Endocrinol. Metab.* **2003**, *88*, 2719–2725. [CrossRef] [PubMed]
57. Horowitz, M.; Harding, P.E.; Maddox, A.F.; Wishart, J.M.; Akkermans, L.M.A.; Chatterton, B.E.; Shearman, D.J.C. Gastric and Oesophageal Emptying in Patients with Type 2 (Non-Insulin-Dependent) Diabetes Mellitus. *Diabetologia* **1989**, *32*, 151–159. [CrossRef] [PubMed]
58. Rijkelijkhuizen, J.M.; McQuarrie, K.; Girman, C.J.; Stein, P.P.; Mari, A.; Holst, J.J.; Nijpels, G.; Dekker, J.M. Effects of Meal Size and Composition on Incretin, α-Cell, and β-Cell Responses. *Metabolism.* **2010**, *59*, 502–511. [CrossRef]
59. Gentilcore, D.; Chaikomin, R.; Jones, K.L.; Russo, A.; Feinle-Bisset, C.; Wishart, J.M.; Rayner, C.K.; Horowitz, M. Effects of Fat on Gastric Emptying of and the Glycemic, Insulin, and Incretin Responses to a Carbohydrate Meal in Type 2 Diabetes. *J. Clin. Endocrinol. Metab.* **2006**, *91*, 2062–2067. [CrossRef]
60. Martens, M.J.I.; Lemmens, S.G.T.; Born, J.M.; Westerterp-Plantenga, M.S. Satiating Capacity and Post-Prandial Relationships between Appetite Parameters and Gut-Peptide Concentrations with Solid and Liquefied Carbohydrate. *PLoS ONE* **2012**, *7*, e42110. [CrossRef]
61. Lachmann, E.H.; Fox, R.A.; Dennison, R.A.; Usher-Smith, J.A.; Meek, C.L.; Aiken, C.E. Barriers to Completing Oral Glucose Tolerance Testing in Women at Risk of Gestational Diabetes. *Diabet. Med.* **2020**, *37*, 1482–1489. [CrossRef]
62. Frid, A.H.; Nilsson, M.; Holst, J.J.; Björck, I.M. Effect of Whey on Blood Glucose and Insulin Responses to Composite Breakfast and Lunch Meals in Type 2 Diabetic Subjects 1–3. 2005. Available online: https://academic.oup.com/ajcn/article-abstract/82/1/69/4863431 (accessed on 2 March 2022).
63. Carr, R.D.; Larsen, M.O.; Winzell, M.S.; Jelic, K.; Lindgren, O.; Deacon, C.F.; Ahrén, B. Incretin and islet hormonal responses to fat and protein ingestion in healthy men. *Am. J. Physiol.-Endocrinol. Metab.* **2008**, *295*, E779–E784. [CrossRef]

64. Vilsbøll, T.; Krarup, T.; Sonne, J.; Madsbad, S.; Vølund, A.; Juul, A.G.; Holst, J.J. Incretin secretion in relation to meal size and body weight in healthy subjects and people with type 1 and type 2 diabetes mellitus. *J. Clin. Endocrinol. Metab.* **2003**, *88*, 2706–2713. [CrossRef]
65. Alssema, M.; Schindhelm, R.K.; Rijkelijkhuizen, J.M.; Kostense, P.J.; Teerlink, T.; Nijpels, G.; Heine, R.J.; Dekker, J.M. Meal composition affects insulin secretion in women with type 2 diabetes: A comparison with healthy controls. The Hoorn prandial study. *Eur. J. Clin. Nutr.* **2009**, *63*, 398–404. [CrossRef]
66. Heinemann, L. Are All Glucose Solutions Used for oGTT Equal? *Diabet. Med.* **2022**, *39*, e14798. [CrossRef] [PubMed]

MDPI  
St. Alban-Anlage 66  
4052 Basel  
Switzerland  
Tel. +41 61 683 77 34  
Fax +41 61 302 89 18  
www.mdpi.com

*Nutrients* Editorial Office  
E-mail: nutrients@mdpi.com  
www.mdpi.com/journal/nutrients

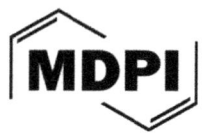

www.ingramcontent.com/pod-product-compliance
Lightning Source LLC
LaVergne TN
LVHW070423100526
838202LV00014B/1517